Fractal Signatures in the Dynamics of an Epidemiology

An Analysis of COVID-19 Transmission

Editors

Santo Banerjee
Dipartimento di Scienze Matematiche
Politecnico di Torino, Torino, Italy

A. Gowrisankar
Department of Mathematics
School of Advanced Sciences
Vellore Institute of Technology
Vellore-632 014, Tamil Nadu, India

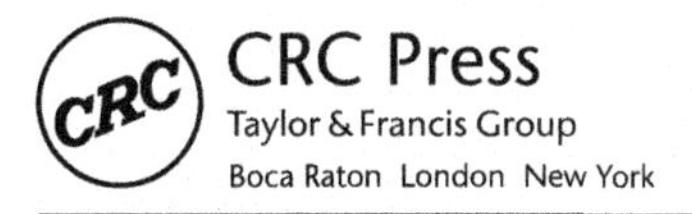

CRC Press is an imprint of the
Taylor & Francis Group, an **informa** business
A SCIENCE PUBLISHERS BOOK

First edition published 2024
by CRC Press
2385 NW Executive Center Drive, Suite 320, Boca Raton FL 33431

and by CRC Press
4 Park Square, Milton Park, Abingdon, Oxon, OX14 4RN

CRC Press is an imprint of Taylor & Francis Group, LLC

Library of Congress Cataloging-in-Publication Data (applied for)

ISBN: 978-1-032-32769-3 (hbk)
ISBN: 978-1-032-32776-1 (pbk)
ISBN: 978-1-003-31664-0 (ebk)

DOI: 10.1201/9781003316640

Typeset in Times New Roman
by Radiant Productions

Preface

Fractals, a vocabulary of irregular patterns, which appear on the coffee table and screen savers have an excellent connection with the pathological architecture of many viruses. Several comprehensive studies are utilizing the fractal dimension as a very effective measure to quantify the degree of randomness of the growth patterns of both communicable and non-communicable diseases. In this respect, this book aims to investigate and examine the COVID-19 epidemic from a broad perspective using fractal and multifractal models. This ongoing pandemic of COVID-19 has drastically collapsed national and international governments across the globe, as a result the entire world is battling to regain its financial and environmental stability. During the last two years, a variety of research articles as well as books have been published to fathom the kinetics of multiple SARS-COV 2 variants. Studies on the epidemiology of COVID-19 in relation with the fractals and fractal functions are being explored due to its irregular dynamical nature. Though, recently the severity of the same disease in a few countries is reduced in small, the consequences from the previous years are still more severe in both developed and developing countries. With the preceding caveats, this book compiles seven chapters describing the construction and application of fractal-based mathematical models for the prognostic purposes of the COVID-19 disease in order to achieve a sustainable environment.

Severe acute respiratory coronavirus 2 (SARS-CoV-2) distribution around the world has led to the global pandemic of coronavirus disease 2019 (COVID-19) since December 2019, which has caused more than 6 million deaths. During the last two years, SARS-CoV-2 has gone through an evolutionary process that has led to the development of several variants and subvariants. These alterations, as well as other factors, have created the spikes of COVID-19. Moreover, with the recent progress made in fractal deep learning and artificial intelligence (AI), several models have been developed to forecast the future of COVID-19. The first chapter aims to review the evolution of SARS-CoV-2 and COVID-19 since 2019. It is also discusses how fractal models have been helping to predict the pandemic behavior and setting strategies by the governments to control the pandemic.

One of the central tools to control the COVID-19 pandemic is the knowledge of its spreading dynamics. In the first chapter, a fractal model capable of describing such transmitting dynamics is constructed, in terms of daily new cases, and provide quantitative criteria for some predictions. In this chapter, a fractal dynamical model using a conformed derivative and fractal time scale is proposed. A Burr-XII shaped solution of the fractal-like equation is obtained. The model is tested using data from several countries, showing that a single function is able to describe very different shapes of the outbreak. The diverse behaviour of the outbreak in those countries is presented and discussed. Moreover, a criterion to determine the existence of the pandemic peak and a expression to find the time to reach herd immunity is also obtained.

The third chapter presents a unique microstrip patch antenna array with a COVID-19 shape designed for both centimeter wave (sub-6 GHz) and millimeter-wave (mm-wave) frequencies for 5G applications. Firstly, a linear-polarized 2 × 4 antenna array that resonates at 3.16 GHz and has a gain of 10.5 dB is discussed. Secondly, a 2 × 2 mm-wave ultra-wideband linear-polarized array operating over the range (22–40) GHz with maximum gain is shown. The produced patch antenna is simulated and optimized by performing parametric studies of the dimensions using the finite element method High-Frequency Structure Stimulator software program, where the array elements have a circular shape surrounded by 5 pairs of crowns. The aforementioned microstrip antenna array for the sub-6 GHz is fabricated on a double-sided copper plate with an FR4-epoxy substrate of 1.6 mm thickness. The printed prototype measured parameters, including S-parameters, polarization, and radiation pattern show a good agreement with simulated results.

The fourth chapter aims to validate the design of a novel unique microstrip fractal patch antenna and its array with a COVID-19 shape designed for wireless applications. The single element patch is a compact, miniature size, multiband, low weight, and low cost patch antenna; the demonstrated patch antenna and its array are simulated using the High-Frequency Structure Stimulator software program. This chapter has productively used the fractal geometry and the COVID-19 shape in order to create a miniature antenna for the implementation of dual-band wireless, satellite, and radar applications (when it is a part of an array) and civil commercial services.

The World Health Organization on Jan 30, 2020 has declared this genomic-virus a 'public health emergency of international concern'. But with time, this phenomenon further spread like a wildfire with no possible anti-viral treatment at the moment due to which it began to be referred as pandemic on 11th March, 2020. Gradually, it has been studied that the entire genomic-sequencing indicated that these viral cells were not at all recombinant. Although, it has been analyzed that relatively much recent corona genomic viral of group-1 category was prevalent. The fifth chapter of the book studies the outbreak of coronavirus towards major parts of United States. With usage of multifractality, self-affinity, narrowing to fractality for time series, the complexity of the situation was dealt with to understand the scenario known as pandemic. Hurst exponent values, multi-fractal, and waveform signal analysis indicate a similar pattern. This study is required as the outliers, or the inaccuracies may keep away the actual picture of the situation. Therefore, it was required to capture this essence related to the pandemic as it had been affecting millions everyday beginning from January in this case of the United States. From the data-driven hybrid analysis, it is observed that Herd immunity started increasing in the society.

In the sixth chapter of this book, the multifractality concepts on the infected cases, death cases, and vaccinated cases of COVID-19 for highly affected countries are investigated through the multifractal detrended fluctuation analysis. This analysis helps us to examine the COVID-19 diffusion process extensively by multifractal spectrum. Further, it may help us to take further actions and also we can increase the vaccinations based on the results obtained from the infected cases and death cases for the representative countries to reduce the rate of infections and the death ratio.

In order to help society towards resilience in the environmentally sustainable public health care system, the seventh chapter focus to provide an integrated fractal based prognostic analysis on the coronavirus transitivity rate. The achievable reconstruction of the epidemic curves based on the fractal interpolation function with variable scaling parameter to construct the predicted data is indulged in this proposed scheme by using the sample COVID-19 datasets with infected and death cases. The improved generalized fractal dimensions of COVID-19 time series are figured out and also the comparative analysis is premeditated between the predicted data interpolated by the fractal interpolation function with the two types of scaling factors. Based on the forecasting results with the sample data set in this integrated research study, the COVID-19 data on any time interval can be taken for the investigation in the similar way. Further, the results suggest the public health care sectors to take effective control measures in order to control the deadly coronavirus diffusion and attain sustainable environment.

The eighth chapter has proposed and analyzed a mathematical model to study the epidemic and economic consequences of novel coronavirus, with special emphasis on the interplays between the disease transmission, the management of pandemic and the socio-economic perspective. Both the asymptomatic and symptomatic individuals are considered and include the effectiveness of disease control into the respective disease transmission rates. The proposed model is analyzed to discuss the feasibility as well as stability of the disease-free and endemic steady states, and an epidemic threshold in the form of basic reproduction number is obtained. Performed as the global asymptotic stability of the disease-free and endemic steady state of the proposed system by constructing suitable Lyapunov function. Through numerical simulations, we observed that to mitigate the direct contacts between susceptible and infected individuals the population must have to maintain the social distances.

The ninth chapter intends to provide a fractal-based approach to analyze a Covid-19 data set in India from June 2020 to May 2022. The entire study period is divided into four half-years, and the analysis is to be carried out separately for each half-year. Covid-19 data analysis begins with the reconstruction of the curves representing the number of daily confirmed cases and the curves for the number of daily tests through the fractal interpolation technique. A linear iterated function system is formulated using the considered data set with a proper vertical scaling factor. Then, the attractor of this iterated function system is the required fractal interpolation curve. Fractal interpolation offers the benefit of minimizing data loss when creating curves. In addition to the reconstruction of the curves, this chapter proposes a more straightforward method to find the cumulative number of Covid-19 cases during each half-year by calculating the area under the curve using fractal numerical integration. It is easier to compute the number of cumulative cases using fractal numerical integration instead of adding up each day's number of cases separately. By determining the ratio of cumulative cases to the entire population, this chapter the analysis the virus' growth rate in the nation.

The tenth chapter discusses the COVID-19 cases from 2020 to 2023 that employ the fractal dimension. This chapter classifies the time series of positive newly confirmed COVID-19 cases, fatality COVID-19 cases from January 2020 to January 2023, and vaccinated and boosted cases from 2021 to 2023 for the world and most affected countries, including the United States, India, the United Kingdom, France, and China. The analysis process has performed by identifying fractal dimension through the Hurst exponent. The year-wise comparison of the aforementioned data is described for both raw data and outcomes.

The countries of the world are still struggling to get rid of the impact of SARS CoV-2. As if this is not enough, different variants of Corona are continuously evolving. These are discovered by analyzing the genetic sequence of the particular virus. Consequently, the eleventh chapter focuses on the various graph interpretations of spike proteins in variants and genetic sequences in subvariants. Furthermore, the variation between the variants and sub-variations of the SARS Cov-2 is investigated by determining the fractal dimension and similarity measures in this chapter.

In the twelfth chapter, a model based on Lambert W function is proposed for analyzing the growth rate of multicellular tumor spheroid. The model is validated with multicellular tumor spheroid data such as 9L, U-87MG and Rat1-T1. Also the model discriminate the growth rate changes in three stages of each tumor data. The obtained results reveal our proposed method is very much suitable for approximating the tumor growth rate for the data which preserves the properties of Gompertz curve.

Contents

Chapter 1

Analysis of the Current, Past, and Future Evolution of COVID-19

Reza Elahi,[1,] Parsa Karami,[1] Mahsa Bazargan,[2] Shahrzad Ahmadi,[3] Arash Azhideh[4] and Abdolreza Esmaeilzadeh[5]*

1.1 Introduction

Since December 2019, the coronavirus disease (COVID-19) pandemic has been a worldwide health concern. COVID-19 is caused by severe acute respiratory syndrome coronavirus 2 (SARS CoV 2), which is a virus from the betacoronaviridae family [1]. As of November 2022, COVID-19 has spread to most countries causing more than 626 million confirmed cases and more than 6.5 million deaths (https://covid19.who.int/ accessed 30 October 2022). Due to the rapid spread and serious health problems caused by the disease, on March 11, 2020, this disease was declared a global pandemic of worldwide importance by the world health organization (WHO) (https://www.who.int/emergencies/diseases/novel-coronavirus-2019).

Major clinical symptoms of COVID-19 include a sore throat, cough, dyspnea, and muscle weakness. In some cases, COVID-19 could also have more aggressive respiratory signs and progress to severe disease with pulmonary distress [2]. Imaging of COVID-19 patients shows patchy ground glass opacifications; however, these signs were reversible and often disappear after recovery [3]. Moreover, other symptoms including vomiting, diarrhea, and mild abdominal discomfort could also be seen [4]–[9]. Major cases of COVID-19-associated mortality are older patients with chronic conditions, including chronic kidney disease, hypertension, diabetes mellitus type II, or cardiopulmonary disease [10]–[12]. Studies have discussed that the mortality rate could increase in the first episodes of a COVID-19 outbreak due to the potential of the virus to infect patients more aggressively and was more pathogenic in first exposures. However, further efforts for a better comprehension of the SARS-CoV-2 pathogenicity, immunization of the population, and proper hygiene observations have led to a significant reduction in mortalities [13].

[1] School of Medicine, Zanjan University of Medical Sciences, Zanjan, Iran.
[2] Virology Research Center, the National Research Institute of Tuberculosis and Lung Diseases (NRITLD), Masih Daneshvari Hospital, Allergy and Immunology Subspecialty Lab, Tehran, Iran.
[3] Department of Immunology, School of Medicine, Sahid Beheshti University of Medical Sciences, Tehran, Iran.
[4] Skull Base Research Center, Sahid Beheshti University of Medical Sciences, Tehran, Iran.
[5] Cancer Gene Therapy Research Center (CGRC), Zanjan University of Medical Sciences, Zanjan, Iran.
* Corresponding author: a46reza@zums.ac.ir

After being declared a pandemic, COVID-19 spread rapidly to most countries around the world. The COVID-19 pandemic has gone through several changes and has experienced an evolutionary process since 2019. Some of these changes could be attributed to the natural behavior of the pandemic, while others are related to worldwide anti-viral vaccination [14]. Mathematical models can study the behavior of a specific disease and can predict its behavior in the future. Understanding the spikes of the COVID-19 pandemic in different countries is a good example of this. Different mathematical models have been proposed for viral spread and other features of the disease [15]–[18]. Based on regression analysis, such models can be used for both monitoring the policies of the governments against the pandemic as well as setting proper policies to control it [19]. Understanding the evolution of past and present evolution of COVID-19 can help predict the future evolution of the disease. In this chapter, we overview the evolution of the SARS-CoV-2 and discuss how new variants affect the pandemic, overview the evolution of the COVID-19 pandemic, and finally discuss the future evolution of COVID-19 based on known mathematical models.

Understanding the evolution of past and present evolution of COVID-19 can help predict the future evolution of the disease. In this chapter, we overview the evolution of the SARS-CoV-2 and discuss how new variants affect the pandemic, overview the evolution of the COVID-19 pandemic, and finally discuss the future evolution of COVID-19 based on known mathematical models.

1.2 An Overview of the Evolution of SARS-CoV-2

In understanding the emergence and evolution of SARS-CoV-2 it is necessary to understand the evolution of COVID-19. In this section, we aim to discuss the current data on the origin of SARS-CoV-2 and its different variants. The Sarbecovirus subgroup of Betacoronavirus contains the coronaviruses that have recently caused pandemic/epidemic outbreaks of infection in human populations. Coronaviruses belonging to this family can be found in large numbers in bats and other animals. This subgroup includes the endemic and low pathogenic coronaviruses, such as HCoV-HKU1, HCoV-NL63, HCoV-OC43, and HCoV-229E, which cause mild symptoms in humans, and SARS-CoV-2, middle-east respiratory coronavirus (MERS-CoV), and severe acute respiratory syndrome coronavirus (SARS-CoV), which cause more severe symptoms [20]. Although the zoonotic transmission mechanism for SARS-CoV-2 is unknown, it is thought to have arisen from Rhinolophus bats [21]. Due to the consistent population growth of coronaviruses (CoVs) and the widespread finding of varied CoVs, bats are thought to be the fundamental hosts for all CoV lineages, in contrast to the epidemic-like growths found in other species [22].

There are beliefs regarding the origin of SARS-CoV-2 that it could be from a seafood market in Wuhan, Hubei Province, China. It is hypothesized that Rhinolophus bats are the natural reservoirs of SARS-CoV-2 [23]. SARS-CoV-2 genomic research uncovered several recombination occasions [24]. Due to the potential for SARS-CoV-2 recombination, virologists have a lot to be concerned about regarding the spread of new and potentially more harmful virus strains. Studies have investigated that SARS-CoV-2 came from the recombination of a coronavirus of bat called RaTG13, although the similarity of these viruses strengthens our guesses about the origin of SARS-CoV-2 the real origin of this virus is still unclear. Viruses could change their genomic structures after their exposure to a new cell, which could improve our hypothesis of several conversions of a bat virus or an unknown-origin virus over the decades turned into the brutal SARS-CoV-2 that cause the recent pandemic and a great number of mortalities around the world [25]. There is a piece of interesting evidence that has been investigated that the flu pandemic that occurred between 1889 and 1891 and caused over a million deaths caused by a member of coronaviruses families was a beta coronavirus called HCoV-OC43 same as the MERS, SARS, and SARS-CoV-2, but it belongs to other subgroups of coronaviruses [26].

Variable changes in transmissibility and virulence follow the formation of a new disease. Regarding SARS-CoV-2, this unpredictability is exacerbated by the fact that it is a unique human illness that has undergone multiple periods of uncontrolled spread throughout the world. It is often wrong to consider that viruses will eventually evolve to become less infectious [24]. Lower virulence of some viruses that have infected humans may be owing to the death of susceptible individuals and/or the survivors' acquisition of partial or complete immunity [27].

Viral variations result from nucleotide alterations that occur spontaneously in the viral genetic sequence along replication, particularly RNA viruses, which exhibit a greater frequency of these changes than DNA viruses [28]. Every time a virus replicates, its genetic material undergoes mutations or changes, producing variations. However, the amount of these nucleotide alterations in coronaviruses is substantially underneath other viruses with RNA genes, due to the presence of a replication-correcting enzyme [29]. The activity of exoribonuclease (ExoN) within SARS-CoV-2 non-structural protein 14 (nsp14) has a "proofreading" impact, and inactivating ExoN is deleterious for the replication of SARS-CoV-2 [30]. The impact of these changes on viral transmission and pathogenicity must be understood. The fact that the identical SARS-CoV-2 mutation has arisen independently in other countries suggests that it may improve the virus's fitness. In addition, there are many mutations across all variations, which points to rapid evolution over brief periods [31].

SARS-CoV-2, similar to other Coronaviruses family members, has a 30kb genome that is responsible for the formation of 4 key structural proteins, including a spike protein (S), an envelope protein (E), a membrane protein (M), and a nucleocapsid protein (N), some other nonstructural genomes. Several recombinations of the genome of coronaviruses are the main cause of the recent global pandemic. S protein is affected by several recombinations in the genome that find a greater ability to bind to its specific receptor in humankind, angiotensin-converting enzyme 2 (ACE2) [20]. The ACE2 receptors on the alveolar epithelial cells, laryngeal, and tracheal epithelial cells are the most host cells for SARS-CoV-2, of which alveolar type II pneumocytes are affected the most [32], [33]. After the entrance of the virus, the viral genome induces replication and production of viral particles, which are released to infect other cells after the host cell death [34]. These events activate the immune response against the virus. The normal activity of the immune system is to prevent the virus from infecting more cells and to recover the damaged organs. However, in some conditions, the self-regulation of the body could be affected by the rapid progression of the disease and the great viral load, which leads to the hyperactivity of the immune response and releasing proinflammatory cytokines and chemokines from the immune and damaged cells, a process called the cytokine storm. The cytokine storm is the leading cause of respiratory distress and death in many cases [35]. Moreover, SARS-CoV-2 can suppress immune activity, which causes severe manifestations of rapid progression disease [36]. These events together caused great waves of mortality around the world during the primary phases of the COVID-19 pandemic (Figure 2) [37].

The WHO divides SARS-CoV-2 strains into two categories: variants of interest (VOI) and variants of concern (VOC). The Centers for Disease Control and Prevention (CDC) characterizes a VOC as an infectious disease exhibiting high transmission and virulence rates, resistance to vaccines and acquired immunity, and the capacity to evade diagnostic identification. Since the initial outbreak in December 2019, the original wild-type strain discovered in Wuhan has given rise to several VOCs (https://www.cdc.gov, cited 2022 Oct 30). Since VOCs have evolved separately in the human population, each pursuing various paths to better achievement relative to early 2020 variations. Although, there is still the risk of new VOCs with distinct virulence features in the future.

Since its emergence, SARS-CoV-2 has undergone many changes, which has led to the development of several variants. Since early 2020, the virus had rapidly evolved into various strains before we were concerned about COVID-19 variations. As COVID-19 began to undergo more powerful mutations, the WHO decided to name each significant variant using the Greek alphabet, beginning with Alpha. Variant Alpha (B.1.1.7) was identified for the first time in late September 2020 and was appointed the prevalent subtype in the UK almost immediately [38]. Nevertheless, the fraction of the Alpha variant exhibited a considerable decrease from April 2021 to June 2021, most notably because Delta variant strains had dramatically grown since April. The Alpha variant has an enormous viral load and is 43 – 90% more contagious than the original wild virus. As a result, those infected with COVID-19 have a 61% – 64% higher chance of death [39], [40]. The B.1.351 lineage, or its Beta form, 20H/501Y.V2, was initially identified in October 2020 in South Africa and has since spread throughout the continent, dominating the second wave in South Africa [41]. The receptor binding domain (RBD) region of the Beta version is mutated in three locations: K417N, E484K, and N501Y. It also has L18F, D80A, D215G, R264I, and A701V alterations in its spike protein. Neutralizing antibodies and vaccinations are less effective due to the presence of mentioned mutations [42]. The Beta version contains 1% of globally found SARS-CoV-2 genomes. Between October 2020 and April 2021, the Beta version spread alarmingly. Like the Alpha type, the Beta variant has declined since April 2021 [43].

On January 6, 2021, the Gamma variant (also called P.1 lineage or the 501Y.V3) was discovered in four Japanese nationals returning to Tokyo after visiting the Brazilian Amazon [44]. The Gamma variant's hallmark collection of distinctive amino acid alterations in the spike protein includes E484K, K417T, and N501Y, among others. The N501Y mutation is shared by the Alpha and Beta versions, whereas the E484K mutation is shared by the Beta and Gamma variants. Human transmission of the Gamma version led to further evolution and the emergence of other variations [45]. Instead of accumulating in a single chronically infected patient, the Gamma variation was acquired through a series of infections, suggesting that it resulted from population-level selection pressure. The global distribution and rapid evolutionary development of the Gamma variant are consistent with a process driven by natural selection under host-virus interaction [46]. There have been about 3% Gamma variant strains in circulation as of September 2021 [43].

Variant Delta (B.1.617.2), initially found in December 2020, caused a significant increase in cases that resulted in the second peak in India and the outbreak of diseases at various events in the United States [47], [48]. Besides the RBD mutations, the Delta version is distinguished from other VOCs by the presence of numerous amino acid changes in the N-terminal domain (NTD) region. B.1.617 is the ancestor of the Delta variety, which evolved into B.1.617.3, B.1.617.2, and B.1.617.1. Due to its fast global spread, the Delta strain was declared a VOC by the WHO on May 11, 2021 [49]. As of September 2021, 29% of all viral genomes uploaded worldwide have been the Delta variety. The majority of documented occurrences of the Delta variation were found in India and Turkey. Delta is also found in Vietnam, the United Kingdom, and Russia. Until June 20, 2021, 76.7 percent (49,407 out of 64,449) of all Delta variations found in the world originated in the UK. Moreover, the new Delta plus variant (B.1.617.2.1 Delta-AY.1) emerged in Louisiana, US, sending infection rates soaring [43]. The replication and spike-mediated entrance rates of the Delta variant are higher than those of B.1.617.1, allowing it to spread more quickly than the Alpha and Kappa variants. These two changes also boost the infectiousness of the virus, facilitate cell fusion, and speed up viral reproduction [50]. In England, Delta variant infections are more likely to result in hospitalization or the need for urgent medical attention [51]. According to data from Public Health England (PHE), the case fatality rate for the Delta version is 0.4% as of September 2021, which is around one-third that of the Alpha form [52].

The most recently recognized VOC is Omicron (B.1.1.529), which was detected for the first time in November 2021 in South Africa and has since been identified in several countries [53]. On November 11, 2021, the first detection of the new Omicron strain (B.1.1.529) occurred in Botswana. Subsequently, it was found in Hong Kong. It was primarily ascribed to the increase in monitoring that the number of cases in these nations climbed dramatically from one week to the next following the disease's identification. The deletions and mutations of the Omicron are linked to improved transmissibility via enhancing the affinity of the S protein for ACE2, as well as host immune evasion and decreased potential of antibodies produced by the vaccine to neutralize the virus [54], [55]. According to studies, Pfizer/BioNTech and Moderna mRNA vaccine's third dosage effectively neutralizes the Omicron variant. However, these vaccinations' first and second doses produced negligible to no neutralization against this variation [56]. Generally, Omicron type infection tends to produce less severe symptoms than other variations. In nations with advanced immunization programs, it is possible to establish wide protection against the virus by vaccination. Nevertheless, in countries with limited vaccination, according to the Omicron variant's low virulence, the dissemination of the Omicron variation can lead to an increase in infection cases but not in fatality rates. Moreover, due to its ineffective cleavage by the host protease, the *in vitro* and *in vivo* replication capacity of Omicron is significantly decreased compared to other SARS-CoV-2 variants such as Delta, Beta, Alpha, and WT [57], [58].

BA.1, BA.2, and BA.3 are Omicron's three separate sub-lineages that were identified nearly simultaneously [59], [60]. Initially, BA.1 was the most prevalent sublineage discovered internationally; however, BA.2 (and it is component sublineages) is currently surpassing BA.1 as the primary form worldwide [60], [61]. Recently, two additional sublineages, BA.5 and BA.4 have been identified in South Africa and have subsequently been recognized in nations such as Australia, Germany, Botswana, China, France, and Belgium [61], [62]. In August of 2022, the Omicron subvariant XBB, a recombinant of the BA.2.75 and BA.2.10.1, was found for the first time. It has produced a minor increase in cases in Singapore and Bangladesh, among other places, and is described as "immune-evasive". However, the severity of the new mutations is unclear (https://fortune.com/2022/10/11/what-is-xbb-variant-covid-singapore-immune-evasive, cited 2022 Nov 1.) [63]. Soumya Swaminathan, a senior scientist at the WHO, issued a warning on October 20, 2022, that the XBB subvariant has been detected in parts of India, including Kerala [64]. BA.5 has two brand-new subtypes: BQ.1 and BQ.1.1 [65]. Two subvariants were detected in the state of New York. BA.2.12.1 (or B.1.1.529.2.12.1) and BA.2.12 (or B.1.1.529.2.12) have 23–27% more growth potential than BA.2 and contributed to an increase in infections in central New York, which dominated by May 24, 2022, in the United States [66]. The emergence of Omicron is expected to have significant consequences for existing measures to manage the SARS-CoV-2 pandemic.

VOIs are variants that probably do not have as much spread and importance, compared to VOCs. Several reports of VOIs are only projected to affect vaccine immunity, transmission, pathogenicity, or acquired immunity. Epsilon (B.1.427/B.1.429) which was found in California is among the VOIs being monitored. Before September 2021, the Epsilon variant included two percent of all SARS-CoV2s and was mostly found in the United States. The Epsilon variation is around 20% more contagious than other variants. However, its pathogenic mechanism is yet unknown [67]. The variant Iota (B.1.526/B.1.526.1) was discovered in New York, Eta (B.1.525) in Nigeria and the United Kingdom, Zeta (P.2) in Brazil, and Theta (P.3) in the Philippines. In August 2020, Lambda (C.37) was discovered for the first time. Since mid-June 2021, the number of Lambda variations has been declining and from April to June 2021, the number of Lambda variants climbed dramatically. As of September 2021, less than 0.5% of all viruses have the Lambda form, mostly disseminated in South America [68]. Delta Plus (B.1.617.2.1) and Kappa (B.1.617) were detected in India. BA.2.75 was discovered in India, and the community of BQ.1 is unclear. Additional research is necessary to understand their effect on the present COVID-19 (cited 2022 Oct 30]. Available from: https://www.who.int/activities/tracking-SARS-CoV-2-variants) [69]. The Kappa variation accounts for fewer than 0.5% of known strains as of September 2021 and is mostly spread in India [70].

It is still being determined if the new variations are more likely to infect children than adults, even though the number of infected youngsters appears to be greater in the UK. It would indicate that both ancient and novel varieties are having an impact on the younger generation. In contrast, younger children and females of Asian origin were shown to be less severely affected by the condition and less susceptible to developing it. This trend may be attributable to increased ACE2 expression among Asians. Children's immune systems are likely to be more robust, which might play an impact. More research is required to pinpoint the transmission's mechanism and its origins. Schools have not been proven to have a role in the viral interpersonal transfer. Therefore, the fact that children continued to attend despite the rest of the area being placed back on lockdown after reopening might be a possible reason [71], [72].

SARS-CoV-2 is regarded as atypical since new human diseases discovered in the last several decades frequently exhibit increased virulence due to a lack of host protection. As the transmission rate of SARS-CoV-2 was already high, it was considered that there was no selection benefit for a drop in virulence. In the case of Omicron, despite its high transmissibility rate, there has been an unexpected and fortunate decrease in the severity of infections due to a shift in the prevalence of upper respiratory infections [73]. Due to the unpredictable nature of SARS-CoV-2 development, it is uncertain whether future variants will be a "milder" version of SARS-CoV-2 or whether a new VOC with unique features and virulence factors will arise [74].

Another crucial concern arises from the ongoing evolutionary trajectory of SARS-CoV-2, given that the virus has been circulating in the human population for over a year and has seen a tremendous population increase by infecting tens of millions of individuals. It has been questioned whether during the epidemic, there have there been any signs of adaptation to human hosts in the SARS-CoV-2 genome. Population genetic investigations of SARS-CoV-2 genomes provide insight into this subject. Such information is still being produced as part of the worldwide effort to comprehend the dynamics of SARS-CoV-2. Since extensive SARS-CoV-2 genome sequence datasets are now available, researchers may track the virus's history in humans to see if any particular locations have undergone adaptive evolution since it was first introduced. In addition to finding targets and candidates for vaccines and treatments, such research will help us distinguish the dynamics of CoVs dissemination and its influence on public health. There is little doubt that this is a vibrant frontier of the current study, with many new understandings likely to be revealed in the weeks and months ahead [75], [76].

1.3 An Overview of the Evolution of COVID-19

The rate at which we are using up the resources of the globe is unsustainable the world's population grew 6 billion in the last century. By the end of the twenty-first century, it is anticipated to be between 14 and 18 billion (https://www.unhcr.org/globaltrends.html, accessed November 5th, 2022) [77], [78]. With over 637,074,723 infected cases and 6,602,220 fatalities (as of 3 November 2022), SARS-CoV-2 has already spread to 216 nations, regions, and territories. The majority of COVID-19-related fatalities happened in countries including Spain, Italy, the United States, the United Kingdom, France, Germany, Brazil, Turkey, Belgium, Iran, etc. [79], [80].

In this section, we aim to overview the past and present evolution of the COVID-19 pandemic (Figure 1). Analysis of the prior outbreaks of other coronaviruses, including SARS and MERS, with mathematic models, showed us the possibility of investigating a pattern of how the disease spreads among the population according to its exposure time. Current findings could consider that by studying and analysing the pattern of infection in the evolution of disease history, we could prevent future catastrophes and improve our decision makings and disease management. Since its evolution, COVID-19 has undergone several changes, which are both related to the physiologic features of the viruses as well as the anti-pandemic policies taken by the governments [81]. Reproductive number (R0) is an epidemiologic determinant of the number of individuals that can be infected by an infected patient. Initial studies on the transmission dynamics of COVID-19 showed that the R0 was 1.4–3.9 (13). Proper vaccination, isolation of patients, and rapid diagnosis of the patients helped to reduce the R0 to less than one [82].

As shown in Figure 1, since the first outbreak of COVID-19 in December 2019, the world has experienced five different peaks. The first peak occurred between October 2020 and February 2021 with the most cases in

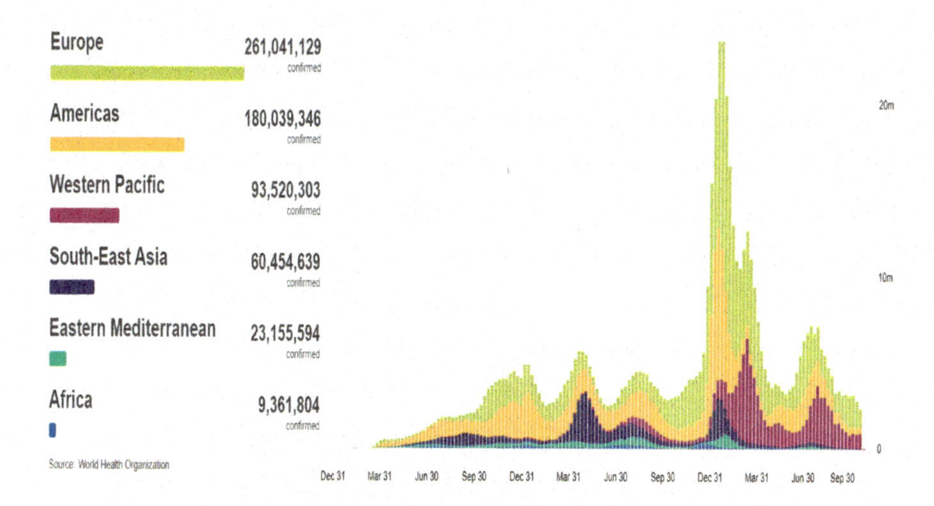

Fig. 1.1: The number-time chart of COVID-19 cases (https://covid19.who.int/).

January 2021. This spike occurred due to inaccessibility to effective protections, medications, and effective vaccines. At the beginning of the outbreak, cases of pneumonia in Wuhan, China, were reported on 8th December 2019. The center for disease control and prevention (CDC) in china enounced the pathogen as a novel coronavirus on 7th January 2020. The first death was reported on 9th January 2020, the first case out of China was reported in Thailand on 13th January 2020, and after one week, WHO reported 282 confirmed positive cases of novel coronavirus disease and 6 deaths. The rapid spread of the disease showed the potential for distribution and severity of the disease. Finally, after one month, on 11th March 2020, the downhill first peak. Later, on December 2020 and January 2021, the 3 most effective vaccines included (Pfizer, Moderna, and AstraZeneca) were used in the UK, Europe, USA, and other countries, which changed the situation and played a key role in future controls of the outbreak [83]–[85].

The second spike occurred between march 2021 and June 2021, during which most cases were found in April 2021. The third one happened between July 2021 and September 2021 and the peak was in august 2021. Due to vaccination and the global protection protocols, the peak number of cases was lower in the third peak. The most dramatic peak was the fourth peak between December 2021 and May 2022. The top peak happened in January 2022, when 23,789,141 cases of COVID-19 around the world were reported. Despite global vaccination, this peak happened due to the new subtype of the virus, named Omicron, which had more transferability but less severity. Therefore, despite the higher number of cases, the mortality was lower than before the peaks. Compared to the first peak, the deaths were lower, and the number of cases decreased faster. The faster decrease of the fourth spike proves that the fourth peak could have predictable data of the finishing downhill of COVID-19 [86]. The final peak of COVID-19 occurred between June 2022 and September 2022. The top spike was in July 2022 which showed a drastic reduction in cases compared with the fourth peak of the disease. During the last two years, researchers have investigated antiviral drugs, anti-inflammation treatments, and alternative medications used for severely ill patients in intensive care units (ICU). Importantly, global efforts to develop vaccines and the efforts made to vaccinate most of the population around the world are other factors contributing to the downhill of COVID-19. Moreover, the restrictions made by the governments, such as the compulsion to use masks and the lockdowns were also other causes of the COVID-19 downhill [87].

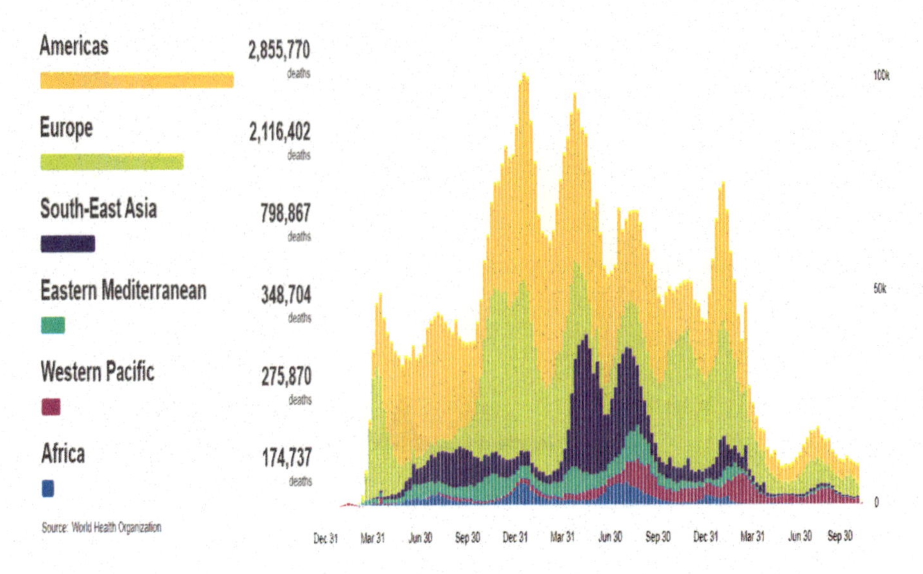

Fig. 1.2: The chart showing the number of COVID-19 deaths per time (https://covid19.who.int/).

Figure 2 presents the death chart of COVID-19. Since 2019, there have been eight spikes which show decreasing trend up to the recent spikes. The first spike occurred between March 2020 and May 2020, the second wave was between June 2020 and august 2020, and the third spike occurred. between October 2020 and February 2021, a dramatic increase happened. This was due to disease spreading, inaccessibility to effective medications for the severe and progressive conditions of disease, and unknown life-saving operations. The fourth spike happened one month after the first one, between March 2021 and June 2021, and because of the similar conditions of inaccessibility to effective disease prevention functions, the second dramatic spike of death occurred similar to the third one. After the fourth wave, the death chart experienced a significant decrease due to the production of vaccines and effective medications for severely ill patients in the ICU. The fifth spike occurred between July 2021 and October 2021, the sixth wave was even lower than the previous wave between October 2021 and December 2021, and the seventh spike happened due to the Omicron and showed a significant increase in death chart between December 2021 and April 2022. Based on the death chart, the duration of this peak was lower than the first high spikes which is because of the higher immunity of the population and the pace of the vaccine production. The last spike occurred between June 2022 and September 2022, which was the lowest spike and showed the effectiveness of the methods of dealing with this disease during these two years.

1.4 Future Evolution of COVID-19 based on Fractal Models

The fractal dimension of the epidemiological curve can help to select the datasets for predicting the behavior of the pandemic. Moreover, the reproduction rate has been shown to have a sensible fractal pattern. Interestingly, Pacurar and colleagues found a correlation coefficient of 0.386 between the new daily cases of COVID-19 and daily global radiation [88]. A supervised learning model can be created to make a prediction based on an unknown input instance. To train the regression model in this learning approach, a dataset of input instances and their matching regressors are used. After that, the trained model makes a forecast for the test dataset or provided unanticipated input data [89]–[91]. The formulation of prediction models using this approach may make use of classification algorithms and regression techniques. The four regression models have been employed for COVID-19 prediction include Exponential Smoothing (ES), Support Vector Machine (SVM), Least Absolute Shrinkage and Selection Operator (LASSO) Regression, and Linear Regression (LR).

Several models have been applied to predict the future death rate of COVID-19. According to the studies' death rate projections, Exponential Smoothing outperforms all other models [92]. However, Linear Regression and LASSO perform similarly well and attain about the same R2 score. SVM, in contrast, performs poorly in this scenario. The ES again outperforms all other models in recovery rate future projection [93]. However, the ES prognosis follows patterns that are incredibly near to the actual scenario when considering the present recovery numbers with some models' forecasts. Regarding the prediction of the uncertainty of A prediction model, the prediction interval is a way to express how uncertain a forecast is. It offers probabilistic lower and upper limits on an outcome variable's estimate. Studies employ prediction intervals on LR to assess this uncertainty since, in general, LR outperforms the other two regression models (LASSO and SVM) in all three scenarios (forecasting death rates, newly confirmed cases, and recovery rates) [94].

One of these models is the Susceptible-Infected-Removed (SIR) model. There are three functions in this model that are based on the time, including susceptible, which means that the individual that is talented for being infected but has not been infected yet, infected i(t): which means the infected individual that could transmit the virus to other non-infected persons, removed R(t), means recovering from virus and immunization against the second infection, and D(t), died individual because of disease. Here is the mathematic formula of the SIRD model:

$$\frac{ds(t)}{dt} = - aS(t)I(t),$$

$$\frac{dI(t)}{dt} = aS(t)I(t) - bI(t),$$

$$\frac{dr(t)}{dt} = bI(t)$$

They have found some issues in this model including, in some populations like India, there could not be homogeneity between infected and susceptible populations. Another major problem with the SIR model is that this model does not present the time and severity of a pick of disease in an active infection period [95]. In a study, a comparison of models including LSTM, stacked LSTM, BiLSTM, and CNN, could predict the COVID-19 spread for 16 days. In addition to the time limitations, their deep learning model could not make comprehensive results and did not include other studies' results [96]. Another study has used the ARIMA model for the prediction of true positive cases in Europe. Although the limitation of this study is the time limitation and did not include other similar studies, they achieved a reasonable RMSE value for France, Italy, and Spain [97].

A good performance model was the deep learning model named, BiLSTM, with a reasonable RMSE value For China. The authors have achieved this result from a comparison of deep learning models including BilSTM, GRU, and LSTM with three statistical models including SVR and ARIMA [98]. In a study from February 2020 to June 2020, an algorithm based on deep LSTM and fractional calculus was hired for predicting COVID-19 spread in eight different countries. The authors concluded that this method could not be extended to every country [99]. In a study, the authors used a complex algorithm based on machine learning methods and they found that when their ES algorithm was combined with other machine learning methods, including LASSO and LR, it could show better performance in predicting the pandemic spread [100].

In a study, for predicting positive cases, they used a simple statistical model which they found positively biased for new peaks and negatively biased for death prediction. The model was applied for the time between January 2020 and May 2020. This model could be disrupted when the disease curve is dynamic [101]. Alzahrani et al reported the confirmed versus predicted cases in Saudi Arabia by using an ARIMA-based statistical model. Their RMSE value has been reported as 21.17 and they did not consider other model analyses compare to their statistical model [102]. Elsheikh et al. evaluated the pandemic spread in Saudi Arabia by using a model based on the LSTM network. This deep-learning algorithm was used between March 2020 and October 2020, and the RMSE value of this algorithm was estimated for death cases and confirmed cases was 100.0239 and 160.608, respectively. In addition to reasonable RMSE value, this study is a comparison of the result of the other statistical models [103].

In another study that included Saudi Arabia in the period of March 2020 to June 2020, the authors used a system based on SIR-F and SIR models. They investigated the SIR parameters included (susceptible, infected, and recover); however, they did not consider similar deep learning or other statistical models analysis [104]. A study based on the fractal-fractional model could predict positive cases in Saudi Arabia, from March 2020 to April 2021, but they have not evaluated this model for other countries [105]. A study used a neural network for their data analysis with the combination of fractal fuzzy technique for their time trends in the United States, Belgium, Mexico, and Italy. The point of this study is the period of their evaluation which was limited to ten days (21 January to 30 January 2021) [106].

Another study in Jordan investigated the hybrid mathematical model, which could not achieve reliable results compared to similar models, this model was performed based on the long-term and short-term forecast models, LTF and STF [107]. In a study that used a fractional SEIR-AHQ model, authors evaluated the data of four cities for 30 days between January 2020 till March 2020. They concluded that non-medical interventions should be considered in the global control of COVID-19 [108]. In a study performed in Egypt, the LSTM model was used to predict cases between February 2020 to August 2020, but the limitation of this study was that they did not evaluate their model function in other countries [109].

AI Shahin et al. performed a study to predict the COVID-19 spread, they used LSTM which showed reasonable results in Saudi Arabia. The point of their study was to investigate the data in a broad period from the first to the end of the COVID-19 spreading wave. They reported that their model could improve the performance of predicting compared to other similar studies based on the deep learning model they have used [110]. Easwaramoorthy et al. produced a fractal-based model to investigate the mortality rate in 5 top countries that were involved with the most progressive rate of COVID-19 spread, including the USA, Brazil, Russia, India, and the UK. They could access reasonable data based on the ARMA that could predict the daily death rate in the first and second waves of the COVID-19 pandemic. This study could suggest a fractal model that has predicted death cases accurately compared to the data released by WHO. Their findings had limitations and variations in some countries, including India and Russia, which could be due to the government politics, operations to control the disease, and their data-gathering performances [111].

Recently, Hadi et al. used a fractional-order COVID-19 model to evaluate the effects of control policies on the pandemic. The authors concluded that control policies, including vaccination, non-pharmaceutical actions, and awareness, all together, can lead to a crucial decrease in the number of infected individuals [112]. In November 2020, Bastos et al. developed a model to forecast the initial evolution of COVID-19, based on Brazilian data from February 25, 2020, to March 30, 2020. They did this based on two SIR model variations and showed that the obligatory social distancing policies were able to flatten the pandemic curve. They also found that asymptomatic infections could affect the symptomatic curve, especially the amplitude of the peak [113].

In 2021, Shahin et al. developed a model based on encoding–decoding deep-learning COVID-19 time series to predict the death, recovered, and confirmed COVID-19 cases. This model had the lowest errors and an R square value of 0.99, compared to other models developed at the time [110]. BeCaked is a combination model of Variational Autoencoder (VAE) and Susceptible-Infectious-Recovered-Deceased (SIRD) which has achieved 0.98 R2 in predicting daily infections and has proposed to have high accuracy to make right-time decisions [114].

To conclude, the future of COVID-19 depends on vaccine development and global vaccination policies, the policies of the governments and people, and the evolution of the SARS-CoV-2. Mutations in the SARS-CoV-2 genome could critically affect the transfection rate and infectivity of the disease, two factors that have the highest impact on the pandemic's spread. Due to incomplete global vaccination, viral genome alterations, variation in the immunologic protection of the individuals, the existence of the virus in animals, and other unknown reasons, the complete eradication of COVID-19 may not be achievable [115].

Established on February 2021, International Science Council (ISC) is a scientific and independent council that aims to predict the future scenarios of the COVID-19 pandemic. Several scenarios could be proposed for COVID-19 in the future. The most optimistic scenario is that by developing next-generation vaccines that would be protective against new viral species, as well as the effective policies taken by the government and community, the pandemic could be taken under control. The other scenario could be the repeated waves of peaks due to several viral genome instabilities that lead to spike protein variations and finally immune escape, where there would be a consistent need for the production of novel vaccines against new variants of SARS-CoV-2 [116]–[118]. Furthermore, since countries can not be isolated for a long time, proper control of the pandemic will require coordinated operations by different countries [119]. Since its emergence in Wuhan, based on the pandemic outbreak and behavior, different models were proposed to predict the outbreaks. The complicated behavior of the COVID-19 pandemic had made it difficult to develop an accurate and effective model. In 2020, Bhardwaj et al. [19] proposed a logistic model for the outbreak of COVID-19 which was validated based on data from China and South Korea. The model showed that in March/April 2020, Sweden, Spain, Germany, and Italy would reach the peak number of infections and proposed lockdown/partial lockdown for these countries at the time.

Pandemic fatigue is another matter of concern in controlling the pandemic and is a term dedicated to the psychological effects of the pandemic on the majority of the population that leads to disobedience of the recommendations by individuals. Recently, in European countries the WHO have reported the emergence of pandemic fatigue. Pandemic fatigue could be of specific importance since people start being demotivated to follow the recommendations of pandemic control. In such cases, it could result in a recurrence of the pandemic or peaks. The proposed strategies to reduce the effect of pandemic fatigue are to keep informing communities about the circumstances and encourage them not to unleash social distancing, washing hands, and vaccinating, with a specific focus on in-danger populations [120], [121].

Numerous possible therapies for this virus have been put up to far, but none of them have received approval. To control the transmission of the virus at the community level, social distance is essential. Lowering the number of infected people and the rate of infection indirectly contributes to preventing the overstretched state of our healthcare systems. Perceived social closeness and stress reactions are correlated. On people who are already lonely or isolated, the impact may be more noticeable. Greater physical health depends on better mental wellness. Putting mental health first is crucial while under a lot of stress. Having said that, a socially distant approach is necessary, and community leaders' participation is essential. Responsible print and electronic media must also play a significant part [122]. To reduce the risk assessment, the virus must be tightly and effectively controlled. To halt this epidemic, everyone should do their part.

1.5 Conclusion

COVID-19 has been a worldwide health problem around the globe. ML-based prediction methods have been used to forecast the likelihood of a COVID-19 epidemic on a worldwide scale. The system uses machine learning methods to analyze a dataset, including day-by-day actual previous data and forecasts future days. ES method has the highest performance in the present forecasting domain. To a certain extent, LASSO and LR also execute competently in predicting mortality rates and confirming cases. These two models' findings indicate that while recovery rates will slow down, mortality rates will rise in the following days. Due to the fluctuations in the dataset values, SVM performs poorly in every case. Setting up a precise hyperplane between the dataset's specified values was challenging. The primary issue that remains unsolved is its viral progress. Even if the infection incidence continues to reduce exponentially, there is still the risk of developing severe disease, an increase in hospitalizations, and a significant strain on health care, even among inoculated individuals. To conclude, prediction models based on the existing circumstances are accurate and may help understand future events. Thus, the study's predictions can also greatly assist the government in terms of prompt action and decision-making to manage the COVID-19 situation.

Conflicts of Interest

The author declares having conflicts of interest.

References

[1] Elahi, R., P. Karami, A.H. Heidary and A. Esmaeilzadeh. 2022. An updated overview of recent advances, challenges, and clinical considerations of IL-6 signaling blockade in severe coronavirus disease 2019 (COVID-19). Int. Immunopharmacol., 105: 108536.

[2] Struyf, T., J.J. Deeks, J. Dinnes, Y. Takwoingi, C. Davenport, M.M. Leeflang, R. Spijker, L. Hooft, D. Emperador, S. Dittrich, J. Domen, S.R.A. Horn and A. Van den Bruel. 2022. Signs and symptoms to determine if a patient presenting in primary care or hospital outpatient settings has COVID-19. Cochrane Database of Systematic Reviews, 5.

[3] Litmanovich, D.E., M. Chung, R.R. Kirkbride, G. Kicska and J.P. Kanne. 2020. Review of chest radiograph findings of COVID-19 pneumonia and suggested reporting language. Journal of Thoracic Imaging, 35(6): 354–60.

[4] Yang Yang, Qing-Bin Lu, Ming-Jin Liu, Yi-Xing Wang, An-Ran Zhang, Neda Jalali, Natalie E. Dean, Ira Longini, M. Elizabeth Halloran, Bo Xu, Xiao-Ai Zhang, Li-Ping Wang, Wei Liu and Li-Qun Fang. 2020. Epidemiological and Clinical Features of the 2019 Novel Coronavirus Outbreak in China, medrxiv.

[5] Holshue, M.L., C. DeBolt, S. Lindquist, K.H. Lofy, J. Wiesman, H. Bruce, C. Spitters, K. Ericson, S. Wilkerson, A. Tural, G. Diaz, A. Cohn, L. Fox, A. Patel, S.I. Gerber, L. Kim, S. Tong, X. Lu, S. Lindstrom, M.A. Pallansch, W.C. Weldon, H.M. Biggs, T.M. Uyeki and S.K. Pillai. Washington State 2019-nCoV Case Investigation Team. 2020. First case of 2019 novel coronavirus in the United States. New England Journal of Medicine.

[6] Pongpirul, W.A., K. Pongpirul, A.C. Ratnarathon and W. Prasithsirikul. 2020. Journey of a Thai taxi driver and novel coronavirus. New England Journal of Medicine, 382(11): 1067–8.

[7] Nanshan Chen, Min Zhou, Xuan Dong, Jieming Qu, Fengyun Gong, Yang Han, Yang Qiu, Jingli Wang, Ying Liu, Yuan Wei, Jia'an Xia, Ting Yu, Xinxin Zhang and Li Zhang. 2020. Epidemiological and clinical characteristics of 99 cases of 2019 novel coronavirus pneumonia in Wuhan, China: A descriptive study. The Lancet, 395(10223): 507–13.

[8] Wang, D., B. Hu, C. Hu, F. Zhu, X. Liu, J. Zhang, B. Wang, H. Xiang, Z. Cheng, Y. Xiong, Y. Zhao, Y. Li, X. Wang and Z. Peng. 2020. Clinical characteristics of 138 hospitalized patients with 2019 novel coronavirus–infected pneumonia in Wuhan, China. Jama, 323(11): 1061–9.

[9] Chen, J., Z.Z. Zhang, Y.K. Chen, Q.X. Long, W.G. Tian, H.J. Deng, J.L. Hu, X.X. Zhang, Pu-Liao, J.L. Xiang, D.X. Wang, P. Hu, F.C. Zhou, Z.J. Li, H.M. Xu, X.F. Cai, D.Q. Wang, Y. Hu, N. Tang, B.Z. Liu, G.C. Wu and

A.L. Huang. 2020. The clinical and immunological features of pediatric COVID-19 patients in China. Genes & diseases, 7(4): 535–41.

[10] Albitar, O., R. Ballouze, J.P. Ooi and S.M.S. Ghadzi. 2020. Risk factors for mortality among COVID-19 patients. Diabetes Research and Clinical Practice, 166: 108293.

[11] Caramelo, F., N. Ferreira and B. Oliveiros. 2020. Estimation of Risk Factors for COVID-19 Mortality-preliminary Results. MedRxiv.

[12] Li, X., S. Xu, M. Yu, K. Wang, Y. Tao, Y. Zhou, J. Shi, M. Zhou, B. Wu, Z. Yang, C. Zhang, J. Yue, Z. Zhang, H. Renz, X. Liu, J. Xie, M. Xie and J. Zhao. 2020. Risk factors for severity and mortality in adult COVID-19 inpatients in Wuhan. Journal of Allergy and Clinical Immunology, 146(1): 110–8.

[13] Li, Q., X. Guan, P. Wu, X. Wang, L. Zhou, Y. Tong, R. Ren, K.S.M. Leung, E.H.Y. Lau, J.Y. Wong, X. Xing, N. Xiang, Y. Wu, C. Li, Q. Chen, D. Li, T. Liu, J. Zhao, M. Liu, W. Tu, C. Chen, L. Jin, R. Yang, Q. Wang, S. Zhou, R. Wang, H. Liu, Y. Luo, Y. Liu, G. Shao, H. Li, Z. Tao, Y. Yang, Z. Deng, B. Liu, Z. Ma, Y. Zhang, G. Shi, T.T.Y. Lam, J.T. Wu, G.F. Gao, B.J. Cowling, B. Yang, G.M. Leung and Z. Feng. 2020. Early transmission dynamics in Wuhan, China, of novel coronavirus–infected pneumonia. New England Journal of Medicine, 2020.

[14] Sun, J., W.T. He, L. Wang, A. Lai, X. Ji, X. Zhai, G. Li, M.A. Suchard, J. Tian, J. Zhou, M. Veit and S. Su. 2020. COVID-19: Epidemiology, evolution, and cross-disciplinary perspectives. Trends in Molecular Medicine, 26(5): 483–95.

[15] Lai, A., A. Bergna, C. Acciarri, M. Galli and G. Zehender. 2020. Early phylogenetic estimate of the effective reproduction number of SARS-CoV-2. J. Med. Virol., 92(6): 675–9.

[16] Castorina, P., A. Iorio and D. Lanteri. 2020. Data analysis on Coronavirus spreading by macroscopic growth laws. International Journal of Modern Physics C, 31(07): 2050103.

[17] Dong, L., J. Zhou, C. Niu, Q. Wang, Y. Pan, S. Sheng, X. Wang, Y. Zhang, J. Yang, M. Liu, Y. Zhao, X. Zhang, T. Zhu, T. Peng, J. Xie, Y. Gao, D. Wang, X. Dai and X. Fang. 2021. Highly accurate and sensitive diagnostic detection of SARS-CoV-2 by digital PCR. Talanta, 224: 121726.

[18] Fanelli, D. and F. Piazza. 2020. Analysis and forecast of COVID-19 spreading in China, Italy and France. Chaos, Solitons & Fractals, 134: 109761.

[19] Bhardwaj, R. 2020. A Predictive Model for the Evolution of COVID-19. Transactions of the Indian National Academy of Engineering, 5(2): 133–40.

[20] Singh, D. and S.V. Yi. 2021. On the origin and evolution of SARS-CoV-2. Experimental & Molecular Medicine, 53(4): 537–47.

[21] Singh, J., P. Pandit, A.G. McArthur, A. Banerjee and K. Mossman. 2021. Evolutionary trajectory of SARS-CoV-2 and emerging variants. Virology Journal, 18(1): 166.

[22] Chen, B., E.K. Tian, B. He, L. Tian, R. Han, S. Wang, Q. Xiang, S. Zhang, T. El Arnaout and W. Cheng. 2020. Overview of lethal human coronaviruses. Signal Transduct. Target Ther., 5(1): 89.

[23] Tian, J., J. Sun, D. Li, N. Wang, L. Wang, C. Zhang, X. Meng, X. Ji, M.A. Suchard, X. Zhang, A. Lai, S. Su and M. Veit. 2022. Emerging viruses: Cross-species transmission of coronaviruses, filoviruses, henipaviruses, and rotaviruses from bats. Cell Rep., 39(11): 110969.

[24] Telenti, A., E.B. Hodcroft and D.L. Robertson. 2022. The evolution and biology of SARS-CoV-2 variants. Cold Spring Harb. Perspect. Med., 12(5).

[25] Voskarides, K. 2022. SARS-CoV-2: Tracing the origin, tracking the evolution. BMC Medical Genomics, 15(1): 1–5.

[26] BrÅNussow, H. and L. BrÅNussow. 2021. Clinical evidence that the pandemic from 1889 to 1891 commonly called the Russian flu might have been an earlier coronavirus pandemic. Microbial Biotechnology, 14(5): 1860–70.

[27] Martin, D.P., S. Weaver, H. Tegally, J.E. San, S.D. Shank, E. Wilkinson, A.G. Lucaci, J. Giandhari, S. Naidoo, Y. Pillay, L. Singh, R.J. Lessells; NGS-SA; COVID-19 Genomics UK (COG-UK); R.K. Gupta, J.O. Wertheim, A. Nekturenko, B. Murrell, G.W. Harkins, P. Lemey, O.A. MacLean, D.L. Robertson, T. de Oliveira and S.L. Kosakovsky Pond. 2021. The emergence and ongoing convergent evolution of the SARS-CoV-2 N501Y lineages. Cell, 184(20): 5189–200.

[28] Lauring, A.S. and E.B. Hodcroft. 2021. Genetic variants of SARS-CoV-2-what do they mean? Jama, 325(6): 529–31.

[29] Denison, M.R., R.L. Graham, E.F. Donaldson, L.D. Eckerle and R.S. Baric. 2011. Coronaviruses: An RNA proofreading machine regulates replication fidelity and diversity. RNA Biol., 8(2): 270–9.

[30] Ogando, N.S., J.C. Zevenhoven-Dobbe, Y. Van der Meer, P.J. Bredenbeek, C.C. Posthuma and E.J. Snijder. 2020. The enzymatic activity of the nsp14 exoribonuclease is critical for replication of MERS-CoV and SARS-CoV-2. J. Virol., 94(23).

[31] Moeller, N.H., K. Shi, OÅN . Demir, S. Banerjee, L. Yin, C. Belica, S. Banerjee, L. Yin, C. Durfee, R.E. Amaro and H. Aihara. 2021. Structure and dynamics of SARS-CoV-2 proofreading exoribonuclease ExoN. bioRxiv.
[32] Blume, C., C.L. Jackson, C.M. Spalluto, J. Legebeke, L. Nazlamova, F. Conforti, J.M. Perotin, M. Frank, J. Butler, M. Crispin, J. Coles, J. Thompson, R.A. Ridley, L.S.N. Dean, M. Loxham, S. Reikine, A. Azim, K. Tariq, D.A. Johnston, P.J. Skipp, R. Djukanovic, D. Baralle, C.J. McCormick, D.E. Davies, J.S. Lucas, G. Wheway and V. Mennella. 2021. A novel ACE2 isoform is expressed in human respiratory epithelia and is upregulated in response to interferons and RNA respiratory virus infection. Nature Genetics, 53(2): 205–14.
[33] Rezaei, M., S.A. Ziai, S. Fakhri and R. Pouriran. 2021. ACE2: Its potential role and regulation in severe acute respiratory syndrome and COVID-19. Journal of Cellular Physiology, 236(4): 2430–42.
[34] Lamers, M.M. and B.L. Haagmans. 2022. SARS-CoV-2 pathogenesis. Nature Reviews Microbiology, 20(5): 270–84.
[35] Esmaeilzadeh, A., D. Jafari, S. Tahmasebi, R. Elahi and E. Khosh. 2021. Immune-Based Therapy for COVID-19. Adv. Exp. Med. Biol., 1318: 449–68.
[36] Taefehshokr, N., S. Taefehshokr, N. Hemmat and B. Heit. 2020. Covid-19: Perspectives on Innate Immune Evasion. Front Immunol., 11: 580641.
[37] Elahi, R., P. Karami, A.H. Heidary and A. Esmaeilzadeh. 2022. An updated overview of recent advances, challenges, and clinical considerations of IL-6 signaling blockade in severe coronavirus disease 2019 (COVID-19). International Immunopharmacology, 108536.
[38] Volz, E., S. Mishra, M. Chand, J.C. Barrett, R. Johnson, L. Geidelberg, W.R. Hinsley, D.J. Laydon, G. Dabrera, Á. O'Toole, R. Amato, M. Ragonnet-Cronin, I. Harrison, B. Jackson, C.V. Ariani, O. Boyd, N.J. Loman, J.T. McCrone, S. Gonçalves, D. Jorgensen, R. Myers, V. Hill, D.K. Jackson, K. Gaythorpe, N. Groves, J. Sillitoe, D.P. Kwiatkowski; COVID-19 Genomics UK (COG-UK) consortium; S. Flaxman, O. Ratmann, S. Bhatt, S. Hopkins, A. Gandy, A. Rambaut and N.M. Ferguson. 2021. Assessing transmissibility of SARS-CoV-2 lineage B.1.1.7 in England. Nature, 593(7858): 266–9.
[39] Davies, N.G., S. Abbott, R.C. Barnard, C.I. Jarvis, A.J. Kucharski, J.D. Munday, C.A.B. Pearson, T.W. Russell, D.C. Tully, A.D. Washburne, T. Wenseleers, A. Gimma, W. Waites, K.L.M. Wong, K. van Zandvoort, J.D. Silverman; CMMID COVID-19 Working Group; COVID-19 Genomics UK (COG-UK) Consortium; K. Diaz-Ordaz, R. Keogh, R.M. Eggo, S. Funk, M. Jit, K.E. Atkins and W.J. Edmunds. 2021. Estimated transmissibility and impact of SARS-CoV-2 lineage B.1.1.7 in England. Science, 372(6538).
[40] Kidd, M., A. Richter, A. Best, N. Cumley, J. Mirza, B. Percival, M. Mayhew, O. Megram, F. Ashford, T. White, E. Moles-Garcia, L. Crawford, A. Bosworth, S.F. Atabani, T. Plant and A. McNally. 2021. S-Variant SARS-CoV-2 Lineage B1.1.7 Is associated with significantly higher viral load in samples tested by TaqPath polymerase chain reaction. J. Infect. Dis., 223(10): 1666–70.
[41] Tegally, H., E. Wilkinson, M. Giovanetti, A. Iranzadeh, V. Fonseca, J. Giandhari et al. 2021. Detection of a SARS-CoV-2 variant of concern in South Africa. Nature, 592(7854): 438–43.
[42] Davies, N.G., C.I. Jarvis, W.J. Edmunds, N.P. Jewell, K. Diaz-Ordaz and R.H. Keogh. 2021. Increased mortality in community-tested cases of SARS-CoV-2 lineage B.1.1.7. Nature, 593(7858): 270–4.
[43] Al Kaabi, N., Y. Zhang, S. Xia, Y. Yang, M.M. Al Qahtani, N. Abdulrazzaq, M. Al Nusair, M. Hassany, J.S. Jawad, J. Abdalla, S.E. Hussein, S.K. Al Mazrouei, M. Al Karam, X. Li, X. Yang, W. Wang, B. Lai, W. Chen, S. Huang, Q. Wang, T. Yang, Y. Liu, R. Ma, Z.M. Hussain, T. Khan, M. Saifuddin Fasihuddin, W. You, Z. Xie, Y. Zhao, Z. Jiang, G. Zhao, Y. Zhang, S. Mahmoud, I. ElTantawy, P. Xiao, A. Koshy, W.A. Zaher, H. Wang, K. Duan, A. Pan and X. Yang. 2021. Effect of 2 inactivated SARS-CoV-2 vaccines on symptomatic COVID-19 infection in adults: A randomized clinical trial. Jama, 326(1): 35–45.
[44] Fujino, T., H. Nomoto, S. Kutsuna, M. Ujiie, T. Suzuki, R. Sato, T. Fujimoto, M. Kuroda, T. Wakita and N. Ohmagari. 2021. Novel SARS-CoV-2 variant in travelers from Brazil to Japan. Emerg. Infect. Dis., 27(4): 1243–5.
[45] GrÅNaf, T., G. Bello, T.M.M. Venas, E.C. Pereira, A.C.D. Paix~ao, L.R. Appolinario, R.S. Lopes, A.C.D.F. Mendonça, A.S.B. da Rocha, F.C. Motta, T.S. Gregianini, R.S. Salvato, S.B. Fernandes, D.B. Rovaris, A.C. Cavalcanti, A.B. Leite, I. Riediger, M.D.C. Debur, A.F.L. Bernardes, R. Ribeiro-Rodrigues, B. Grinsztejn, V. Alves do Nascimento, V.C. de Souza, L. Gonçalves, C.F. da Costa, T. Mattos, F.Z. Dezordi, G.L. Wallau, F.G. Naveca, E. Delatorre, M.M. Siqueira and P.C. Resende. 2021. Identification of a novel SARS-CoV-2 P.1 sub-lineage in Brazil provides new insights about the mechanisms of emergence of variants of concern. Virus Evol., 7(2): veab091.
[46] Naveca, F.G., V. Nascimento, V.C. De Souza, A.L. Corado, F. Nascimento, G. Silva, Á. Costa, D. Duarte, K. Pessoa, M. Mejía, M.J. Brandão, M. Jesus, L. Gonçalves, C.F. da Costa, V. Sampaio, D. Barros, M. Silva, T. Mattos, G. Pontes, L. Abdalla, J.H. Santos, I. Arantes, F.Z. Dezordi, M.M. Siqueira, G.L. Wallau, P.C. Resende, E. Delatorre,

T. Gräf and G. Bello. 2021. COVID-19 in Amazonas, Brazil, was driven by the persistence of endemic lineages and P.1 emergence. Nat. Med., 27(7): 1230--8.
[47] Brown, C.M., J. Vostok, H. Johnson, M. Burns, R. Gharpure, S. Sami, R.T. Sabo, N. Hall, A. Foreman, P.L. Schubert, G.R. Gallagher, T. Fink, L.C. Madoff, S.B. Gabriel, B. MacInnis, D.J. Park, K.J. Siddle, V. Harik, D. Arvidson, T. Brock-Fisher, M. Dunn, A. Kearns and A.S. Laney. 2021. Outbreak of SARS-CoV-2 infections, including COVID-19 vaccine breakthrough infections, associated with large public gatherings - Barnstable County, Massachusetts, July 2021. MMWR Morb. Mortal Wkly. Rep., 70(31): 1059–62.
[48] Cherian, S., V. Potdar, S. Jadhav, P. Yadav, N. Gupta, M. Das, P. Rakshit, S. Singh, P. Abraham, S. Panda and N. Team. 2021. SARS-CoV-2 Spike Mutations, L452R, T478K, E484Q and P681R, in the Second Wave of COVID-19 in Maharashtra, India. Microorganisms, 9(7).
[49] Mlcochova, P., S.A. Kemp, M.S. Dhar, G. Papa, B. Meng, I. Ferreira, Datir R, D.A. Collier, A. Albecka, S. Singh, R. Pandey, J. Brown, J. Zhou, N. Goonawardane, S. Mishra, C. Whittaker, T. Mellan, R. Marwal, M. Datta, S. Sengupta, K. Ponnusamy, V.S. Radhakrishnan, A. Abdullahi, O. Charles, P. Chattopadhyay, P. Devi, D. Caputo, T. Peacock, C. Wattal, N. Goel, A. Satwik, R. Vaishya, M. Agarwal; Indian SARS-CoV-2 Genomics Consortium (INSACOG); Genotype to Phenotype Japan (G2P-Japan) Consortium; CITIID-NIHR BioResource COVID-19 Collaboration; A. Mavousian, J.H. Lee, J. Bassi, C. Silacci-Fegni, C. Saliba, D. Pinto, T. Irie, I. Yoshida, W.L. Hamilton, K. Sato, S. Bhatt, S. Flaxman, L.C. James, D. Corti, L. Piccoli, W.S. Barclay, P. Rakshit, A. Agrawal and R.K. Gupta. 2021. SARS-CoV-2 B.1.617.2 Delta variant replication and immune evasion. Nature, 599(7883): 114–9.
[50] Shiehzadegan, S., N. Alaghemand, M. Fox and V. Venketaraman. 2021. Analysis of the delta variant B. 1.617. 2 COVID-19. Clinics and Practice, 11(4): 778–84.
[51] Robert Challen, Louise Dyson, Christopher E. Overton, Laura M. Guzman-Rincon, Edward M. Hill, Helena, B. Stage, Ellen Brooks-Pollock, Lorenzo Pellis, Francesca Scarabel, David J. Pascall, Paula Blomquist, Michael Tildesley, Daniel Williamson, Stefan Siegert, Xiaoyu Xiong, Ben Youngman, Juniper, Jonathan M. Read, Julia R. Gog, Matthew J. Keeling and Leon Danon. 2021. Early epidemiological signatures of novel SARS-CoV-2 variants: Establishment of B. 1.617. 2 in England. MedRxiv, 2021.
[52] SARS-CoV P. variants of concern and variants under investigation in England. 2021. Available from: https://assets. publishing. service. gov. uk/government/uploads/system/uploads/attachmentdata/file/988619. Variants-of-Concern-VOC-Technical-Briefing-12-England pdf.
[53] Bazargan, M., R. Elahi and A. Esmaeilzadeh. 2022. OMICRON: Virology, immunopathogenesis, and laboratory diagnosis. J. Gene Med., 24(7): e3435.
[54] Karim, S.S.A. and Q.A. Karim. 2021. Omicron SARS-CoV-2 variant: A new chapter in the COVID-19 pandemic. Lancet, 398(10317): 2126–8.
[55] Greaney, A.J., T.N. Starr, P. Gilchuk, S.J. Zost, E. Binshtein, A.N. Loes, S.K. Hilton, J. Huddleston, R. Eguia, K.H.D. Crawford, A.S. Dingens, R.S. Nargi, R.E. Sutton, N. Suryadevara, P.W. Rothlauf, Z. Liu, S.P.J. Whelan, R.H. Carnahan, J.E. Jr. Crowe and J.D. Bloom. 2021. Complete mapping of mutations to the SARS-CoV-2 spike receptor-binding domain that escape antibody recognition. Cell Host Microbe., 29(1): 44–57, e9.
[56] Garcia-Beltran, W.F., K.J. St Denis, A. Hoelzemer, E.C. Lam, A.D. Nitido, M.L. Sheehan, C. Berrios, O. Ofoman, C.C. Chang, B.M. Hauser, J. Feldman, A.L. Roederer, D.J. Gregory, M.C. Poznansky, A.G. Schmidt, A.J. Iafrate, V. Naranbhai and A.B. Balazs. 2021. mRNAbased COVID-19 vaccine boosters induce neutralizing immunity against SARS-CoV-2 Omicron variant. MedRxiv, 2021.
[57] Andrews, N., J. Stowe, F. Kirsebom, S. Toffa, T. Rickeard, E. Gallagher, C. Gower, M. Kall, N. Groves, A.M. O'Connell, D. Simons, P.B. Blomquist, A. Zaidi, S. Nash, N. Iwani Binti Abdul Aziz, S. Thelwall, G. Dabrera, R. Myers, G. Amirthalingam, S. Gharbia, J.C. Barrett, R. Elson, S.N. Ladhani, N. Ferguson, M. Zambon, C.N.J. Campbell, K. Brown, S. Hopkins, M. Chand, M. Ramsay and J. Lopez Bernal. 2022. Covid-19 vaccine effectiveness against the Omicron (B.1.1.529) variant. N. Engl. J. Med., 386(16): 1532–46.
[58] Shuai, H., J.F. Chan, B. Hu, Y. Chai, T.T. Yuen, F. Yin, X. Huang, C. Yoon, J.C. Hu, H. Liu, J. Shi, Y. Liu, T. Zhu, J. Zhang, Y. Hou, Y. Wang, L. Lu, J.P. Cai, A.J. Zhang, J. Zhou, S. Yuan, M.A. Brindley, B.Z. Zhang, J.D. Huang, K.K. To, K.Y. Yuen and H. Chu. 2022. Attenuated replication and pathogenicity of SARS-CoV-2 B.1.1.529 Omicron. Nature, 603(7902): 693–9.
[59] Berkhout, B. and E. Herrera-Carrillom. 2022. SARS-CoV-2 evolution: On the sudden appearance of the Omicron variant. J. Virol., 96(7): e0009022.
[60] Haseltine, W. 2022. Birth of the Omicron Family: BA. 1, BA. 2, BA. 3 each as different as Alpha is from Delta, Forbes.

[61] Yu, J., A.Y. Collier, M. Rowe, F. Mardas, J.D. Ventura, H. Wan, J. Miller, O. Powers, B. Chung, M. Siamatu, N.P. Hachmann, N. Surve, F. Nampanya, A. Chandrashekar and D.H. Barouch. 2022. Neutralization of the SARS-CoV-2 Omicron BA.1 and BA.2 variants. N. Engl. J. Med., 386(16): 1579–80.
[62] Maxmen, A. 2022. Are new Omicron subvariants a threat? Here's how scientists are keeping watch. Nature, 604(7907): 605–6.
[63] World Health Organization. 2022. COVID-19 Weekly Epidemiological Update, edition 115, 26 October 2022.
[64] Chen, J., R. Wang, Y. Hozumi, G. Liu, Y. Qiu, X. Wei and G.W. Wei. 2022. Emerging dominant SARS-CoV-2 variants. arXiv preprint arXiv, 221009485.
[65] Mustafa, M. and A. Makhawi. 2022. What Learned from Omicron Sub-Variants BQ. 1 and BQ. 1.1.
[66] Del Rio, C. and P.N. Malani. 2022. COVID-19 in 2022-The beginning of the end or the end of the beginning? JAMA, 327(24): 2389–90.
[67] Marjanovic, S., R.J. Romanelli, G.C. Ali, B. Leach, M. Bonsu, D. Rodriguez-Rincon and T. Ling. 2022. COVID-19 Genomics UK (COG-UK) Consortium: final report. Rand Health Q, 9(4): 24.
[68] Romero, P.E., A. Dávila-Barclay, G. Salvatierra, L. González, D. Cuicapuza, L. Solís, P. Marcos-Carbajal, J. Huancachoque, L. Maturrano and P. Tsukayama. 2021. The emergence of SARS-CoV-2 variant lambda (C. 37) in South America. Microbiology Spectrum, 9(2): e00789–21.
[69] O'Toole, Á., E. Scher, A. Underwood, B. Jackson, V. Hill, J.T. McCrone, R. Colquhoun, C. Ruis, K. Abu-Dahab, B. Taylor, C. Yeats, L. du Plessis, D. Maloney, N. Medd, S.W. Attwood, D.M. Aanensen, E.C. Holmes, O.G. Pybus and A. Rambaut. 2021. Assignment of epidemiological lineages in an emerging pandemic using the pangolin tool. Virus Evol., 7(2): veab064.
[70] Singh, J., A.G. Malhotra, D. Biswas, P. Shankar, L. Lokhande, A.K. Yadav, A. Raghuvanshi, D. Kale, S. Nema, S. Saigal and S. Singh. 2021. Relative consolidation of the Kappa variant pre-dates the Massive second wave of COVID-19 in India. Genes, 12(11): 1803.
[71] Chen, J., Q. Jiang, X. Xia, K. Liu, Z. Yu, W. Tao, W. Gong and J.J. Han. 2020. Individual variation of the SARS-CoV-2 receptor ACE2 gene expression and regulation. Aging Cell, 19(7).
[72] Zimmermann, P., L.F. Pittet, A. Finn, A.J. Pollard and N. Curtis. 2022. Should children be vaccinated against COVID-19? Arch. Dis. Child., 107(3): e1.
[73] Meng, B., A. Abdullahi, I. Ferreira, N. Goonawardane, A. Saito, I. Kimura, D. Yamasoba, P.P. Gerber, S. Fatihi, S. Rathore, S.K. Zepeda, G. Papa, S.A. Kemp, T. Ikeda, M. Toyoda, T.S. Tan, J. Kuramochi, S. Mitsunaga, T. Ueno, K. Shirakawa, A. Takaori-Kondo, T. Brevini, D.L. Mallery, O.J. Charles; CITIID-NIHR BioResource COVID-19 Collaboration; Genotype to Phenotype Japan (G2P-Japan) Consortium; Ecuador-COVID19 Consortium; J.E. Bowen, A. Joshi, A.C. Walls, L. Jackson, D. Martin, K.G.C. Smith, J. Bradley, J.A.G. Briggs, J. Choi, E. Madissoon, K.B. Meyer, P. Mlcochova, L. Ceron-Gutierrez, R. Doffinger, S.A. Teichmann, A.J. Fisher, M.S. Pizzuto, A. de Marco, D. Corti, M. Hosmillo, J.H. Lee, L.C. James, L. Thukral, D. Veesler, A. Sigal, F. Sampaziotis, I.G. Goodfellow, N.J. Matheson, K. Sato and R.K. Gupta. 2022. Altered TMPRSS2 usage by SARS-CoV-2 Omicron impacts infectivity and fusogenicity. Nature, 603(7902): 706–14.
[74] Willett, B.J., J. Grove, O.A. MacLean, C. Wilkie, G. De Lorenzo, W. Furnon, D. Cantoni, S. Scott, N. Logan, S. Ashraf, M. Manali, A. Szemiel, V. Cowton, E. Vink, W.T. Harvey, C. Davis, P. Asamaphan, K. Smollett, L. Tong, R. Orton, J. Hughes, P. Holland, V. Silva, D.J. Pascall, K. Puxty, A. da Silva Filipe, G. Yebra, S. Shaaban, M.T.G. Holden, R.M. Pinto, R. Gunson, K. Templeton, P.R. Murcia, A.H. Patel, P. Klenerman, S. Dunachie; PITCH Consortium; COVID-19 Genomics UK (COG-UK) Consortium; J. Haughney, D.L. Robertson, M. Palmarini, S. Ray and E.C. Thomson. 2022. SARS-CoV-2 Omicron is an immune escape variant with an altered cell entry pathway. Nat. Microbiol., 7(8): 1161–79.
[75] Jogalekar, M.P., A. Veerabathini and P. Gangadaran. 2021. SARS-CoV-2 variants: A double-edged sword? Exp. Biol. Med. (Maywood), 246(15): 1721–6.
[76] Mistry, P., F. Barmania, J. Mellet, K. Peta, A. Strydom, I.M. Viljoen, W. James, S. Gordon and M.S. Pepper. 2021. SARS-CoV-2 variants, vaccines, and host immunity. Front. Immunol., 12: 809244.
[77] Esmaeilzadeh, A., A.J. Maleki, A. Moradi, A. Siahmansouri, M.J. Yavari, P. Karami and R. Elahi. 2022. Major severe acute respiratory coronavirus-2 (SARS-CoV-2) vaccine-associated adverse effects; benefits outweigh the risks. Expert Rev. Vaccines, 21(10): 1377–94.
[78] Heidary, A., R. Elahi and M. Nazari. 2021. Benign Cerebral Edema and Increased Intracranial Pressure (ICP) as manifestations of COVID-19 reinfection; A case report. J. Clin. Lab. Med., 6(1).
[79] Gallotti, R., F. Valle, N. Castaldo, P. Sacco and M. De Domenico. 2020. Assessing the risks of 'infodemics' in response to COVID-19 epidemics. Nature Human Behaviour, 4(12): 1285–93.

[80] Wong, M.Y.Z., D.V. Gunasekeran, S. Nusinovici, C. Sabanayagam, K.K. Yeo, C.Y. Cheng and Y.C. Tham. 2021. Telehealth demand trends during the COVID-19 pandemic in the top 50 most affected countries: Infodemiological evaluation. JMIR Public Health and Surveillance, 7(2): e24445.

[81] Le, T.T., J.P. Cramer, R. Chen and S. Mayhew. 2020. Evolution of the COVID-19 vaccine development landscape. Nat. Rev. Drug Discov., 19(10): 667–8.

[82] Swerdlow, D.L. and L. Finelli. 2020. Preparation for possible sustained transmission of 2019 novel coronavirus: Lessons from previous epidemics. Jama, 323(12): 1129–30.

[83] Carvalho, T., F. Krammer and A. Iwasaki. 2021. The first 12 months of COVID-19: A timeline of immunological insights. Nature Reviews Immunology, 21(4): 245–56.

[84] Singh, S., C. Mcnab, R.M. Olson, N. Bristol, C. Nolan, E. Bergstrøm, M. Bartos, S. Mabuchi, R. Panjabi, A. Karan, S.M. Abdalla, M. Bonk, M. Jamieson, G.K. Werner, A. Nordström, H. Legido-Quigley and A. Phelan. 2021. How an outbreak became a pandemic: A chronological analysis of crucial junctures and international obligations in the early months of the COVID-19 pandemic. The Lancet, 398(10316): 2109–24.

[85] Allam, Z. 2020. The first 50 days of COVID-19: a detailed chronological timeline and extensive review of literature documenting the pandemic. Surveying the Covid-19 Pandemic and its Implications, 1.

[86] Wiegand, T., A. Nemudryi, A. Nemudraia, A. McVey, A. Little, D.N. Taylor, S.T. Walk and B. Wiedenheft. 2022. The rise and fall of SARS-CoV-2 variants and ongoing diversification of Omicron. Viruses, 14(9): 2009.

[87] Felsenstein, S., J.A. Herbert, P.S. McNamara and C.M. Hedrich. 2020. COVID-19: Immunology and treatment options. Clinical Immunology, 215: 108448.

[88] Pacurar, C.M., V.D. Păcurar and M. Paun. 2021. An Analysis of COVID-19 in Europe Based on Fractal Dimension and Meteorological Data.

[89] Baran, S. and D. Nemoda. 2016. Censored and shifted gamma distribution based EMOS model for probabilistic quantitative precipitation forecasting. Environmetrics, 27(5): 280–92.

[90] Grushka-Cockayne, Y. and V.R.R. Jose. 2020. Combining prediction intervals in the M4 competition. International Journal of Forecasting, 36(1): 178–85.

[91] Nash, C.M. 2020. Harvard Professor Sounds Alarm on 'Likely' Coronavirus Pandemic: 40% to 70% of World Could Be Infected This Year.

[92] Safi, S.K. and O.I. Sanusi. 2021. A hybrid of artificial neural network, exponential smoothing, and ARIMA models for COVID-19 time series forecasting. Model Assisted Statistics and Applications, 16(1): 25–35.

[93] Khan, M.A., R. Khan, F. Algarni, I. Kumar, A. Choudhary and A. Srivastava. 2022. Performance evaluation of regression models for COVID-19: A statistical and predictive perspective. Ain Shams Engineering Journal, 13(2): 101574.

[94] Hwang, E. 2022. Prediction intervals of the COVID-19 cases by HAR models with growth rates and vaccination rates in top eight affected countries: Bootstrap improvement. Chaos, Solitons & Fractals, 155: 111789.

[95] Cooper, I., A. Mondal and C.G. Antonopoulos. 2020. Dynamic tracking with model-based forecasting for the spread of the COVID-19 pandemic. Chaos, Solitons & Fractals, 139: 110298.

[96] Zeroual, A., F. Harrou, A. Dairi and Y. Sun. 2020. Deep learning methods for forecasting COVID-19 time-Series data: A Comparative study. Chaos, Solitons & Fractals, 140: 110121.

[97] Ceylan, Z. 2020. Estimation of COVID-19 prevalence in Italy, Spain, and France. Science of The Total Environment, 729: 138817.

[98] Shahid, F., A. Zameer and M. Muneeb. 2020. Predictions for COVID-19 with deep learning models of LSTM, GRU and Bi-LSTM. Chaos, Solitons & Fractals, 140: 110212.

[99] Karaçuha, E., N.Ö. Önal, E. Ergün, V. Tabatadze, H. Alkaş, K. Karaçuha, H.O. Tontus and N.V.N. Nu. 2020. Modeling and prediction of the covid-19 cases with deep assessment methodology and fractional Calculus. IEEE Access, 8: 164012–34.

[100] Rustam, Furqan, Reshi, Aijaz Ahmad, Mehmood, Arif, Ullah, Saleem, On, Byung-Won, Aslam, Waqar and Choi, Gyu Sang. 2020. COVID-19 future forecasting using supervised machine learning models. IEEE Access, 8: 101489–99.

[101] Petropoulos, F., S. Makridakis and N. Stylianou. 2020. COVID-19: Forecasting confirmed cases and deaths with a simple time series model. International Journal of Forecasting.

[102] Alzahrani, S.I., I.A. Aljamaan and E.A. Al-Fakih. 2020. Forecasting the spread of the COVID-19 pandemic in Saudi Arabia using ARIMA prediction model under current public health interventions. J. Infect. Public Health, 13(7): 914–9.

[103] Elsheikh, A.H., A.I. Saba, M. Abd Elaziz, S. Lu, S. Shanmugan, T. Muthuramalingam, R. Kumar, A.O. Mosleh, F.A. Essa and T.A. Shehabeldeen. 2021. Deep learning-based forecasting model for COVID-19 outbreak in Saudi Arabia. Process Safety and Environmental Protection, 149: 223–33.
[104] Alanazi, S.A., M. Kamruzzaman, M. Alruwaili, N. Alshammari, S.A. Alqahtani and A. Karime. 2020. Measuring and preventing COVID-19 using the SIR model and machine learning in smart health care. Journal of Healthcare Engineering, 2020.
[105] Jeelani, M.B., A.S. Alnahdi, M.S. Abdo, M.A. Abdulwasaa, K. Shah and H.A. Wahash. 2021. Mathematical modeling and forecasting of COVID-19 in Saudi Arabia under fractal-fractional derivative in Caputo sense with power-law. Axioms, 10(3): 228.
[106] Melin, P. and O. Castillo. 2021. Spatial and temporal spread of the COVID-19 pandemic using self organizing neural networks and a fuzzy fractal approach. Sustainability, 13(15): 8295.
[107] Hussein, T., M.H. Hammad, P.L. Fung, M. Al-Kloub, I. Odeh, M.A. Zaidan and D. Wraith. 2021. COVID-19 pandemic development in Jordan—short-term and long-term forecasting. Vaccines, 9(7): 728.
[108] Ma, N., W. Ma and Z. Li. 2021. Multi-model selection and analysis for COVID-19. Fractal and Fractional, 5(3): 120.
[109] Marzouk, M., N. Elshaboury, A. Abdel-Latif and S. Azab. 2021. Deep learning model for forecasting COVID-19 outbreak in Egypt. Process Safety and Environmental Protection, 153: 363–75.
[110] Shahin, A.I. and S. Almotairi. 2021. A deep learning BiLSTM encoding-decoding model for COVID-19 pandemic spread forecasting. Fractal and Fractional, 5(4): 175.
[111] Easwaramoorthy, D., A. Gowrisankar, A. Manimaran, S. Nandhini, L. Rondoni and S. Banerjee. 2021. An exploration of fractal-based prognostic model and comparative analysis for second wave of COVID-19 diffusion. Nonlinear Dynamics, 106(2): 1375–95.
[112] Hadi, M.S. and B. Bilgehan. 2022. Fractional COVID-19 modeling and analysis on successive optimal control policies. Fractal and Fractional, 6(10): 533.
[113] Bastos, S.B. and D.O. Cajueiro. 2020. Modeling and forecasting the early evolution of the Covid-19 pandemic in Brazil. Scientific Reports, 10(1): 19457.
[114] Nguyen, D.Q., N.Q. Vo, T.T. Nguyen, K. Nguyen-An, Q.H. Nguyen, D.N. Tran and T.T. Quan. 2022. BeCaked: An explainable artificial intelligence model for COVID-19 forecasting. Sci. Rep., 12(1): 7969.
[115] Sun, J., W.T. He, L. Wang, A. Lai, X. Ji, X. Zhai, G. Li, M.A. Suchard, J. Tian, J. Zhou, M. Veit and S. Su. 2020. COVID-19: Epidemiology, evolution, and cross-disciplinary perspectives. Trends in Molecular Medicine, 26(5): 483–95.
[116] Skegg, D., P. Gluckman, G. Boulton, H. Hackmann, S.S.A. Karim, P. Piot and C. Woopen. 2021. Future scenarios for the COVID-19 pandemic. The Lancet, 397(10276): 777–8.
[117] Nugent, M.A. 2022. The future of the COVID-19 Pandemic: How good (or bad) can the SARS-CoV2 spike protein get? Cells, 11(5).
[118] Baloch, Z., A. Ikram, S. Shamim, A. Obaid, F.M. Awan, A. Naz, B. Rauff, K. Gilani and J.A. Qureshi. 2022. Human coronavirus spike protein based multi-epitope vaccine against COVID-19 and potential future zoonotic coronaviruses by using immunoinformatic approaches. Vaccines (Basel), 10(7).
[119] Kristiann Allen, Tatjana Buklijas, Andrew Chen, Naomi Simon-Kumar, Lara Cowen, James Wilsdon and Peter Gluckman. 2020. Tracking global evidence-to-policy pathways in the coronavirus crisis: A preliminary report.
[120] Reicher, S. and J. Drury. 2021. Pandemic fatigue? How adherence to Covid-19 regulations has been misrepresented and why it matters. BMJ, 372.
[121] Haktanir, A., N. Can, T. Seki, M.F. Kurnaz and B. Dilmaç. 2021. Do we experience pandemic fatigue? current state, predictors, and prevention. Current Psychology, 1–12.
[122] Aquino, E.M.L., I.H. Silveira, J.M. Pescarini, R. Aquino, J.A. Souza-Filho, A.S. Rocha, A. Ferreira, A. Victor, C. Teixeira, D.B. Machado, E. Paixão, F.J.O. Alves, F. Pilecco, G. Menezes, L. Gabrielli, L. Leite, M.C.C. Almeida, N. Ortelan, Q.H.R.F. Fernandes, R.J.F. Ortiz, R.N. Palmeira, E.P.P. Junior, E. Aragão, L.E.P.F. Souza, M.B. Netto, M.G. Teixeira, M.L. Barreto, M.Y. Ichihara and R.T.R.S. Lima. 2020. Social distancing measures to control the COVID-19 pandemic: Potential impacts and challenges in Brazil. Ciencia & Saude Coletiva, 25: 2423–46.

Chapter 2

A Fractal Viewpoint to Covid-19 Infection

Oscar Sotolongo-Costa,[1] *José Weberszpil*[2,*] and *Oscar Sotolongo-Grau*[3]

2.1 Introduction

The worldwide pandemic caused by the SARS-CoV-2 coronavirus outbreak has attracted the attention of the scientific community due to, among other factors, its fast spread. Its strong contamination capacity has created a fast growing population of people enduring COVID-19, its related disease, and a non small peak of mortality. The temporal evolution of contagion over different countries and worldwide brings up a common dynamic characteristic, in particular, its fast rise to reach a maximum followed by a slow decrease (incidentally, very similar to other epidemic processes) suggesting some kind of relaxation process, which we try to deal with, since relaxation is, essentially, a process where the parameters characterizing a system are altered, followed by a tendency to equilibrium values. In Physics, clear examples are, among others, dielectric or mechanical relaxation. In other fields (psychology, economy, etc.) there are also phenomena in which an analogy with "common" relaxation can be established. In relaxation, temporal behavior of parameters is of medular methodological interest. That is why pandemics can be conceived as one in which this behavior is also present. For this reason, we are interested, despite the existence of statistical or dynamical systems method, in the introduction of a phenomenological equation containing parameters that reflect the system´s behavior, from which its dynamics emerges. We are interested in studying the daily presented new cases, not the current cases by day. This must be noted to avoid confusion in the interpretation, i.e., we study not the cumulative number of infected patients reported in databases, but its derivative. This relaxation process in this case is, for us, an scenario that, by analogy, will serve to model the dynamics of the pandemics. This is not an ordinary process. Due to the concurrence of many factors that make this a very complex study its description must turn out to be a non classical description. So, we will consider that the dynamics of this

[1] Cátedra Henri Poincaré de sistemas complejos, Universidad de La Habana, Habana 10400 Cuba.
Email: osotolongo@gmail.com

[2] Universidade Federal Rural do Rio de Janeiro, UFRRJ-IM/DTL; Av. Governador Roberto Silveira s/n- Nova Iguaçú, Rio de Janeiro, Brasil 695014.

[3] Alzheimer Research Center and Memory Clinic, Fundació ACE, Institut Català de Neurociències Aplicades; 08029 Barcelona, Spain.
Email: osotolongo@fundacioace.com

* Corresponding author: josewebe@gmail.com

pandemic as described by a "fractal" or internal time [21]. The network formed by the people in its daily activity forms a complex field of links which are very difficult, if not impossible, to describe. However, we can take a simplified model where all the nodes belong to a small world network, but the time of transmission from one node to other differs for each link. So, in order to study this process let us assume that spread occurs in "fractal time" or internal time [9, 21]. This is not a new tool in physics. In Refs. [6, 7, 13] this concept has been successfully introduced and here, we keep in mind the possibility of a fractal-like kinetics [12], but generalizing as a nonlinear kinetic process. Here we will follow to what we refer as a "relaxation-like" approach, to model the dynamics of the pandemic and that justify the fractal time. By analogy with relaxation, an anomalous relaxation, we build up a simple nonlinear equation with fractal-time. We also regain the analytical results using a deformed derivative approach, using conformable derivative (CD) [10]. In Ref. [17] one of the authors (J.W.) have shown intimate relation of this derivative with complex systems and nonadditive statistical mechanics. This was done without resort to details of any kind of specific entropy definition.

This chapter is outlined in sections as follows: In Section 2, we present the fractal model formulated in terms of conformable derivatives, to develop the relevant expressions to adjust data of COVID-19. In Section 3, we show the results and discussion referring to the data fitting along with discussions. In Section 4, we finally cast our general conclusions and possible paths for further investigations.

2.2 Fractal Model

Let us denote by $F(t)$ the number of contagions up to time t. The CD is defined as [10]

$$D_x^\alpha f(x) = \lim_{\epsilon \to 0} \frac{f(x + \epsilon x^{1-\alpha}) - f(x)}{\epsilon}. \tag{2.1}$$

Note that the deformation is placed in the independent variable. For differentiable functions, the CD can be written as

$$D_x^\alpha f = x^{1-\alpha} \frac{df}{dx}. \tag{2.2}$$

An important point to be noticed here is that the deformations affect different functional spaces, depending on the problem under consideration. For the conformable derivative [16–20], the deformations are put in the independent variable, which can be a space coordinate, in the case of, e.g., mass position dependent problems, or even time or spacetime variables, for temporal dependent parameter or relativistic problems. Since we are dealing with a complex system, a search for a mathematical approach that could take into account some fractality or hidden variables seems to be adequate. This idea is also based in the fact that we do not have full information about the system under study. In this case, deformed derivatives with fractal time seems to be a good option to deal with this kind of system. Deformed derivatives, in the context of generalized statistical mechanics are present and connected [17]. There, the authors have also shown that the $q-deformed$ derivative also has a dual derivative and a $q-exponential$ related function [11]. Here, in the case under study, the deformation is considered for the solutions-space or dependent variable, that is, the number $F(t)$ of contagions up to time t. One should also consider that justification for the use of deformed derivatives finds its physical basis on the mapping into the fractal continuum [4, 5, 17]. That is, one considers a mapping from a fractal coarse grained (fractal porous) space, which is essentially discontinuous in the embedding Euclidean space, to a continuous one [19]. In our case the fractality lies in the temporal variable. Then the CD is with respect to time.

A nonlinear relaxation model can be proposed here, again based on a generalization of Brouers-Sotolongo fractal kinetic model (BSf) [6, 7], but here represented by a nonlinear equation written in terms of CD:

$$D_t^\alpha F = \frac{1}{\tau^\alpha} F^q, \tag{2.3}$$

where τ is our "relaxation time"and q and α here are real parameters. We do not impose any limit for the parameters. Equation (2.3) has as a well known solution a function with the shape of Burr XII [8], with :

$$F = F_0 \left[1 + (1-q) \frac{(t^\alpha - t_0^\alpha)}{\tau^\alpha \alpha F_0^{1-q}} \right]^{\frac{1}{1-q}}. \tag{2.4}$$

The density (in a similar form of a PDF, but here it is not a PDF) is, then:

$$f(t) = \frac{F_0^q}{\tau^\alpha} \left[C + (1-q) \frac{t^\alpha}{\tau^\alpha \alpha F_0^{1-q}} \right]^{\frac{q}{1-q}} t^{\alpha-1}, \tag{2.5}$$

where $C = 1 - \frac{(1-q)t_0^\alpha}{\tau^\alpha \alpha F_0^{1-q}}$,which can be expressed as:

$$f(t) = A'[C + B't^\alpha]^{-b} t^{a-1} \tag{2.6}$$

where the parameter are $A' = \frac{F_0^q}{\tau^\alpha}$, $B' = (1-q)\frac{1}{\tau^\alpha \alpha F_0^{1-q}}$, $b = \frac{q}{q-1}$, $a = \alpha$.

Or, in a simpler form for data adjustment purposes

$$f(t) = A[1 + Bt^\alpha]^{-b} t^{a-1}, \tag{2.7}$$

with $A = \frac{A'}{C^b}$, $B = \frac{B'}{C}$.

This is very similar, though not equal, to the function proposed by Tsallis [14, 15] in an ad hoc way. Here, however, a physical representation by the method of analogy is proposed to describe the evolution of the pandemics. Though we have introduced A, B, C, b, and a as parameters to simplify the fitting, the true adjustment constants are, clearly, q, τ and α. Note that we do not impose any restrictive values to the parameters.

There is no need to demand that the solution always converge. The equation to obtain Burr XII has to impose restrictions but this is not the case. In Burr XII the function was used as a probability distribution. But here the function describes a dynamic, which can be explosive, as shown for the curves of Brazil and Mexico. Therefore, if we consider infinite population, a peak will never be reached unless the circumstances change (treatments, vaccines, isolation, etc.). Our model does not impose finiteness of the solution. The possibility for a decay of the pandemic in a given region in this model requires the fulfillment of the condition

$$a(1-b) - 1 < 0, \tag{2.8}$$

what expresses the property that

$$\lim_{t \to \infty} f(t) = 0, \tag{2.9}$$

what means that the function has a local maximum. If this condition is not accomplished, the pandemic does not have a peak and, therefore, the number of cases increases forever in this model.

In this case there is, apart from the change of propagation and development conditions, the possibility for a given country that does not satisfies condition (2.8), to reach "herd immunity", i.e., when the number of contagions has reached about 60% of population, in which case we may calculate the time to reach such state using (2.4), assuming $t_0 = 0$:

$$T_{hi} = [(0.6P)^{1/(1-b)} - 1)/B]^{1/a}. \tag{2.10}$$

We will work with what we will call T_{1000} ahead and that seems to make more sense and bring more information.

2.3 Results and Discussion

With Eq. (2.7) let us fit the data of the epidemic worldwide. The data was extracted from Johns Hopkins University [1] and the website [2] to process the data for several countries.

We covered the infected cases taken at Jan 22 as day 1, up to June 13. The behavior of new infected cases by day is shown in Figure 2.1. The fitting was made with gnuplot 5.2. As it seems, the pandemic shows some sort of "plateau", so the present measures of prevention are not able to eliminate the infection propagation in a short term, but it can be seen that condition (2.8) is weakly fulfilled. In the particular case of Mexico the fitting is shown in Figure 2.2. In this case condition (2.8) is not fulfilled. In terms of our model this means that the peak is not predictable within the present dynamics. Something similar occurs with Brazil, as shown in Figure 2.3. The data for Brazil neither fulfills the condition (2.8). In this case there is neither the prevision of a peak and we can say that the data for Mexico and Brazil reveals a dynamics where the peak seems to be quite far if it exists. But there are some illustrative cases where the peak is reached. Progression of the outbreak in Cuba and Iceland are shown in Figures 2.4 and 2.5 respectively. Condition (2.8) is satisfied for both countries and we can see that the curve of infection rate descends at a good speed after past the peak. Now let us take a look at United States data, shown in Figure 2.6. The USA outbreak is characterized by a very fast growth until the peak and, then, very slow decay of the infection rate is evident. As discussed above,

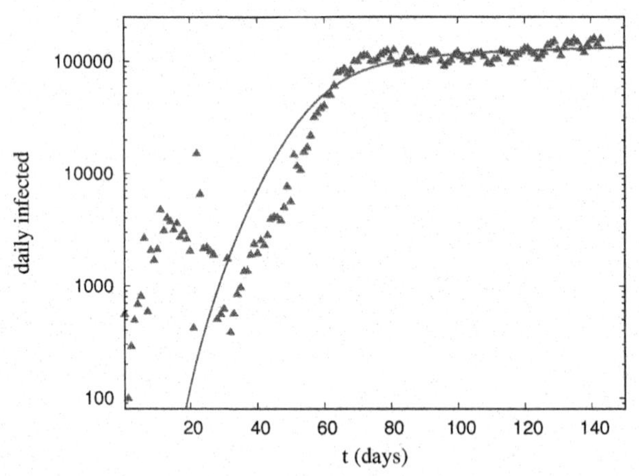

Fig. 2.1: Worldwide infections from Jan, 22 to June 13 and fitting with Eq. (2.7). The behavior fits well with parameters in Table 2.1. Condition (2.8) is satisfied.

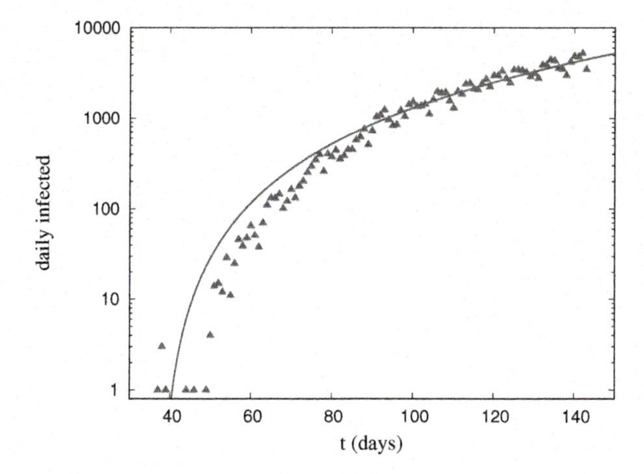

Fig. 2.2: Daily infections in Mexico and fitting with Eq. (2.7) for parameters in Table 2.1. T_{hi} = 778 days. Condition (2.8) is not satisfied.

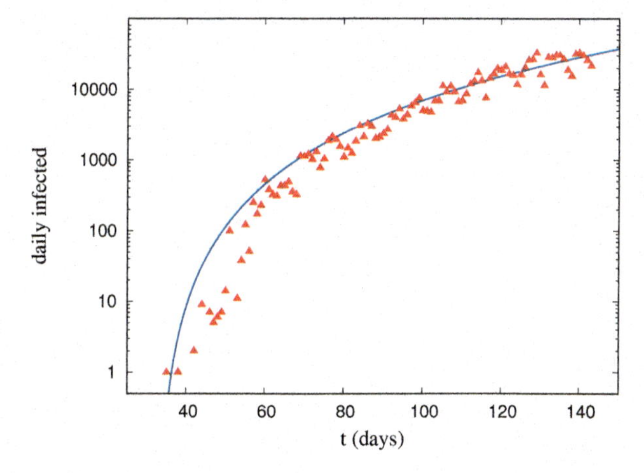

Fig. 2.3: Evolution of daily cases in Brazil and fitting with Eq. (2.7) for parameters in Table 2.1. T_{hi} = 298 days. Condition (2.8) is not satisfied.

the outbreak will be controlled for almost infinite time in this dynamics. There is also some intermediate cases as Spain and Italy, shown in Figures 2.7 and 2.8. In this case the data exhibits the same behavior as in USA, a fast initial growth and a very slow decay after the peak. However, the outbreak is controlled in a finite amount of time. In Table 2.1 we present the relevant fitting parameters, including herdimmunity time, T_{hi} and T_{1000}, the time to reach a rate of 1000 infections daily. This, for countries that have not reached the epidemic peak, Mexico and Brazil. We also include the population, P; of each country. As can be seen from fitting coefficients, the exponent b drives the behavior of infections in every country. Those countries that manage well the disease expansion have b values wide larger than 1. Countries with b values close to one, as Italy and Spain, have managed the pandemics but poorly and at high costs. The recovery in both countries will be long. The same is valid for USA, that managed the outbreak poorly and its struggle with an even longer recovery to normal life. Even the worst case scenario has taken place in Mexico and Brazil, with very

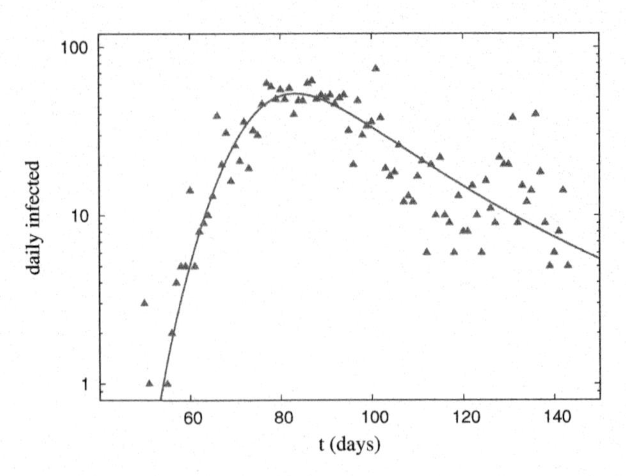

Fig. 2.4: Daily infections in Cuba. The theoretical curve fits with data though with a poor correlation due to the dispersion. See fitting parameters in Table 2.1. Condition(2.8) is satisfied.

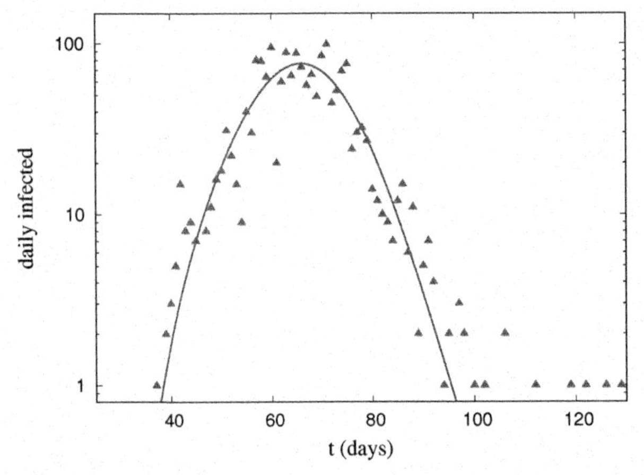

Fig. 2.5: Daily infections in Iceland, where the pandemic seems to have ceased. Here again, in spite of the relatively small correlation coefficient, the behavior of the pandemic in this country looks well described by Eq. (2.7). See fitting parameters in Table 2.1. Condition (2.8) is satisfied.

low values of b. Those countries are experiencing a big outbreak where even they can get herd immunity. This, however, implies very high values of infections and mortality for the near future.

But let us briefly comment on herd immunity. Those countries that have managed to stop the outbreak, even with relative high mortality as Spain and Italy, will not reach the herd immunity. As a matter of fact, This can not be calculated for those countries. Then, we can see countries like Brazil where, if the way to deal with the outbreak does not change, the herd immunity will be reached. Even when it seems desirable, the ability to reach the herd immunity brings with it a high payload. That is, for a country like Brazil the herd immunity would require more than 100 million of infected people. That is, much the same as if a war devastates the country. There is a similar scenario in Mexico, but the difference here is that the value for T_{hi}

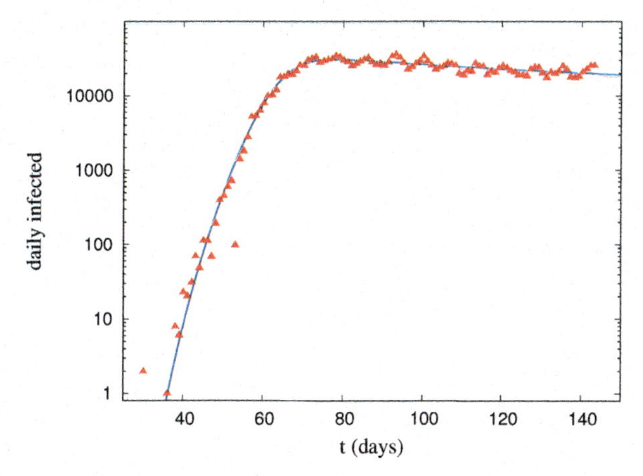

Fig. 2.6: Daily infections in USA, where the peak looks already surpassed. Here again, the behavior of the pandemic in this country looks well described by Eq. (2.7). See fitting parameters in Table 2.1. Condition (2.8) is satisfied.

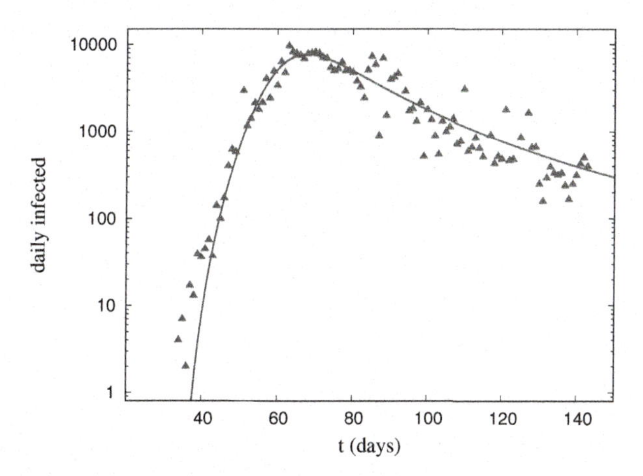

Fig. 2.7: Daily infections in Spain. the data shows a large dispersion but the curve describes well the behavior. See fitting parameters in Table 2.1. Condition (2.8) is satisfied.

is so high that SARS-CoV-2 could even turn into a seasonal virus, at least for some years. We can expect around the same mortality but scattered over a few years.

A special observation deserves USA, where T_{hi} tends to infinity. Here we can expect a continuous infection rate for a very long time. The outbreak is controlled but not enough to eradicate the virus. The virus will not disappear in several years but maybe the healthcare system could manage it. The virus will get endemic, and immunity will never be reached. However the infections and mortality rate associated with it, can be, hypothetically, small if compared with Mexico and Brazil. We can also compare the speed of the outbreak in different countries. As we already said in Table 2.1 we calculated T_{1000} for some countries. However, it should be noticed that this time is not calculated from day 0, which is always January 22, but for the approximated day when the outbreak began in the correspondent country. By example, in Brazil there was no cases at January, 22 but the first cases were detected around March, 10. So both, data fitting and T_{1000}, were calculated

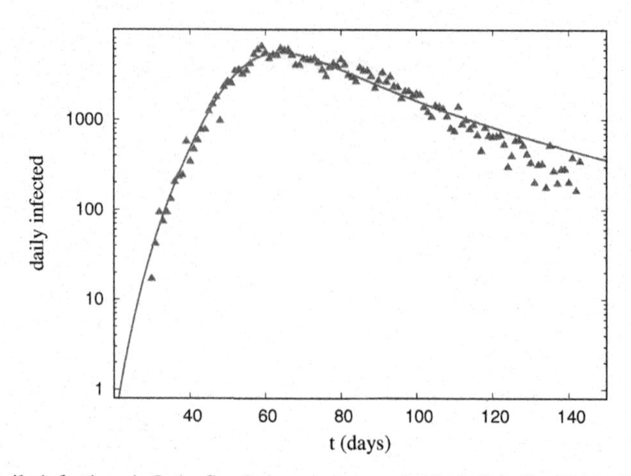

Fig. 2.8: Daily infections in Italy. See fitting parameters in Table 2.1. Condition (2.8) is satisfied.

Table 2.1: Relevant fitting parameters for each country.

Country	A	B	a	b	P	T_{hi}(days)	T_{1000}
Brazil	0.0152828	0.0104434	4.31197	0.0671095	212559417	298	36
Cuba	1.80E-05	3.30E-09	5.31906	1.40779	11326616	-	-
Iceland	6.08E-05	1.69E-09	5.09845	4.94326	341243	-	-
Italy	1.20E-07	1.85E-13	7.50956	1.32858	60461826	-	34
Mexico	0.0541958	0.0104956	3.60005	0.0641971	128932753	778	56
Spain	0.000170317	2.75E-10	6.31706	1.35476	46754778	-	19
USA	1.09E-13	5.99E-20	11.5099	0.973087	331002651	-	34
Worldwide	3.18E-06	4.65E-13	6.84834	0.816744	7786246434	-	29

from March, 10. As can be seen from fitting coefficients, the exponent b drives the behavior of infections in every country. Those countries that manage well the disease expansion have b values wide larger than 1. Countries with b values close to one, as Italy and Spain, have managed the pandemic but poorly and at high costs. The recovery in both countries will be long. The same is valid for USA, that managed the outbreak poorly and is struggling with an even longer recovery to normal life. Even worst scenario has taken place in Mexico and Brazil, with very low values of b. Those countries are experiencing a big outbreak where even can get herd immunity. This, however, implies very high values of infections and mortality for the near future.

2.4 Conclusions and Outlook for Further Investigations

In this chapter, for the first time, we presented a model built using the method of analogy, in this case with a nonlinear relaxation-like behavior. With this, a decent fit with the observed behavior of the daily number of cases over time is obtained. The explicit expressions obtained may be used as a tool to approximately forecast the development of the COVID-19 pandemic in different countries and worldwide. In principle, this model can be used as a help to elaborate or change actions. This model does not incorporate any particular property of this pandemic, so we think it could be used to study pandemics with different sources. With the collected data of the pandemics at early times, using this model, it can be predicted the possibility of a peak, indefinite growth, time for herd immunity, etc.

What seems to be clear from the COVID-19 data, the fitting and the values shown in the Table 2.1, is that SARS-CoV-2 is far from being controlled at the world level. Even when some countries appear to control the outbreak, the virus is still a menace for its health system. Furthermore, nowadays in the interconnected world it is impossible for any country to keep closed borders and pay attention to what happens only inside. All isolation measures should be halted at some time and we can expect new outbreaks in countries like Spain or Italy even after the current one could be controlled. The only way to control the spread of SARS-CoV-2 seems to be the development of a vaccine that provides the so much desired herd immunity. Indeed, the model made it possible to make an approximate forecast of the time to reach the herd immunity. This may be useful in the design of actions and policies about the pandemic. We have introduced the T_{1000}, that gives information about the early infection behavior in populous countries. A possible improvement of this model is the formal inclusion of a formulation including the dual conformable derivative [11, 16].

Acknowledgments

One of the authors, José Weberszpil, would like to thank to FAPERJ (the Carlos Chagas Filho Research Support Foundation of the State of Rio de Janeiro, FAPERJ), for the research support, APQ1. $E_2 7/2021$ AUXÍLIO BÁSICO À PESQUISA (APQ1) EM ICTs SEDIADAS NO ESTADO DO RIO DE JANEIRO 2021. Nº DO PROCESSO SEI-260003/015164/2021 - APQ1.

References

[1] https://coronavirus.jhu.edu/data/new-cases.

[2] https://www.worldometers.info/.to.

[3] Balankin, A.S., J. Bory-Reyes and M. Shapiro. 2016. Towards a physics on fractals: Differential vector calculus in three-dimensional continuum with fractal metric. Physica A: Statistical Mechanics and its Applications, 444: 345-–359.

[4] Balankin, A.S. and B.E. Elizarraraz. 2012. Hydrodynamics of fractal continuum flow. Physical Review E, 85(2): 025302.

[5] Balankin, A.S. and B.E. Elizarraraz. 2012. Map of fluid flow in fractal porous medium into fractal continuum flow. Physical Review E, 85(5): 056314.

[6] Brouers, F. 2014. The fractal (BSf) kinetics equation and its approximations. Journal of Modern Physics, 5(16): 1594.

[7] Brouers, F. and O. Sotolongo-Costa. 2006. Generalized fractal kinetics in complex systems (application to biophysics and biotechnology). Physica A: Statistical Mechanics and its Applications, 368(1): 165-–175.

[8] Burr, I.W. 1942. Cumulative frequency functions. The Annals of mathematical statistics, 13(2): 215-–232.

[9] Jonscher, A.K. 1994. All forms of relaxation take place in fractal time. Proceedings of IEEE Conference on Electrical Insulation and Dielectric Phenomena-(CEIDP'94), IEEE, 755–760.

[10] Khalil, R., M. Al Horani, A. Yousef and M. Sababheh. 2014. A new definition of fractional derivative. Journal of Computational and Applied Mathematics, 264: 65-–70.

[11] Wanderson, R. and J. Weberszpil. 2018. Dual conformable derivative: Definition, simple properties and perspectives for applications. Chaos, Solitons & Fractals, 117: 137–141.

[12] Schnell, S. and T.E. Turner. 2004. Reaction kinetics in intracellular environments with macromolecular crowding: Simulations and rate laws. Progress in Biophysics and Molecular Biology, 85: 235-–260.

[13] Sotolongo-Costa, O., L.M. Gaggero-Sager and M.E. Mora-Ramos. 2015. A non-extensive statistical model for time-dependent multiple breakage particle-size distribution. Physica A: Statistical Mechanics and its Applications, 438: 74–80.

[14] Tsallis, C. and U. Tirnakli. 2020. Predicting COVID-19 peaks around the world, medExiv.

[15] Tsallis, C. and U. Tirnakli. 2020. Predicting COVID-19 peaks around the world. Frontiers in Physics, 8: 217.

[16] Weberszpil, J., C.F.L. Godinho and Y. Liang. 2020. Dual conformable derivative: Variational approach and nonlinear equations. EPL (Europhysics Letters), 128(3): 31001.

[17] Weberszpil, J., M. Jatkoske Lazo and J.A. Helayël-Neto. 2015. On a connection between a class of q-deformed algebras and the Hausdorff derivative in a medium with fractal metric. Physica A: Statistical Mechanics and its Applications, 436: 399–404.

[18] Weberszpil, J. and W. Chen. 2017. Generalized Maxwell relations in thermodynamics with metric derivatives. Entropy, 19(8): 407.

[19] Weberszpil, J. and J.A. Helayël-Neto. 2016. Variational approach and deformed derivatives. Physica A: Statistical Mechanics and its Applications, 450: 217–227.

[20] Weberszpil, J. and J.A. Helayël-Neto. 2017. Structural scale q-derivative and the LLG equation in a scenario with fractionality. EPL (Europhysics Letters), 117(5): 50006.

[21] Weberszpil, J. and O. Sotolongo-Costa. 2017. Structural derivative model for tissue radiation response. Journal of Advances in Physics, 13(4): 4779–4785.

Chapter 3

Design of Covid-19 Fractal Antenna Array for 5G and mm-WAVE Wireless Application

J.S. Abdaljabar,[1,*] *M. Madi,*[2] *A. Al-Hindawi*[3] and *K. Kabalan*[4]

3.1 Design of COVID-19 Antenna Array for Centimeter Wave Band

It is well known that microstrip patch antenna arrays have the positive characteristics of small size, various shapes, low fabrication cost, as well as being lightweight, which makes them widely used in many applications such as the WiMAX, Global Position System (GPS), and weather radar devices. Examples of microstrip antennas include the design and realization of radar antenna patch array at 9.4 GHz frequency with coaxial probe feeding [1] and making microstrip patch antenna using inset raising technique feed for weather radar applications at S-band frequencies [2]. In the studies above there are several drawbacks such as complex feeding techniques, and low gain considering the number of antenna elements.

To overcome these obstacles an antenna array is used, where the gain and the beam width of the radiation pattern is increased dramatically. Much research has been done in this area, for instance, to overcome the low gain, an application for weather radar systems with a rectangular microstrip patch antenna was designed in [3] it is a 2×4 array has a microstrip line rationing technique, that works at frequencies from 2.7 GHz to 2.9 GHz uses FR-4 substrate material. Another antenna array design suitable for GPS application is described in [27] which is designed to function in the C-band used to receive signals from the telemetry link of an Unmanned Air Vehicle.

Building a dual-band, and high-efficiency circular patch has become very popular and feasible to be utilized in microstrip antenna array. They are simple and inexpensive to manufacture and are suitable for planar and non-planar configurations [5]. The design and characteristics of the double sided microstrip circular antenna array is presented in [10], for dual bands at 6.05–7 GHz and 9–10 GHz to support weather radar applications and directional radiation pattern with gain of 3.12 dB 3.8 dB at 6.5 GHz and 9.5 GHz

[1] Communication Engineering Department, Sulaimaniya Polytechnic University (SPU), in Sulaymaniyah, Kurdistan Region, Iraq.
[2] HCT (Higher colleges of Technology) Abu Dhabi, UAE.
Email: mervatmadi@icloud.com
[3] Communication Engineering Department, Technical College of Engineering, Sulaimaniya Polytechnic University, Sulay-maniyah, Kurdistan Region, Iraq.
Email: assad.jasim@spu.edu.iq
[4] Department of Engineering and Architecture, American University of Beirut.
Email: kabalan@aub.edu.lb
* Corresponding author: jihan.salah@spu.edu.iq

respectively. In [7], high gain 2×4 circular patch antenna array is designed on an FR4 substrate of standard thickness 1.5 mm. The proposed antenna arrays use probe feeding technique, and are designed for 2.4 GHz resonant frequency suitable for WLAN applications.

Although the above antenna array solved the issue of low gain and poor radiation efficiency, they are still suffering from its relatively large size and narrow bandwidth, especially for thin substrates. Many techniques have been introduced to improve the characteristics of the patch antenna, one of these techniques is using fractal geometry. Fractal geometry is an efficient technique for fabricating multi-band, low-profile antennas [8, 9]. The scaling and self-similarity in fractal shape antennas facilitate multi-band and broadband properties along with the reduced dimensions of the antennas. Koch, Sierpinski, Minkowski, Hilbert, and Cantor arrays are recent examples of multi-band antenna configurations based on fractal geometries.

This chapter deals with two types of arrays simulated in HFSS software using fractal geometry and microstrip antenna technology. Arrays allow smaller area higher gain/efficiency, multi-band/broadband characteristics, and larger directivity while fractal geometry increase electrical length and hence reduces the frequency of the patch. Fractal geometry is applied by adding discs around one larger disc to mimic COVID-19 shape. The first array is suitable for WiMAX, GPS, and weather radar applications, centimeter sub-6GHz frequency. The second array is for mm-wave 5G wireless systems. Fabrication and measurement was done in the American University of Beirut labs. The design steps of the first array shall be explained thoroughly in next section.

3.1.1 Single Element Design

Regarding the one element design, an FR4-epoxy substrate with permittivity of 4.4 is used to construct the COVID-19 patch antenna, and this material is utilized due to its low cost and effectiveness in reproducing the simulated designs. The 2D and 3D simulated models with dimensions are shown in Figure 3.1. The overall dimensions of the substrate (L, W, h) are $(4 \times 3 \times 0.16)\text{cm}^3$. The main patch antenna is circular with a radius of 10 mm. The patch antenna is fed using the microstrip line method. It forms the unique shape of the coronavirus for the patch and constitutes the basic element for building the antenna array.

The design steps are similar to those used in the previous chapter, however, the resonance frequency and consequently the patch dimensions are different according to Balanis [26] equations for designing the radius of the circular patch, by setting the frequency to 3.2 GHz. On the other hand, the crowns in this design contribute to improving the reflection coefficient and reducing the resonance frequency. Figure 3.2 shows a comparison for single element circular patch with and without crowns to show the positive effects of adding the crowns.

As shown in Figure 3.1, the microstrip feeding line is a series of two transmission lines: The first one is matched to 50Ω, its width is calculated according to equation (4) in the previous chapter to be 3 mm and it's length is is obtained using the optimization technique in HFSS to be 6 mm. The second 100Ω transmission line, which is directly connected to the patch (Figure 3.1), has a width and length of 5 mm, and 0.15 mm respectively. Note the optimization method here is done using trial and error in changing dimensions to achieve the targeted design. The final results of the single elements are shown in Figure 3.3, with resonance frequency of 3.4 GHz, and directional radiation pattern, and showing E and H-planes.

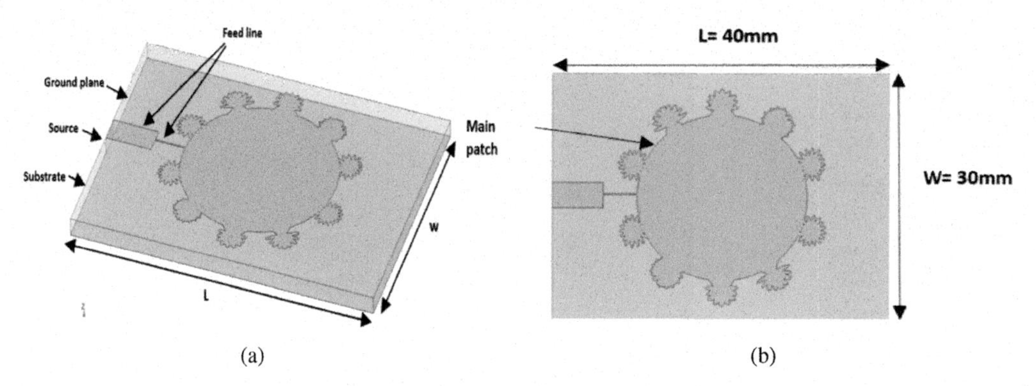

Fig. 3.1: (a) Three-dimensional patch antenna. (b) Two-dimensional structure of the simulated patch antenna.

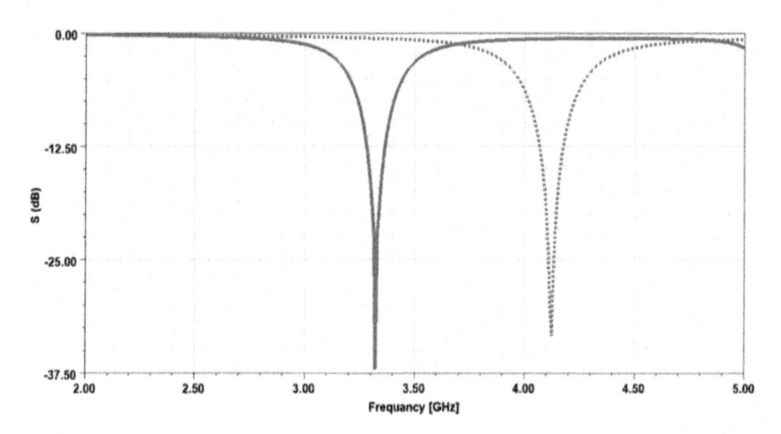

Fig. 3.2: Comparison between the S-parameters for the single element with crowns (solid line) and without crowns (dotted line).

3.1.2 Design of 2 × 1 Array

The layout of the antenna array structure of 2×1 was composed of two identical elements of the basic element patch which was simulated in the previous section. Firstly, two elements were connected in parallel; when the resonance frequency was 3.16 GHz the optimized results were measured when the distance between the two patches is 0.55λ which is equal to 54 mm.

In this case, a parallel network feeding line connection was used to supply a uniform distribution of power to all the elements. The feeding line consists of 100Ω transmission line (TL) which is directly connected to the patch with a length of 13 mm and a width of 0.1 mm. The two patches are connected with another 100Ω line with dimensions of (L, W) (54.2 mm, 0.1 mm) which is connected to the 50Ω TL. The 50Ω TL has (5 mm× 3 mm) (length, width) and it is connected directly to the input power entire network. The dimensions of the patch elements, such as width and length, were calculated using equation (4). The 3D radiation pattern, reflection coefficient, and the 2D structure of this array are shown in Figure 3.4. Note that the antenna has a high gain of 5.32 dB for a $6 \times 8\text{cm}^2$ area and has a directional radiation pattern.

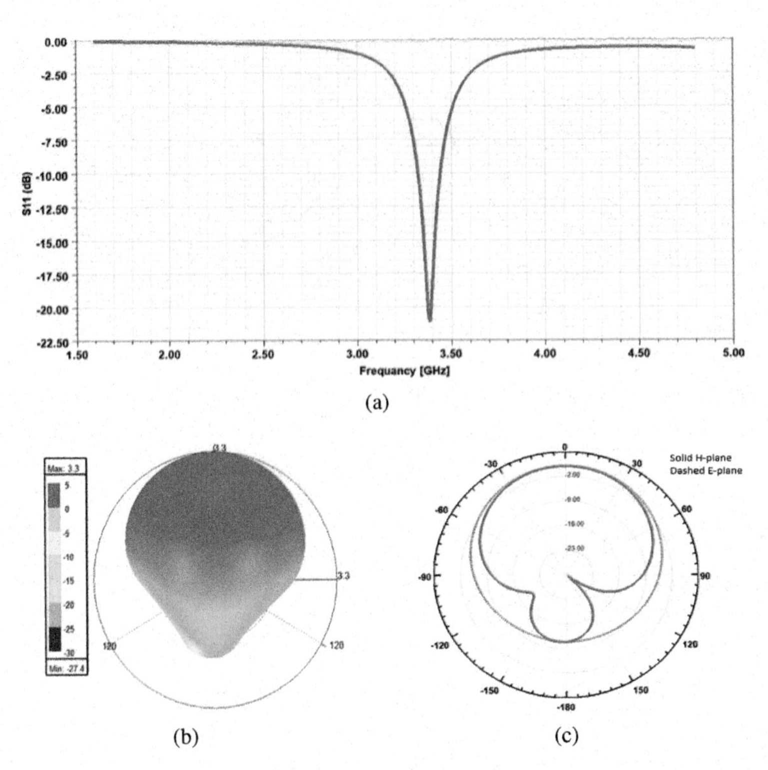

(a)

(b) (c)

Fig. 3.3: (a) Reflection coefficient curve concerning the frequency, (b) 3D radiation pattern, and (c) 2D radiation pattern.

3.1.3 Design of 2 × 2 Array

The proposed design procedure continues and a 2 × 2 antenna array is proposed in a square shape to reduce the feeding TL dimensions used and to occupy a small size of 38 mm × 38 mm. The patch is printed at the top layer of the substrate and the bottom layer of the substrate consist of a full ground plane. The configuration follows the same procedure of the 2 × 1 array. A coaxial prob feeding in the center of the array is connected to provide equalized electrical power for every patch in the network. In this design, the distance between the patch is changed to find the best radiation efficiency, and the results for this design are shown in Figure 3.5. The simulated antenna array is designed to resonate at 3.26 GHz, and the feeding lines were calculated according to the equation (4). The 70Ω TL has a width and length 2mm and 18 mm respectively, and the 50Ω TL width, length has 3 mm, 5 mm respectively. Clearly, according to Figure (5), the operating frequency is reduced from 3.4 to 3.26 GHz, the area dropped from $6 \times 8\text{cm}^2$, to less than $4 \times 4\text{cm}^2$, the radiation pattern has a more regular directive shape, and the gain increased from 5.32 dB to 7.8 dB, compared to the older 2 × 1 array.

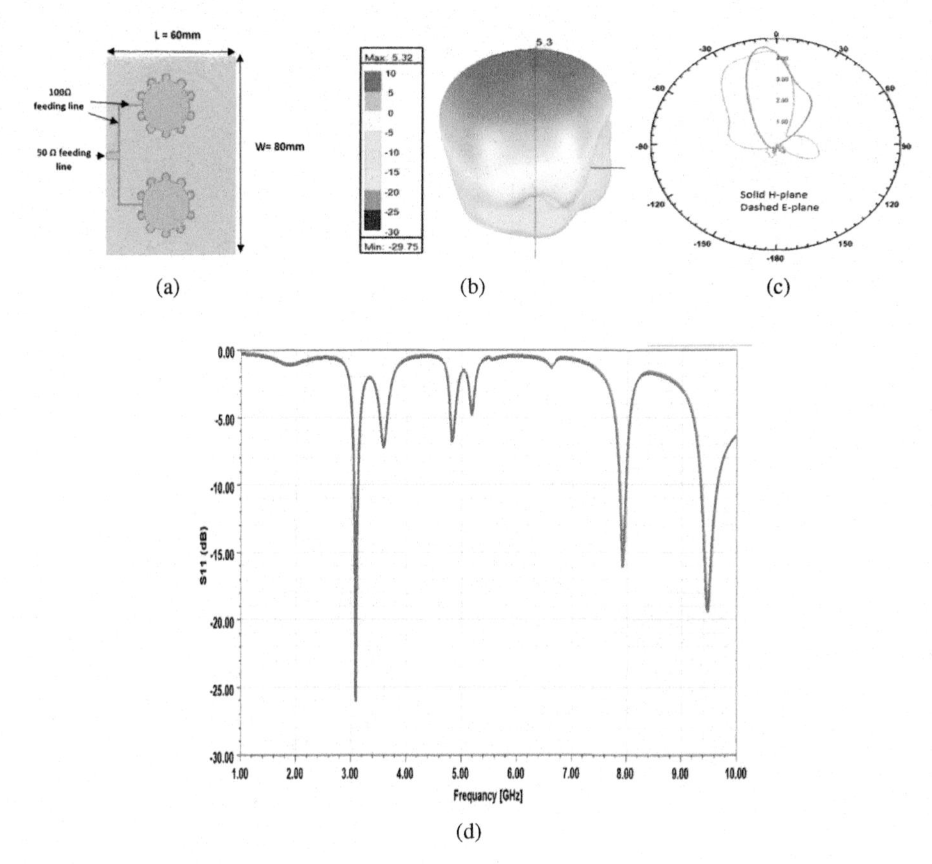

(a) (b) (c)

(d)

Fig. 3.4: Results for the 2 × 1 antenna array when the resonance frequency is 3.1 GHz. (a) 2D structure and (b) 3D radiation pattern, (c) E-plane and H-plane radiation pattern, (d) S-parameter curve.

3.1.4 Design of 2 × 4 Array

When the 2×2 array is finalized, the 2×4 array is set to study. This type of array is simulated on a rectangular substrate with overall dimensions of (L, W, h) to be $(26 \times 10 \times 0.16)\text{cm}^3$ as shown in Figure 3.6. The patch antenna is fed using the coaxial probe feed method which is connected at the center of the antenna array to provide similar feeding for every element in the array. After using the optimization technique of the HFSS program the best dimensions of the substrate was found, where the vertical distance between two elements is 53mm and horizontal distance is 55 mm and the TLs have width and length of $(3.5, 10)\text{mm}^2$, $(1.2, 67)\text{mm}^2$ and $(0.3, 161.5)\text{mm}^2$ for the 50Ω, 70Ω, and 100Ω lines respectively. It is remarkable to notice the current distribution density on the 2 × 4 antenna array surface. Different colors are shown in Figure 3.7, and they represent different current density values: the blue color has the least current density and the red color has the highest value. The design shows that the current distribution reached the far edge of the crowns at every patch in the array, hence explaining the obtained increased gain and the reduced frequency compared to the previous 2 × 2 array, where the gain jumped to 10.1 dB and the lowest operating frequency dropped to 2.08 GHz compared to 7.8 dB and 3.26 GHz for the previous 2×2 array. The S11 curve is shown in Figure 3.8, it is clear from this figure that this antenna array is resonating on four different frequencies 2.09GHz, 3.1 GHz,

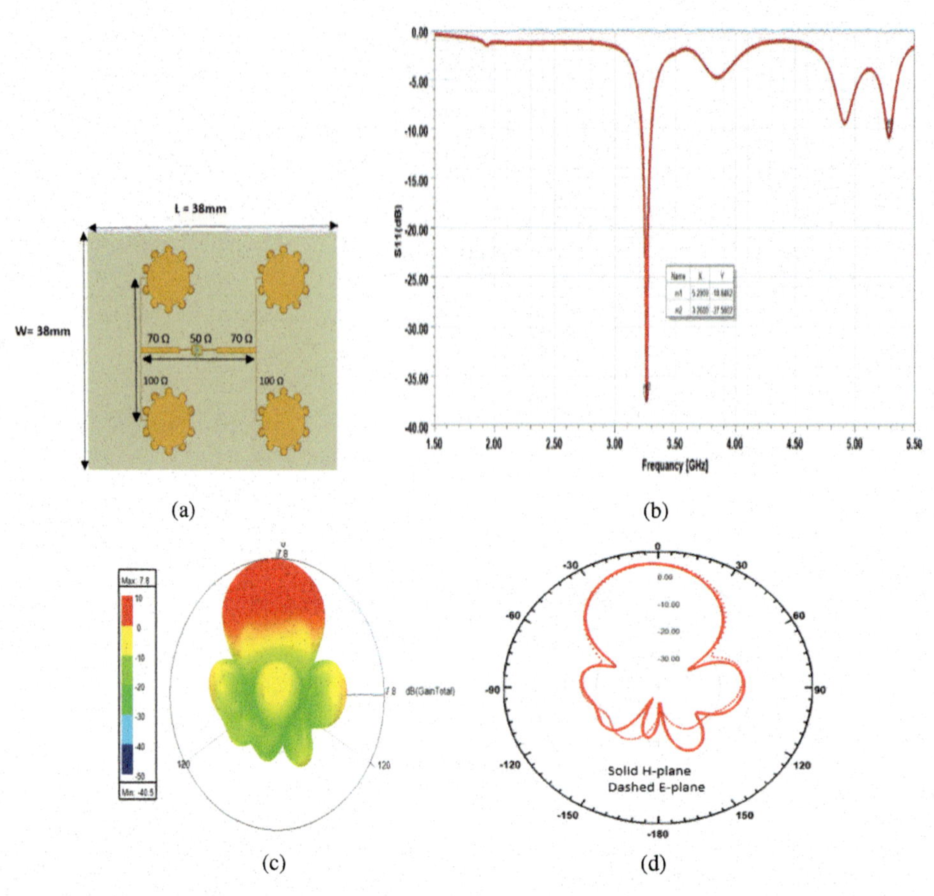

Fig. 3.5: Results for the 2 × 2 antenna array, where (a) structure of the array, (b) radiation coefficient curve, (c) 3D gain plot at 3.26 GHz, (d) 2D radiation pattern at the resonance frequency.

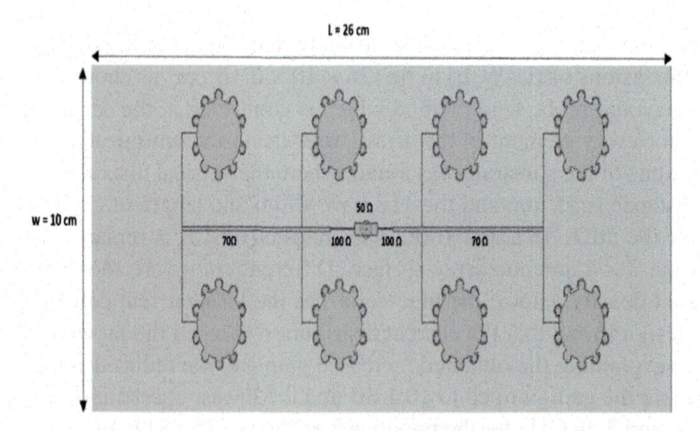

Fig. 3.6: The two-dimensional structure of the simulated patch antenna.

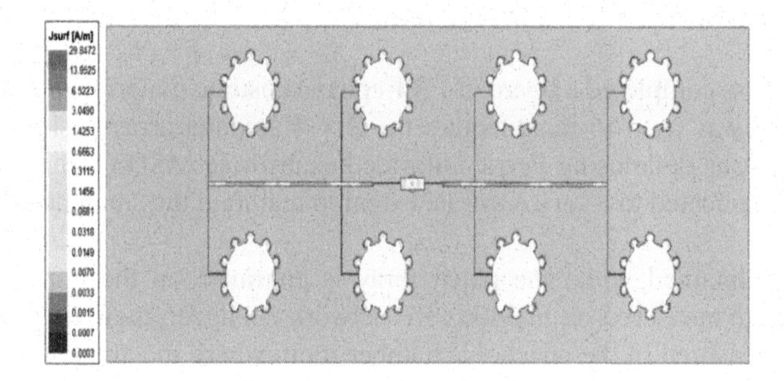

Fig. 3.7: The current distribution density on the surface of the 2 × 4 antenna array.

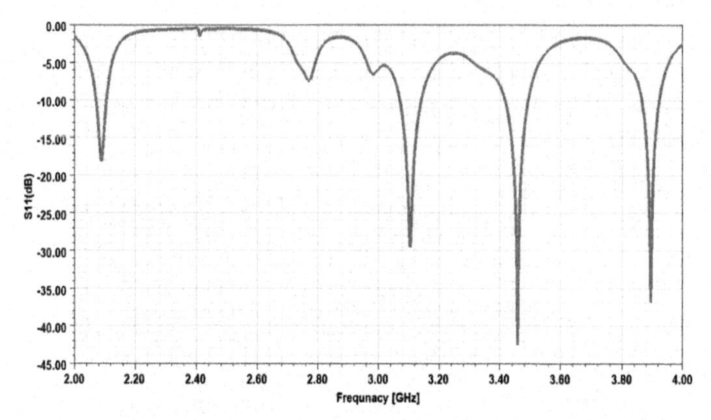

Fig. 3.8: S_{11} parameter curve for the 2 × 4 antenna array.

3.4 GHz and 3,8 GHz with reflection coefficient of 17.7dB, -28.8 dB, -42.45 dB, and -36.7 dB respectively. The maximum gain is obtained at 3.16GHz which is 10.1 dB. The optimized results of this array at 3.16 GHz are shown in Figure 3.9.

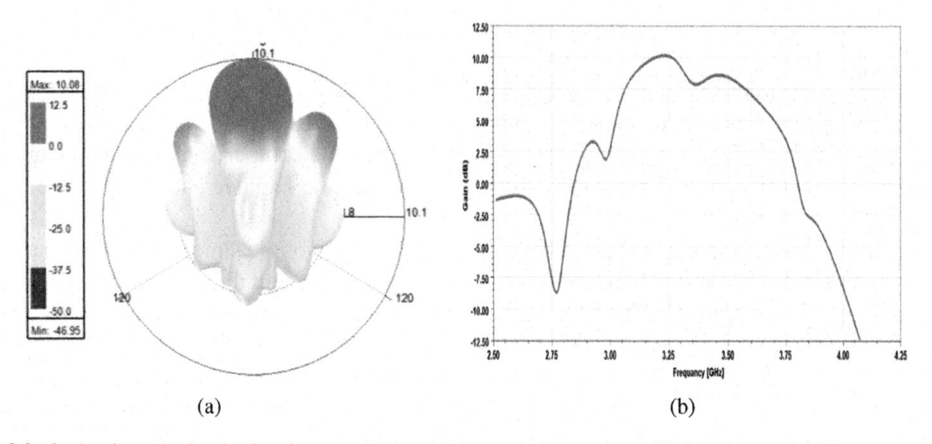

(a) (b)

Fig. 3.9: Optimal results for the 2 × 4 antenna array. (a) 3D radiation pattern, (b) Gain versus frequency curves.

3.2 Antenna Fabrication and Measurements

When the simulation process completed a board of FR4-epoxy substrate material with a double-sided copper plate of 1.6mm thickness was used to manufacture the 2 × 4 antenna arrays using the chemical etching method. The etching step was done using Ferric chloride hexahydrate MSDS (which is commonly used to etch copper), and it was duplicated to a very accurate extent to maintain the small details of the spikes on the crowns of every patch.

A full ground was maintained while the patch array is engraved on the upper copper side. The S-parameters of the arrays are measured on FieldFox RF network Analyzer, then the radiation efficiency, and the gain parameters are measured in the anechoic chamber room where the antenna is the transmitter and a horn antenna is the receiver. The distance between the transmitter and the receiver is 4 m. This multi-band frequency low-cost patch antenna array prototype is shown in Figure 3.10. The S_{11}-parameter of this array is measured on the network analyzer as shown in Figure 3.11. This figure also shows good consistency between the measured and the simulated reflection coefficient curves. The discrepancy of the S11 parameter between simulated and measured plots is maximum 80 MHz and is interpreted to be resulting from errors in fabrication, measurements being done on a network analyzer hence not in free space, and due to SMA connectors matching fabrication errors.

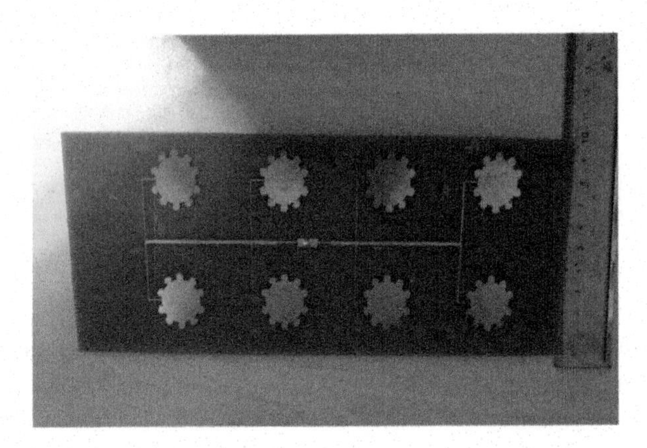

Fig. 3.10: The two-dimensional structure for a 2 × 4 antenna simulated and manufactured array.

Following the measurements of the S-parameter for the 2 × 4 patch antenna array, the polarization was measured in the anechoic chamber. Figure 3.12 shows the photos of this room when the antenna array was connected to the rotating table as a transmitter. Figure 3.13 shows the comparison between the measured and the simulated results of the co-polar and the cross-polar for both the E-plane and the H-plane of the 2 × 4 antenna array.

In the first and second images of Figure 3.13, the radiation pattern of the simulated and measured curve at 3.16 GHz was depicted. The red and black lines represent the simulated and the measured results respectively. The co-polar and cross-polar radiations give us the polarization characteristics of the studied antenna. It is also found that the maximum measured gain of the designed antenna is 9 dB at the resonant frequency. In Figure 3.13, it is clear that the difference between the co-polar and cross-polar radiations is around than 26 dB in the direction of maximum radiations, hence the antenna is linearly polarized. It was found that the maximum simulated and measured gain of the designed antenna was 10.25 dB and 9dB respectively. Table 3.1 shows the improvements of the gain value when the number of elements are increased.

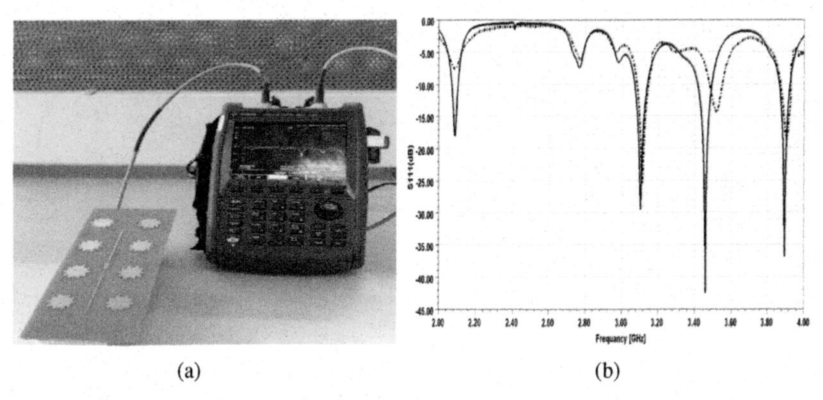

(a) (b)

Fig. 3.11: (a) Photo of the measured S11 on the network analyzer. (b) Reflection coefficient curves for a 2×4 antenna array. Solid line is the simulated curve and dashed line is the measured curve.

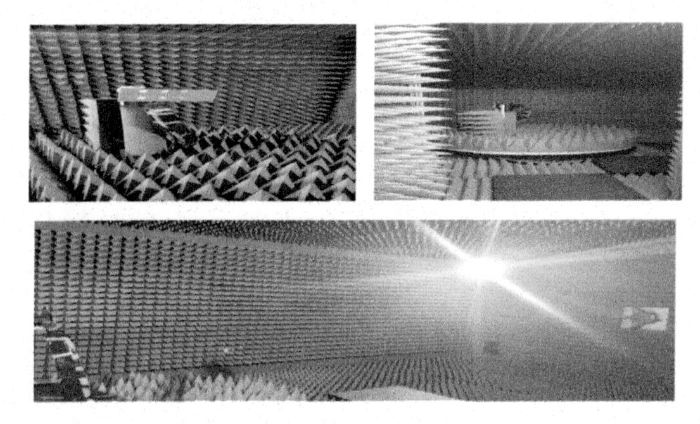

Fig. 3.12: Photos of the anechoic chamber room when the 2×4 antenna array polarizations were measured.

Table 3.1: Comparison between the proposed work and other antenna arrays.

Type of array	$S_{11}(GHz)$	Resonance frequency (GHz)	Gain (dB)
One element	-21.7	3.4	3.3
Two elements	-26,-16,-19	3.1,7.9,9.5	5.3,4,2.6
Four elements	-37.5,-10.8	3.2,5.2	7.8,4
Eight elements	-18,-29.8,-43,-36	2.05,3.1,3.49,3.9	-2.4,10.1,7,6.6

3.3 Design of COVID-19 Antenna Array for Millimeter Wave Band

Recently, the number of smart devices that people require has been dramatically increasing, the objective of the future generations of mobile communications 5G and 6G are to look for advanced technology to provide an increase in capacity, bandwidth, and energy efficiency, compared with 4G. Several techniques are used to improve the data rate; where mm-wave is one of the most essential solutions for the next generation. This technique expands the bandwidth, and thus improves the data transmission capacity. For instance, a study

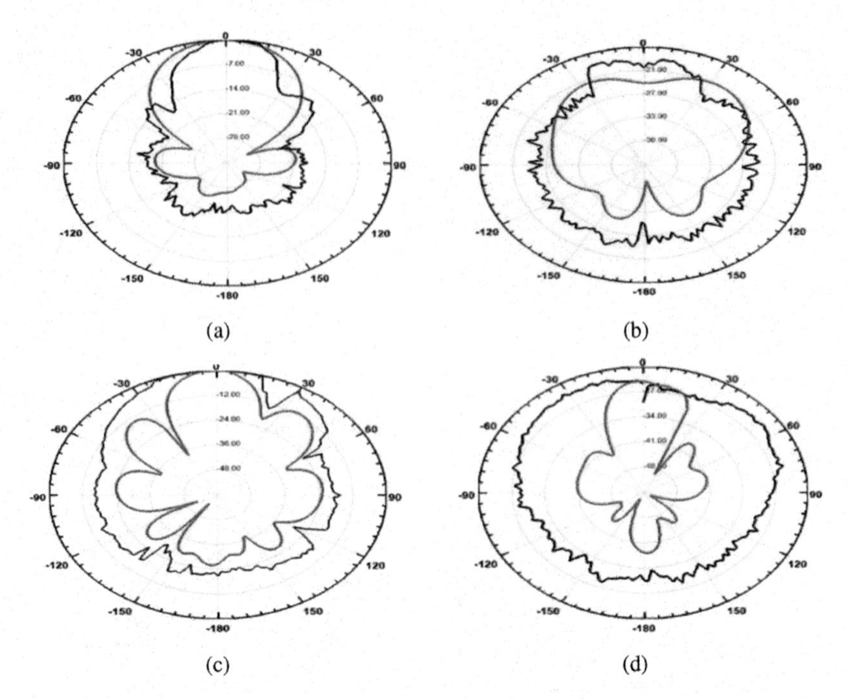

Fig. 3.13: Comparison between the simulated and the measured 2D radiation pattern for the 2 × 4 antenna array, where the red color represents the simulated results and the black represents the measured results.

released in 2019 [26] illustrated the modification of conventional circular patches where an FR-4 epoxy substrate with dimension of 40mm × 40mm × 1.6mm was designed to improve the antenna gain.

Another study published in [11] in 2022 manufactured a *T* and *L* slotted microstrip patch antenna used for future mobile and wireless communication. The size of the antenna is 10 × 10mm^2 with thickness of 1.6 mm and the dielectric constant of substrate 4.4 with FR-4 epoxy material is used. This antenna is fed by the 50Ω microstrip (TL) and T and L slotted radiating patch is used [12]. A 4-port MIMO antenna array operating in the mm-wave band for 5G applications is presented in [13]. The array elements are rectangular-shaped slotted patch antennas, while the ground plane is made defected with rectangular, circular, and a zigzag-shaped slotted structure to enhance the radiation characteristics of the antenna.

The proposed structure can operate in a 25.5–29.6 GHz frequency with peak gain of 8.3 dB. The array is designed on RO4350B with dimensions of the substrate are 130 × 68 × 0.76mm^3 with bandwidth of 1 GHz from 27.5 to 28.5 GHz., which matches the dimensions of modern smart phones. A single antenna with 3 × 3 metamaterial unit cells is proposed in [16] to operate at a frequency band (24–30) GHz, this antenna is characterized with 6 GHz bandwidth, and maximum peak gain of 12.4 dB.

Unfortunately, the limitation of using mm-wave frequencies is the high loss of free space patch which is mainly caused by high operating frequencies, Therefore, an antenna array with high gain and wide bandwidth becomes a requirement. To reap the best benefits from the performance of the COVID-19 patch shape, and to design a model with ultra-wide bandwidth another configuration was built to serve the requirements of the mm-wave band. In this section the main contribution is to design a serial antenna array, operating at 28 GHz with high gain and ultra-wide bandwidth of 18 GHz proposed for the second band of the 5G wireless mobile applications.

3.3.1 Design of Single-Element Antenna

The COVD-19 patch antenna which was presented in the past chapters, it is redesigned at resonance frequency of 28 GHz on the FR4-epoxy with h = 1.6mm. Figure 3.14 shows the optimized dimensions of the 2D and 3D patch and Table 3.2 represents the optimal dimensions for this unique patch antenna.

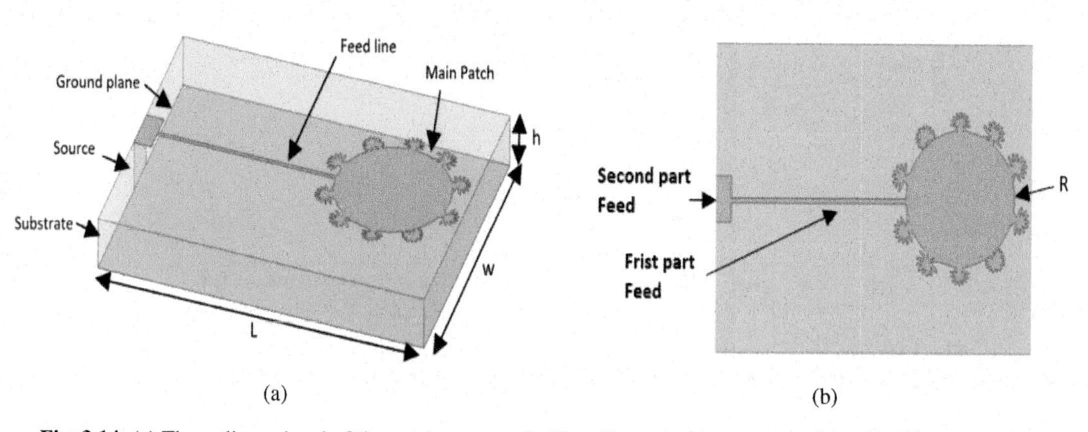

Fig. 3.14: (a) Three-dimensional of the patch antenna. (b) Two-dimensional prototype of the simulated patch antenna.

Table 3.2: Parameter descriptions of the simulated patch antenna at the mm-wave band.

Decryptions	**Symbols**	**Values in (mm)**
Length of the substrate	L	20
Width of the substrate	W	10
Radius of the main patch	R	2.2
Height of the substrate	h	1.6
first feeding part	(L,W)	(1,0.15)
Second feeding part	(L,W)	(1.5,0.7)

The overall dimensions of the substrate (L, W, h) are $(2 \times 1 \times 0.16)\text{cm}^3$. The main circular patch antenna radius is 2.2 mm which is calculated according to Balanis equations [10] of designing the circular patch at resonance frequency 28 GHz. The patch antenna was fed using the strip feed line method. The feeding line consists of two parts: the first is directly connected to the left side of the patch with a length and width of (1 mm, 0.15 mm).The second part has a length and width of (1.5 mm, 0.7 mm). Adding the crowns around the main circular patch improves the reflection coefficient, and the resonance frequency, as shown in Figure 3.15. In this figure, two curves show the S11 results of the circular patch with and without crowns to take note of the effects of the crowns on the main patch antenna. Initially, when a simple circular patch with a radius of 2.2 mm and operating frequency of 28 GHz was designed without crowns, it resonated at 28.9 GHz with a reflection coefficient of -27 dB.

After adding the crowns to the circular patch, the resonance frequency and the reflection coefficient improve to be 28.3 GHz, -34 dB respectively.

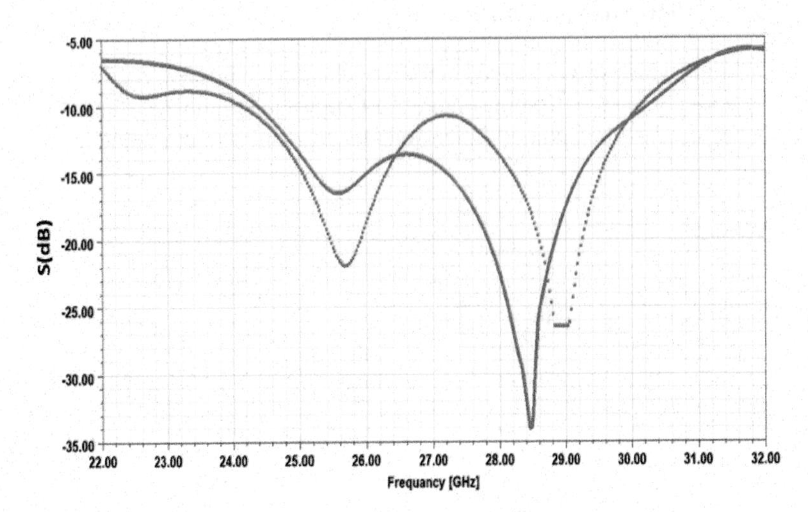

Fig. 3.15: (dot line) Circular patch without crowns, (solid line) circular patch with crowns.

From this comparison, it becomes apparent that adding the crowns around the main circular patch not only gives the patch its unique shape but also progresses the reflection coefficient and the resonance frequency of the miniature antenna. The 3D radiation pattern was plotted and the maximum gain was measured to be 5.4 dB at 28.3 GHz. Furthermore, the radiation efficiency for the E-plane and H-plane curves is drawn in Figure 3.16.

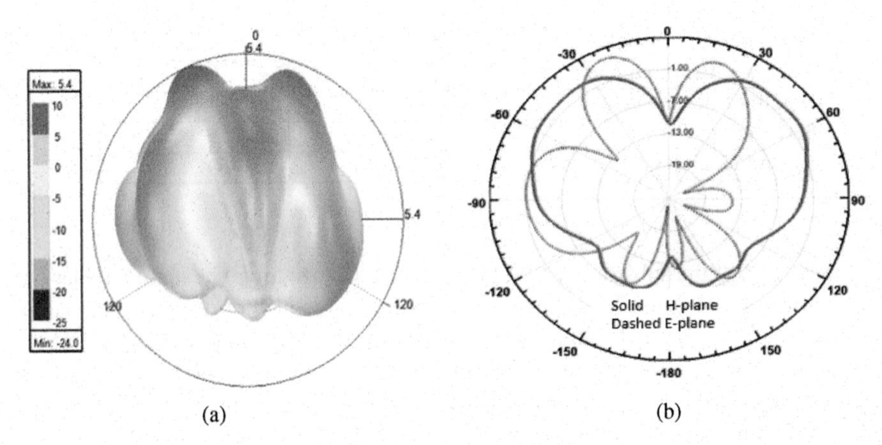

Fig. 3.16: (a) 3D radiation pattern, (b) 2D radiation pattern, the dotted line is the H-plane and the solid line is the E-plane.

3.3.2 Design of Two-Element Antenna Array (2 × 1)

When the simulation of a single element of the patch was finalized, an array was built from this patch. Firstly, two elements were connected in parallel, and the spacing distance is changing to obtain the resonance frequency of 26.7 GHz. The optimal results, considering the gain, the reflection coefficient, and the bandwidth, were obtained at distance between elements (from center to center) of 0.55λ as shown in Table 3.3 and Figure 3.17. The feed line consists of two parts: The first one was connected directly to the source with 0.9 mm as a length and 1.5mm as a width. The second TL, connected to the patch has (8mm × 0.1mm) for (length, width). The optimal 3D radiation pattern and reflection coefficient are shown in Figures 3.18a and 3.18b respectively. The reflection coefficient curve is illustrated in Figure 3.19. The gain value in this array is increased to be 7.8 dB whereas in the single element it was only 5.4 dB.

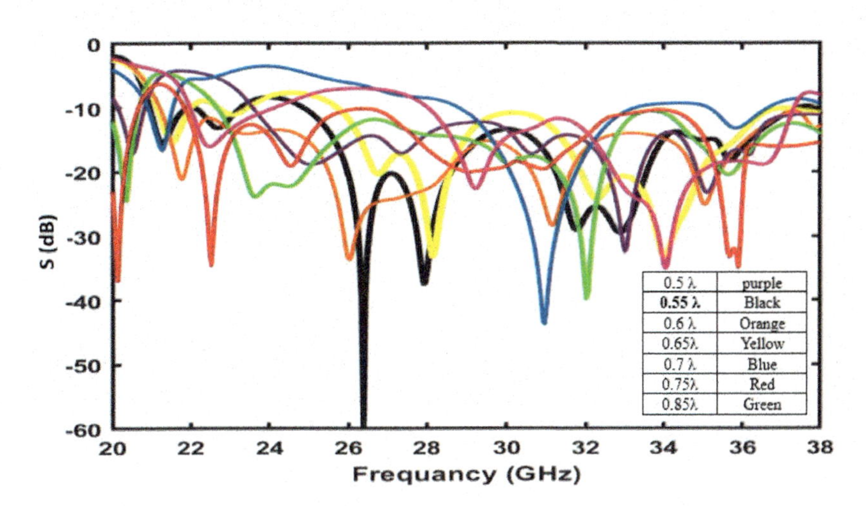

Fig. 3.17: Different reflection coefficient curves for different distance (from center to center) values.

Table 3.3: Comparison between the reflection coefficient, gain, and bandwidth concerning the spacing distance changes when the resonance frequency is 26.7 GHz.

Spacing distance (mm)	Curve color	Gain (dB)	Percentage Bandwidth
0.5λ	Purple	7.2	25.7-37
0.55λ	Black	7.8	25.4-38
0.6λ	Orange	7.3	23-30
0.65λ	Yellow	7	24-37
0.7λ	Blue	7.2	26-30 30-38
0.75λ	Red	7.5	29-33
0.85λ	Green	6.9	23-32

3.3.3 Design of Four-Element Antenna Array (2 × 2)

One of the simplest methods of feeding for the linear antenna array is serial feeding, and it is compact because of the space improvement compared with parallel feeding because the input power of the antenna was provided from one end of the array. When the optimal results of the 2 × 1 array are achieved, a 2 × 2 array is demonstrated. In this array, two series elements were connected with the 2 × 1 array and the distance

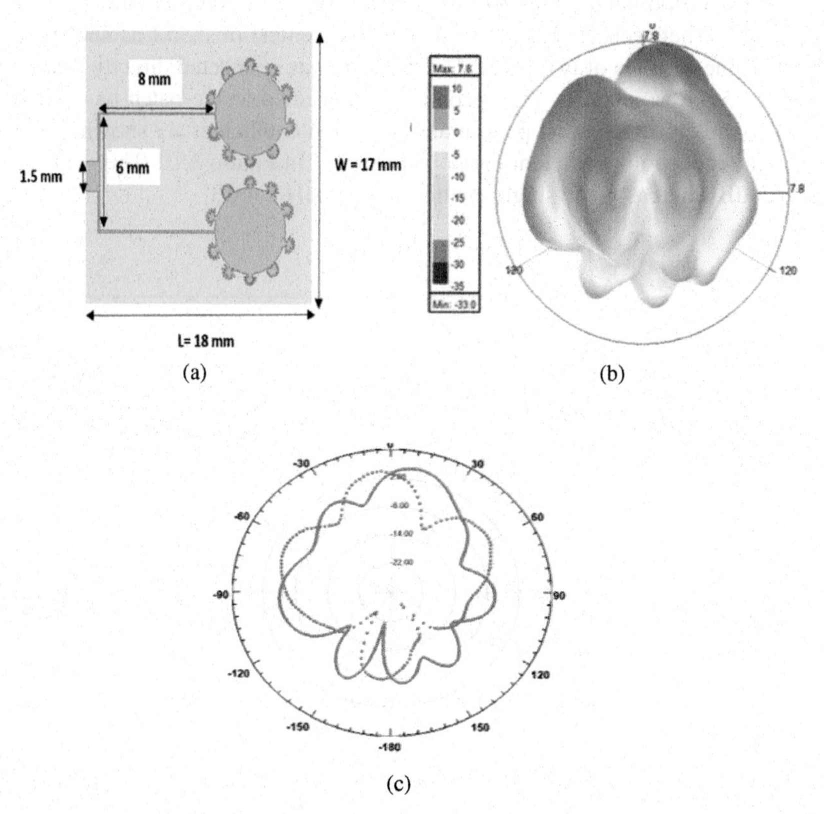

Fig. 3.18: (a) The 2 × 1 antenna array model with dimensions, (b) 3D radiation pattern at the resonance frequency, (C) 2D radiation pattern, solid line is the H-plane, the dashed line is the E-plane.

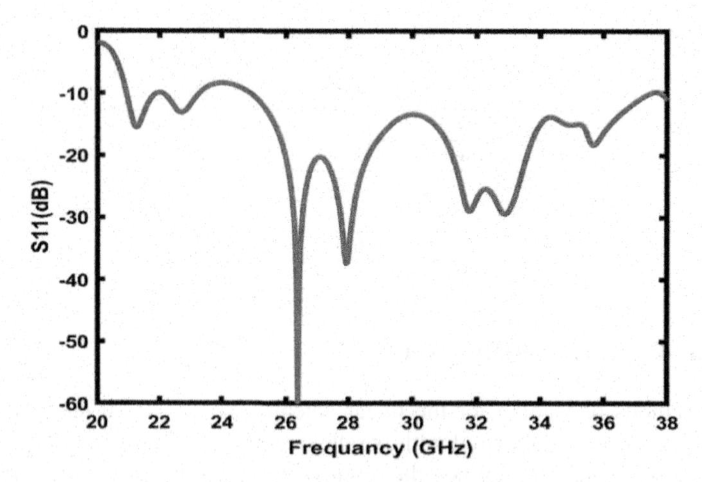

Fig. 3.19: Reflection coefficient curve for the 2 × 1 antenna array.

Table 3.4: Results for the 2 × 2 patch array resonate at 28 GHz.

Spacing distance with respect to λ	Curve color	Gain (dB)	Bandwidth percentage (%)	Lowest Resonance frequency (GHz)	Reflection coefficient (dB)
0.65λ	Dark blue	8.53	46.4	28.5	-32
0.7λ	Dark orange	8.9	57.14	29	-40
0.75λ	Orange	9.1	46.4	28.2	-45
0.8λ	Purple	9.3	64.2	28.7	-40
0.85λ	Green	9.2	28	34	-49
0.9λ	Light blue	9	35.7	28.5	-37
λ	Red	8.8	50	34.6	-48

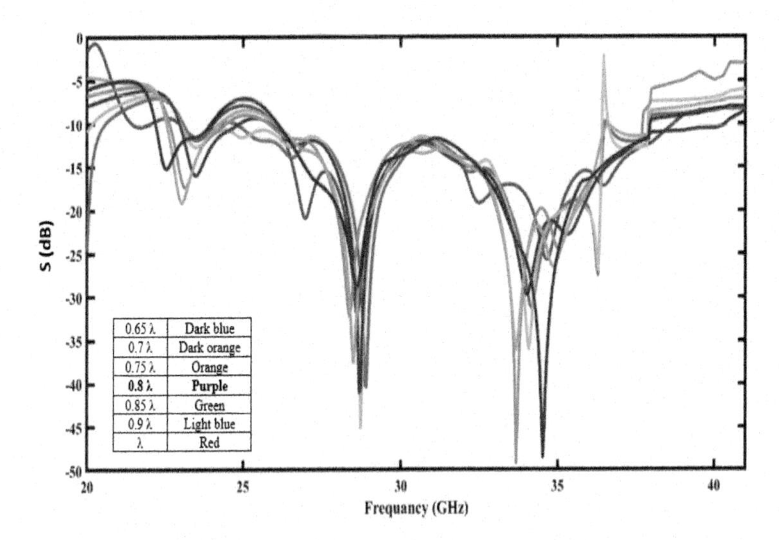

Fig. 3.20: Reflection coefficient curves with different spacing distances.

between the horizontal patches has been varied from 0.65λ (7 mm) to λ (10 mm) to find the best results for this array. Table 3.4 shows the changes in the gain, the bandwidth, resonance frequency, and the reflection coefficient concerning the distance changes. Figure 3.20 shows the S11 curves that were measured concerning the distance changes.

From the previous results, the best values are found when the distance between the parallel array and the additional two series array elements is 8.25 mm (0.8λ), (see Figure 3.21) the gain is 9.3 dB and an ultra-wide bandwidth is measured to be from 22 GHz to 40 GHz. The 2D structure with its dimensions is shown in Figure 3.21. The optimal results of the 2 × 2 patch antenna array from the 3D, 2D radiation efficiency, the reflection coefficient curves, and the corresponding simulated results at the desired frequency band are demonstrated in Figure 3.22. For a better understanding of the advantages of this type of array, a comparison of the proposed antenna array with another state of arts was tabulated in Table 3.5. The proposed antenna is superior to the recent studies in terms of bandwidth, and small size.

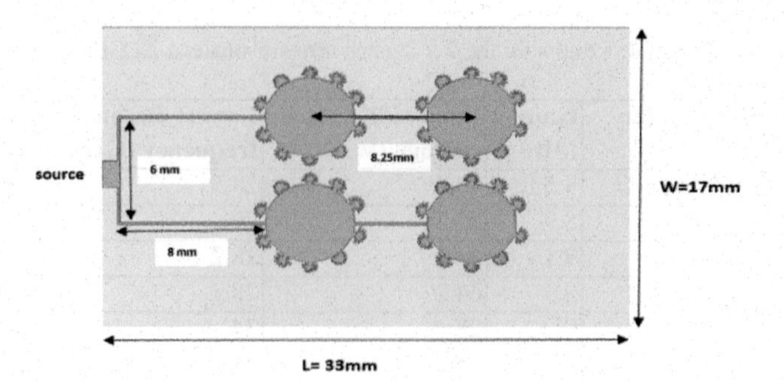

Fig. 3.21: 2D structure for the 2×2 antenna array.

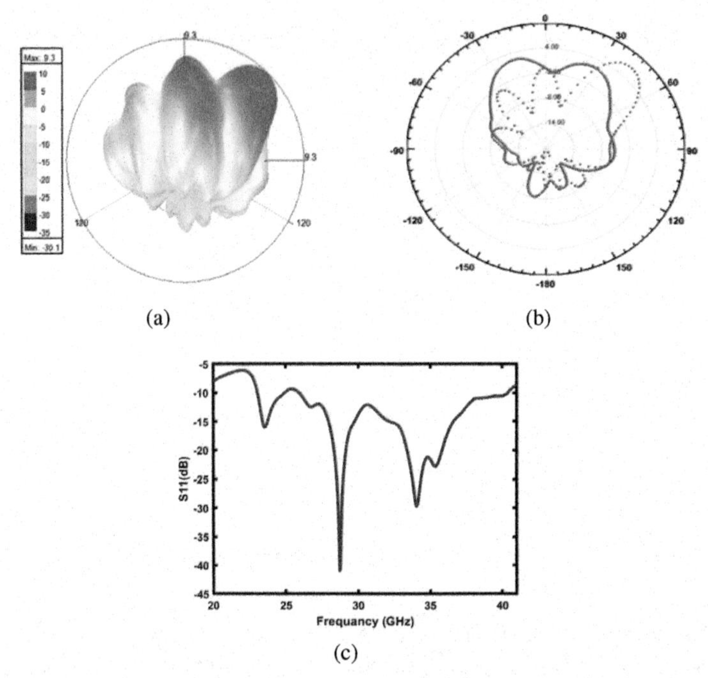

Fig. 3.22: (a) 3D radiation pattern resonated at 28 GHz.(b) 2D radiation pattern, the dotted line is the H-plane and the sold line is the E-plane, (c) Reflection coefficient curve.

Table 3.5: Comparison between the proposed work and other antenna arrays in the mm-wave band.

References	Size (mm^2)$(L \times W)$	**Resonance frequency (GHz)**	**Gain (dB)**	**Bandwidth (GHz)**	**No. of ports**
[13]	30×35	28	8.4	4.1	4
[14]	28×30	28	12	1	4
[15]	20×20	28	8	0.87	2
[16]	52×23	27	13	5	2
[17]	30×23	27	4	5	2
Proposed work	33×17	28	9.3	18	1

3.4 Conclusion

A COVID-19 patch antenna is constructed in the centimeter wave band suitable for WiMAX, GPS and radar applications. An array was created from this patch which was printed on an FR4-epoxy material with 0.16 cm height. This array is a 2×4 single polarized antenna with 21cm × 10cm length and width respectively. At 3.16 GHz operating frequency, the maximum simulated and measured gain are 10.25 dB and 9 dB respectively. There is an acceptable agreement between the simulated and measured results for the S_{11} parameters where the discrepancy in the results is explained by errors in exact duplication of the design due to miniature detailed dimensions and mismatches or reflection in SMA and coaxial feed connection. Moreover, another COVID-19 patch was created for the mm-wave band. An antenna array of 2×2 was also designed with area of 3.3cm × 1.7cm, this array resonates at 28 GHz and has an ultra-wide bandwidth extended from 22 to 40 GHz with a maximum measure gain of 9.3 dB. These results allow this array to perform in an extremely wide band of applications, especially in the second range of the new radio (NR) 5G wireless applications. Even though the design of COVID-19 patch antenna elements and arrays faced many challenges, there are very important potentials harvested from it to support the reality of the 5G cellular networks, and without doubt, this technology will stay the main field for researchers to develop the next generation of the mobile network and cellular services systems and applications.

References

[1] Purba, B.M. 2013. Design and realization of Patch Array FMCW Radar antenna in 9.4 GHz frequency with recommendations coaxial prob. IEEE European Radar Conference, 2(3): 7065.

[2] Agnesya, C.D. 2016. Making the patch microstrip antenna using inset feed recoding technique for application of Radar Wither in S-band frequency. Padang State Polytechnic.

[3] Elisma, N. and H. Madiawati. 2021. Realization of rectangular patch 2×4 microstrip array antennas at frequency 2.7 GHZ-2.9 GHZ for weather radar applications. Journal of Electronics and Communication Engineering, 16(1): 8–26.

[4] Sharma, M., P. Bagri and N. Desbmukya. 2013. Design of 2×4 microstrip patch antenna in *C*-band. International Conference on Electrical, Electronics and Computer Engineering.

[5] Taylor Rayon, J. and S.K. Sharma. 2012. Compact spirograph planar monopole antenna covering C/X band with invariant radiation pattern characteristics. IEEE Transactions on Antennas and Propagation, 60(12).

[6] Harane, M. and H. Ammor. 2018. Design & development of 4×2 microstrip patch antenna array with circular polarized elements for satellite application. International Symposium on Advanced Electrical and Communication Technologies (ISAECT), 1–4.

[7] Ayn, Q., P.A.N. Rao, P.M. Rao and B.S. Prasad. 2018. Design and analysis of high gain 2×2 and 2×4 circular patch antenna arrays with and without air-gap for WLAN applications. 2018 Conference on Signal Processing and Communication Engineering Systems (SPACES), 41–44.

[8] Jang, H.A., D.O. Kim and C.Y. Kim. 2012. Size reduction of patch antenna array using CSRRs loaded ground plane. PIERS Proceedings, 1487–1489, Kuala Lumpur, Malaysia, 27–30.

[9] Goodwill, K., V.N. Saxena and M.V. Kartikeyan. 2013. Dual–band CSSRR inspired microstrip patch antenna for enhancing antenna performance and size reduction. 2013 International Conference on Signal Processing and Communication (ICSC), 495–497.

[10] Balanis, C.A. 2005. Antenna Theory: Analysis and Design, 3rd Edition, John Wiley and Sons Inc., New York.

[11] Saini, J. and S.K. Agarwal. 2017. T and L slotted patch antenna for future mobile and wireless communication. 2017 8th International Conference on Computing, Communication and Networking Technologies (ICCCNT), 1–5.

[12] Panda, R.A., P. Dash, K. Mandi and D. Mishra. 2019. Gain enhancement of a biconvex patch antenna using metallic rings for 5G application. 2019 6th International Conference on Signal Processing and Integrated Networks (SPIN), 840–844.

[13] Khalid, M., S. Iffat Naqvi, N. Hussain, M. Rahman, S.S. Mirjavadi and M.J. Khan. 2020. 4-port MIMO antenna with defected ground structure for 5G millimeter-wave applications. Electronics, 9(1): 6–9.

[14] Ikram, M., Y. Wang, M.S. Sharawi and A. Abbosh. 2018. A novel connected PIFA array with MIMO configuration for 5G mobile applications. 2018 Australian Microwave Symposium (AMS), 19–20, Brisbane, QLD.

[15] Zhang, Y., J. Deng, M. Li, D. Sun and L. Guo. 2019. A MIMO dielectric resonator antenna with improved isolation for 5G mm-wave applications. IEEE Antennas and Wireless Propagation Letters, 18(4): 747–751.

[16] Salemal-Bawri, S., M.T. Islam, T. Shabbir and G. Mohamad. 2020. Hexagonal shaped NZI MTM based MIMO antenna for mm-Wave application. IEEE Access.

[17] Alekhya, B., N.A. Murugan, B.T.P. Madhav and N. Kartheek. 2021. Millimeter-wave reconfigurable antenna for 5G wireless communications. Electromagnetics Research Letters, 101(1): 107–115.

Chapter 4

Design of Fractal COVID-19 Microstrip Patch Antenna Array for Wireless Applications

J.S. Abdaljabar,[1,*] *M. Madi,*[2] *A. Al-Hindawi*[3] and *K. Kabalan*[4]

4.1 Introduction and Preliminaries

In February 2002, the Federal Communications Commission (FCC) in the United States authorized the frequency range from 3.1 to 10 GHz since it can be used in civil commercial services. Since then the researchers are factoring in this in designing their antennas with this frequency band in mind. The most significant kind of antenna which becomes the most widely used technology in the mobile communication system is the microstrip patch antenna because of its lightweight, low power consumption, and ease of integration and fabrication. There are many possible patch shapes used in practice, the circular and the rectangular are the most commonly used shapes, the researchers are paying attention to building an array with less space by concentrating on the geometry of the patch, this makes the circular patch the most favourable in some array implementations since it needs less spacing than the rectangular patch antenna operating at the same frequency band.

In specific applications like satellite communications and radar applications, there has been a demand for reducing the size of the ordinary patch and having a patch antenna operating in several discrete frequency bands. For instance, mobile phones have rapidly faced a reduction in size resulting and having a multiband cellular phone in a new evolution of patch antennas that are utilized in mobile communication to replace the traditional ones.

[1] Communication Engineering Department, Sulaimaniya Polytechnic University (SPU), in Sulaymaniyah, Kurdistan Region, Iraq.
[2] HCT (Higher colleges of Technology) Abu Dhabi, UAE.
Email: mervatmadi@icloud.com
[3] Communication Engineering Department, Technical College of Engineering, Sulaimaniya Polytechnic University, Sulay-maniyah, Kurdistan Region, Iraq.
Email: assad.jasim@spu.edu.iq
[4] Department of Engineering and Architecture, American University of Beirut.
Email: kabalan@aub.edu.lb
* Corresponding author: jihan.salah@spu.edu.i

Various techniques were proposed to have an effective small size multiband antenna by the designers such as:

- using a metamaterial superstrate [1–3].
- using a high permittivity dielectric substrate [4].
- using a substrate with a relatively high permittivity [5].
- the use of reshaping or adding slots to the patch [6, 7].
- using modification method on the ground plane [8, 9].
- using the shorting pin [10].
- placing notches near to the pin or the feeding point [11].
- and finally using the Fractal technique [12, 13].

4.2 Fractal Geometry

Recently, fractal geometry technology has been implemented in many science and engineering branches. The fractal geometry in antenna engineering explored special characteristics, where the fractal antenna becomes an efficient technique used for designing wideband, high gain, small size, and small side lobe array.

The word fractal was first explained by Benoit Mandelbrot in 1975, where the word fractal came from the Latin word fractus which means "to break" in order to create irregular fragment shapes [14].

One of the most essential properties of the geometry in the fractal antenna is made aiming for maximizing the perimeter of the material used in the antenna in order to improve the electromagnetic radiation in the transition and the receiving process within a specific volume or area. Furthermore, the standard antenna can be operating with only a single frequency band meanwhile the fractal antenna operates in multiband frequency, which controls the space limitation problem, especially in the antenna array [15].

The geometrical configuration of the fractal antennas can be split up into two main configurations: random and deterministic. Sierpinski gaskets and von Koch snowflakes are the main objects in deterministic configuration, as proposed in [15, 16]. It is used to improve the efficiency and the gain of the overall antenna. Random configuration, on the other hand, is represented by natural phenomena like lightning bolts [17]. There are many microstrip patch antennas, beyond these configurations, that were demonstrated to demonstrate the fractal geometry in order to implement special irregular, miniaturized patch antennas. Such a good example is the flower shape patch which was operating at 2.4 GHz as illustrated in [18, 26]. Another interesting shape is a wheel-shaped antenna which was constructed in 2017 with $32 \times 36\text{mm}^2$ at the frequency band 3 GHz. Further research in this area includes a sphere shape antenna; in 2018 it was printed on RT Doroid substrate with 14 mm length and 18 mm width [20]. In biomedical applications, a $10 \times 10\text{mm}^2$ antenna is demonstrated to detect breast cancer, as shown in [21].

The COVID-19 virus has spread around the world, since 2020, and it has become a major public health pandemic that is still changing lives and daily habits. Recently, due to an increasing interest in this virus, the pictures of COVID-19 have been published in most scientific and non-scientific journals. The inspiration for the antenna patch shape of this chapter was taken from the silhouette of a COVID-19 virus. This chapter will adopt the design of the COVID-19 patch antenna and use the advantages of fractal geometry features to design a very small size prototype and its array that are suitable for dual-band wireless applications. The single patch resonates at 7.5 GHz (in C-band) and 17 GHz (in K_u-band) which makes the proposed patch suitable for the downlink of satellite communication systems, breast cancer detection, and smart home concept (at 7.5 GHz) [22–24], and its also used in the transmission of direct broadcast services (DBS) and Fixed Satellite Service (at 17 GHz) [25]. The application of fractal geometry on the planar structure of the COVID-19 circular patch antenna results in enhancing the resonance frequency and the reflection coefficient of the antenna. This design is analysed using the finite element method-based software, ANSYS HFSS simulator.

4.3 Antenna Configuration

The configuration of the proposed COVID-19 antenna model and the actual virus image are represented in Figure 4.1. The structure of the 2D and 3D COVID-19 model and its dimensions are illustrated in Figure 4.2. According to the structure of this model, an FR4-epoxy substrate with relative permittivity of 4.4 is used to build the microstrip patch antenna. This material is used in fabrication because of its low cost and availability in the market. The overall dimensions of the substrate (L, W, h) are $(1 \times 1 \times 0.16)\text{cm}^3$. The main patch antenna is a circular patch with a radius of 4 mm. The coaxial probe feeding method is used to excite the antenna, and the pin of the coaxial feed is placed at a point (0 mm, –1.18 mm) when the center of the patch is considered as the origin.

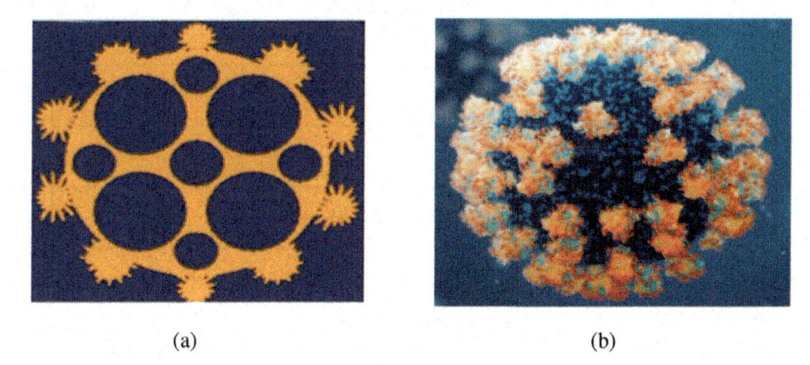

(a) (b)

Fig. 4.1: (a) The simulated COVID-19 antenna. (b) The image of the actual virus.

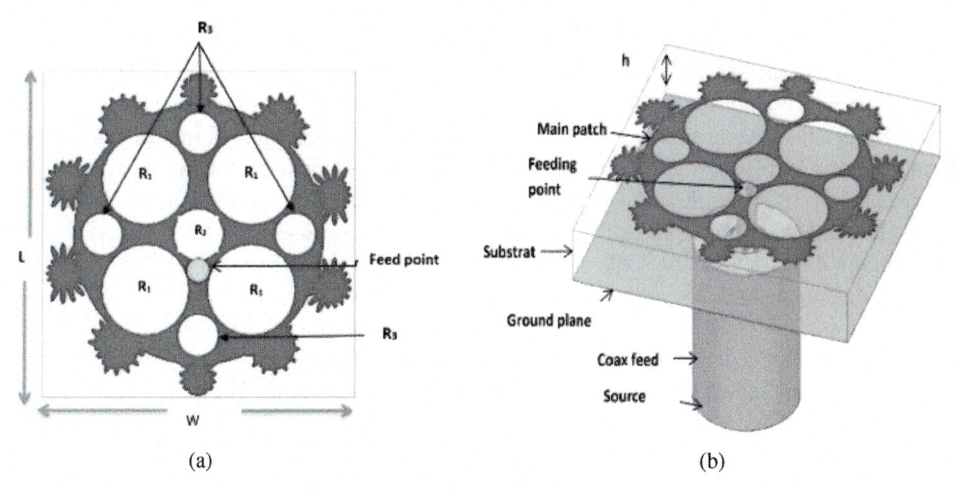

(a) (b)

Fig. 4.2: (a) Shows a two-dimensional prototype of the simulated COVID-19 patch antenna. (b) Shows the three-dimensional COVID-19 patch antenna.

The coaxial feed consists of three parts: the inner conductor, which is connected sprightly to the patch with a 0.735 mm radius, the insulator of Teflon with a radius of 1.2 mm, and the outer conductor connected to the ground with a 2.5 mm radius. This feeding method is considered the best because it gives the overall patch the same shape as the COVID-19 virus shape. The main circular patch antenna is firstly built without fractals; however, the electrical length of the antenna was low which leads to an extremely high resonance frequency. Different fractal shapes have been demonstrated to improve the resonance frequency. The best results are optimized when nine circles were inserted; one of them is at the center of the patch of radius R_2, four small circles of radius R_3 were distributed equally around the center with 90° rotation, while the other four big circles of radius R_1 were distributed equally around the center with rotation of 45°. Further optimizations are used using trial and error to estimate the radius of the fractal circles that obtain the optimal resonance frequency and reflection coefficient. The finalized dimensions of these circles are illustrated in Table 4.1.

Table 4.1: Parameter descriptions of the simulated COVID-19 patch antenna.

Decryptions	Symbols	Values in (mm)
Length of the substrate	L	10
Width of the substrate	W	10
Radius of the main patch	R	4
Radius of the big fractal circle	R_1	1.4
Radius of middle fractal circle	R_2	0.8
Radius of the small fractal circle	R_3	0.65
Height of the substrate	h	1.6

When the main circular patch is optimized, the crowns are drawn around the main circular patch to obtain the unique shape of the COVID-19 virus. Ten crowns are surrounded the main patch with a 36° angle between each adjacent crown. The first crown on top of the main patch was initially created, four ellipses with a major radius of 0.33 mm and a minor radius of 0.24 mm were used to make the original spike, see Figure 4.3a, (Figure 4.3b is the magnified picture of Figure 4.3a). Next, two copies of this spike were rotated and duplicated around itself with an angle of 26° firstly (light blue color) in Figure 4.3c, and −26° secondly (green color) to have 5 spikes in total, which were eventually united to demonstrate the first crown, as shown in Figure 4.3d. Similarly, more spikes were added to the other pair of crowns to make each pair with its own unique shape to provide the similarity with the original virus. This crown was rotated and duplicated with 180° around the origin to have the second crown diametrically opposite as shown in Figure 4.3e. Next, by leaving a distance of 36° from the top crown, another crown with more spikes is implemented. This crown was also rotated and mirrored to have the fourth crown as shown in Figure 4.3f. The same procedure is followed in Figure 4.3g, and Figure 4.3h, to have six and eight crowns respectively. The final shape of the COVID-19 patch antenna with five pairs of crowns is deployed in Figure 4.3i.

It has been chosen to simulate the COVID-19 patch antenna with only five pairs of crowns; because this number gives the resonance frequency and the reflection coefficient curves (S_{11}). Firstly, when the number of crowns was only 8 the reflection coefficient was almost -10 dB (as shown in Figure 4.4); The next step was building 12 crowns surrounding the central patch; however, the resonance frequency was completely lost. Therefore, 10 crowns were chosen to have double band frequencies with wide bandwidth, and the reflection coefficient curves at 7.5 GHz and 17 GHz are found in Figure 4.2.

After finalizing the size of the substrate, the circular patch radius, and the number of crowns, it is essential to add the fractal geometry on the main circular patch to determine whether a miniaturized patch can

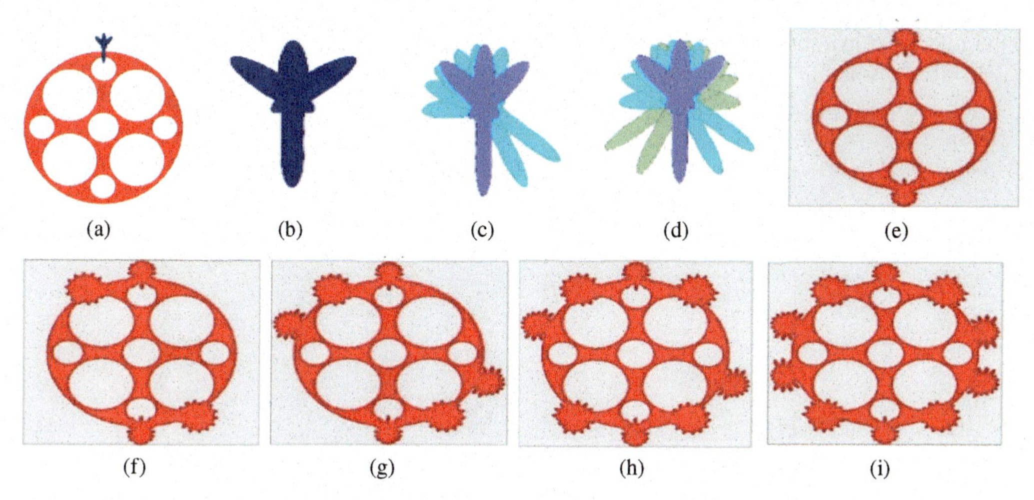

Fig. 4.3: Steps of drawing the crowns around the main circular.

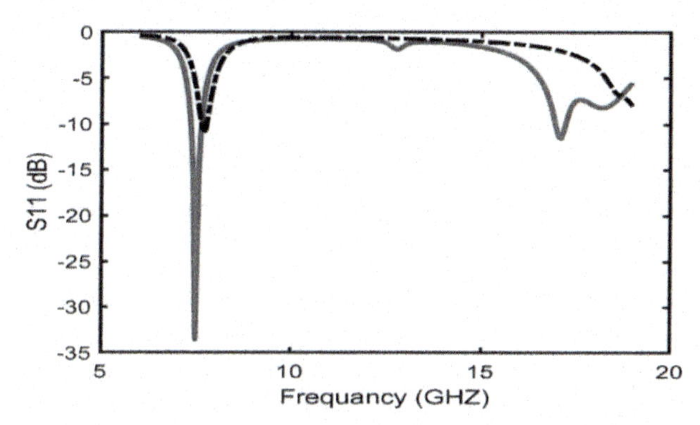

Fig. 4.4: Simulated S_{11} curves: black line when there are 8 crowns on the antenna. Red line when there are 10 crowns on the antenna.

resonate at 7.5 GHz. According to Figure 4.5, six different images have been investigated to represent the current distribution density on the COVID-19 patch surface. Different current distribution density values are represented with different colours as shown in Figure 4.5; where the red color has the highest current density, as the colours change from red to blue, the current density decreased gradually until it reaches its least value at the red colour. Therefore, it is important to notice the changes in increasing the red surface area of the patch since with better current distribution (the red surface area) best resonant frequency is obtained.

The COVID-19 patch was designed firstly without any fractal shapes on its surface, as shown in Figure 4.5a; yet, the current distribution density was only concentrated around the position of the feed point. When the first circle was iterated from the centre of the patch (as shown in Figure 4.5b), the distribution of the current density extended to a wider area far away from the feed position. In Figure 4.5c, after iterating four more circles, the current distribution density improved drastically and reached the edge crowns. Despite this, the resonance frequency was far from the accepted value and even when four more circles were iterated, no significant difference in the resonance frequency was detected. Ultimately, new fractal geometry is adopted

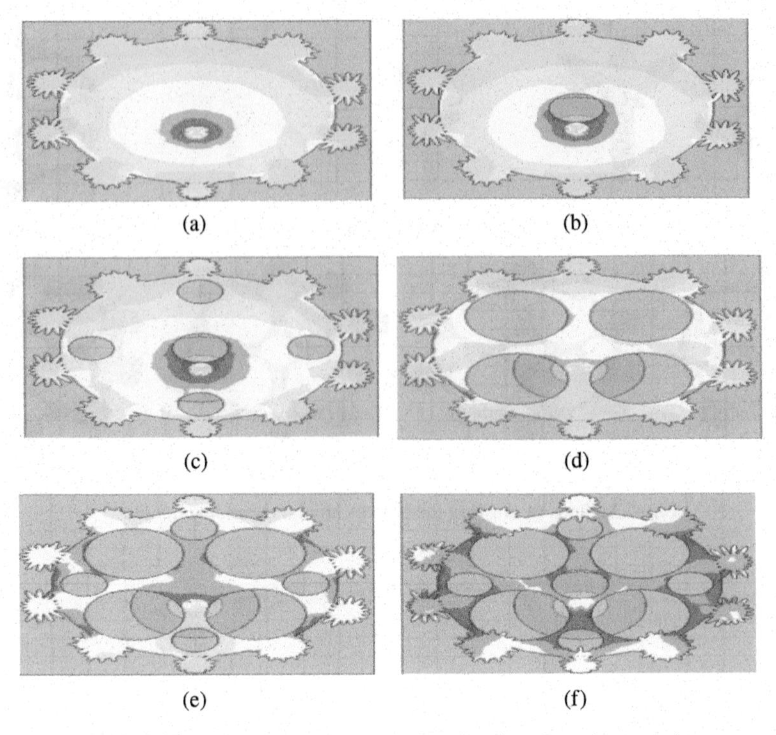

Fig. 4.5: The current distribution density of various fractal geometries.

as shown in Figure 4.5d, the current distribution density expanded and reached the crowns, however, the resonance frequency did not progress. Interestingly, when both of the fractal geometries of Figure 4.5c and Figure 4.5d were used together on the patch surface, the results improved significantly. Two fractal geometries were designed, firstly the fractal geometry of Figure 4.5e, and secondly the geometry of Figure 4.5f. Finally, depending on improving the current distribution density and the resonance frequency results, the decision was to have the COVID-19 patch of Figure 4.5f as the final simulation of the COVID-19 patch shape.

4.4 Some of Related Formula

Before fulfilling the design of the patch antenna, the following equations are used to find the dimensions of the circular patch antenna [26].

$$F = \frac{(8.791 \times 10^{9})}{f_r \sqrt{\varepsilon_r}} \tag{4.1}$$

Where F is the fringing factor, f_r is the resonance frequency, c is the free space velocity of light and ε_r is the dielectric constant of the substrate. The main radius of the patch (R) is calculated as follows:

$$R = F \times \left\{1 + \left(\frac{2h}{\pi \varepsilon_r F}\right)\left[ln\left(\frac{\pi F}{2h}\right) + 1.7726\right]\right\}^{\frac{-1}{2}} \tag{4.2}$$

The resonance frequency corresponds to any TM_{mn0} mode is given as

$$f_{rmn0} = \left(\frac{c}{2\sqrt{\varepsilon_r}}\right)\left[\frac{X_{mn}}{R}\right] \tag{4.3}$$

Here, n and m are modes concerning R, and X_{mn} is the derivative of the Bessel function.

Initially, when f_r = 7.5 GHz, h = 1.6 mm, and ε_r = 4.4, the radius of the main patch is calculated to be 5.21 mm according to Eqs. (1) and (2). Upon doing an extensive literature review different fractal geometries are simulated to minimize the antenna radius size and increase its electrical length. It was observed that after using nine slotted circles the main radius of the patch is reduced to 4mm and a dual-frequency band is achieved. Finally, 10 crowns of crowns are inserted to give the patch its last shape of COVID-19 virus.

The process of adding fractal circles and crowns around the main patch helped to improve both the reflection coefficient and the resonance frequency. Figure 4.6 shows a comparison between three curves, first of all, when a simple circular patch with a radius of 4mm and operating frequency of 7.5 GHz was designed without crowns and fractals it resonated at 9.9 GHz with a reflection coefficient of -11 dB. The second step was simulating the main patch with fractals, the results further developed to become (8.8 GHz, - 11.4 dB) for the lower band and (18.8 GHz, -21 dB) for the higher band. Finally, when 5 pairs of crowns are drawn around the fractal patch the resonance frequency and the reflection coefficient improve dramatically to be (7.5 GHz, -37dB) for the lower band and (17 GHz, -11.5 dB) for the higher band. It becomes apparent from this comparison; that adding the crowns around the main circular patch not only gives the patch its unique shape of the COVID-19 virus but also improves the reflection coefficient and the resonance frequency of the miniature patch antenna.

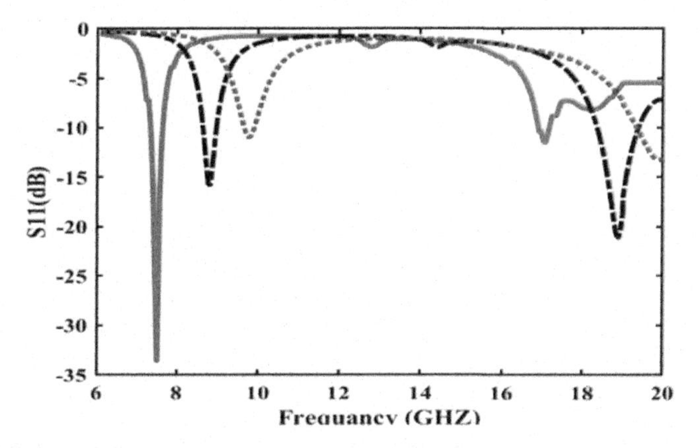

Fig. 4.6: Blue dot line: circular patch without fractal without crowns. Black dash line: circular patch with fractals without crowns. Red solid line: circular patch with fractals with crowns.

4.5 Results and Discussion

The three-dimensional radiation pattern was plotted and the maximum gain was simulated to be 0.8 dB at the 7.5 GHz and 2.21 dB at 17 GHz as illustrated in Figure 4.7. Moreover, the gain and radiation efficiency are drawn concerning the frequency as shown in Figure 4.8.

When the simulation of the miniaturized patch is completed, the prototype is fabricated using a double-sided copper plate (FR-4 epoxy) material for the substrate with a thickness of 1.6 mm. A chemical etching

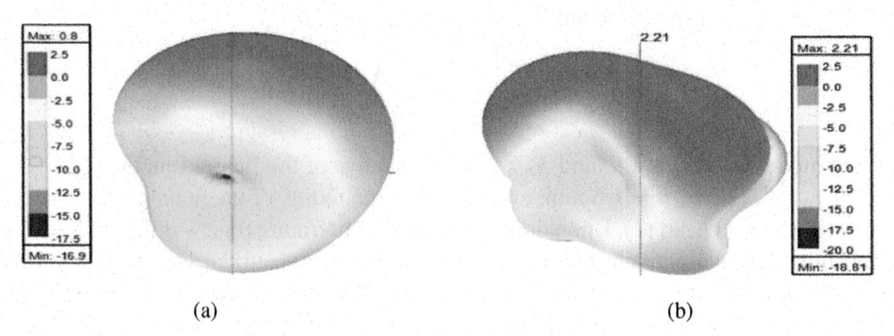

Fig. 4.7: 3D radiation pattern of the simulated COVID-19 antenna: (a) is at 7.5 GHz. (b) is at 17 GHz.

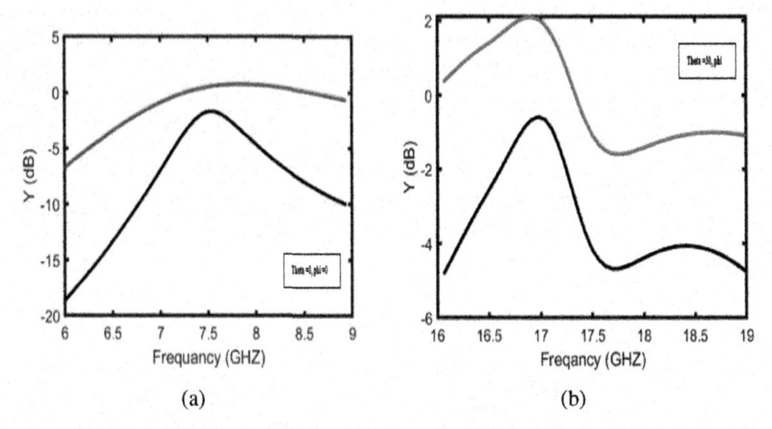

Fig. 4.8: Simulated gain (upper red line) and radiation efficiency (lower black line) at (a) is at 7.5 GHz. (b) is at 17 GHz.

method is used to print the patch on the substrate and maintain a full ground for the antenna when the patch is engraved on the top layer, this procedure is duplicated to a very accurate extent to have the small details of the small spikes of the crowns which surround the main patch. The multi-band frequency with low weight and small size prototype is demonstrated in Figure 4.9. The measured and the simulated reflection coefficient curves are compared and plotted in Figure 4.10.

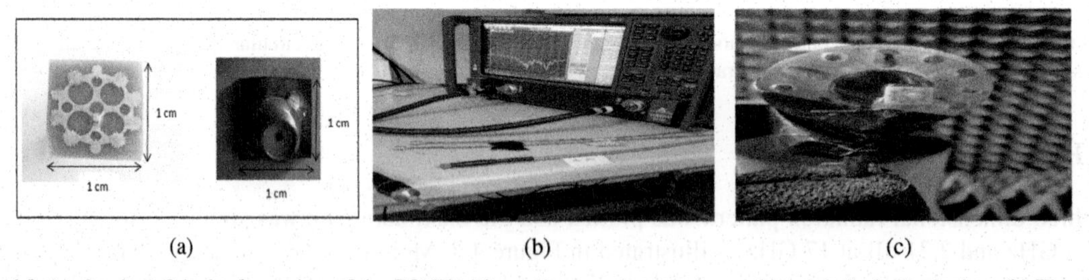

Fig. 4.9: (a) On the left is the front view of the COVID-19 patch antenna prototype, and on right is the back view. (b) The single patch connected to the network analyser. (c) The same patch is in the anechoic chamber room.

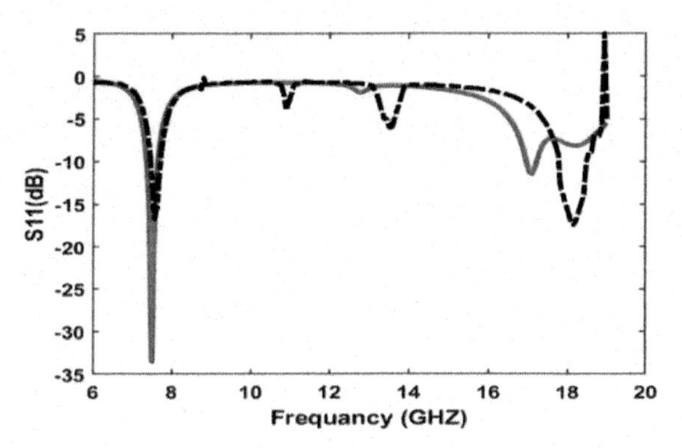

Fig. 4.10: Comparison of the reflection coefficient of both the simulated (red solid line) and the measured (black dash line) results.

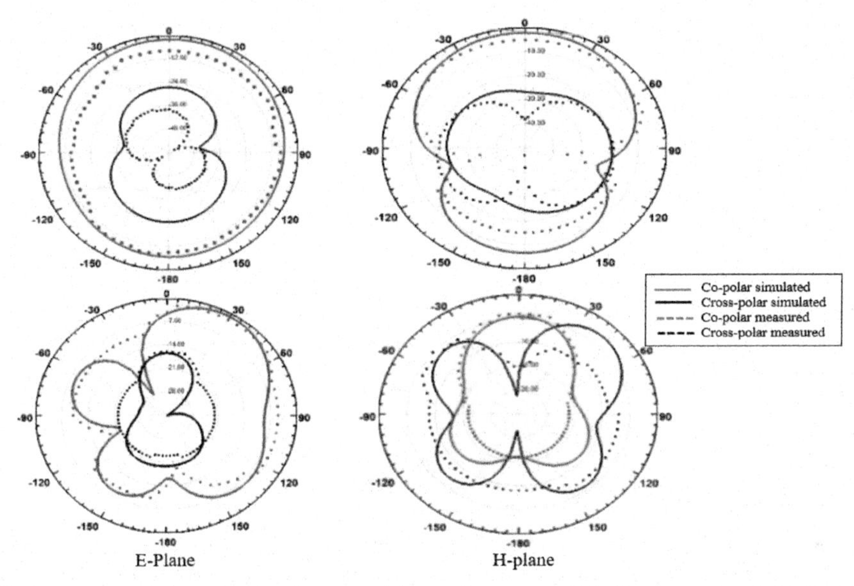

Fig. 4.11: Radiation patterns for simulated and measured (dashed) curves at 7.5 GHz (on top) and 17 GHz (on the bottom) respectively.

The simulated and the measured radiation characteristics of the designed antenna are shown in Figure 4.11. The E-plane and the H-plane for both co-polarization and cross-polarization radiation patterns are represented. The top images of Figure 4.11, show the radiation pattern of the simulated and the measured curve at 7.5 GHz, while the bottom images depicted the radiation patterns for the simulated and the measured results at 17 GHz. The simulated results are represented in a solid line and the dashed results represented the measured results. The polarization characteristics of the studies antenna are given by the co-polar and the cross-polar curves, its obvious that the difference between the co polar and the cross-polar radiation is greater than 30 dB for the lower band the 20 dB for the higher band in the maximum direction of the radiations, then the antenna is considered as a linearly polarized antenna. The maximum measured gain of the designed antenna was 0.2 dB at 7.5 GHz and 2 dB at 17 GHz. Table 4.2 shows a comparison between the proposed work and other irregularly shaped patch antennas according to their sizes and operating band frequency. The demonstrated antenna is compared with other different design antennas which have almost the same size as the proposed antenna, as shown in Table 4.3. From the results, we examine that our antenna is easy to fabricate according to its miniature size and the layers used for the antenna works in dual-band resonance frequency.

Table 4.2: Comparison between COVID-19 patch antenna and other irregular shape patch antennas.

Reference number	**Antenna volume $(cm)^3$**	**Resonance frequency (GHz)**	**Gain (dB)**
[8]	69	1.28	4
[10]	17	0.193,0.22	1.91,2.07
[14]	24.3	1.5, 2.6	5.3, not given
[16]	6.4	2.4	2.5
[18]	5.76	3.14,4.28, 5.1,6.9	1.9,10.9,1.8,9.3,4
[26]	1.44	2.9, 9.5	2.8, 4.11
[20]	0.252	6	10
Proposed work	0.16	7.5,17	0.2,2

Table 4.3: Comparison between the proposed work and other miniature patch antennas.

Reference	**Layers used**	**Patch area (mm^2)**	**Resonance frequency (GHz)**
[21]	2	10×10	7.7
[23]	2	20×20	12.25,14.16
[25]	3	9.5×8	15.33, 17.6
[26]	1	22×21	12.07, 14.44
[27]	1	20×20	12.38, 14.4
Proposed work	1	10×10	7.5, 17

4.6 Antenna Array Design Using Miniaturized Patch Element

A single element microstrip-patch antenna has the positive points of small size, various shapes, low cost of fabrication, dual-polarization, and being lightweight. Usually, the radiation pattern of the single element is relatively wide and each element has a low value of gain, low efficiency, and cross-polarization. To overcome these obstacles, the electrical size of the antenna must be increased leading to more directive characteristics. Another approach is to provide an assembly of radiation antennas in an electrical and geometrical configuration known as antenna array. These arrays are characterized by high gain that can be long-distance beam.

4.6.1 Single Element Design using Microstrip Feeding Line

In the previous sections, the single miniaturized antenna patch simulation was optimized; it used the coax prob feed method to find the results. In this section, the COVID-19 patch antenna is fed using the microstrip feeding line method to make the simulation process of the single element and the double elements easier. The 2D and 3D simulated COVID-19 models with dimensions are shown in Figure 4.12.

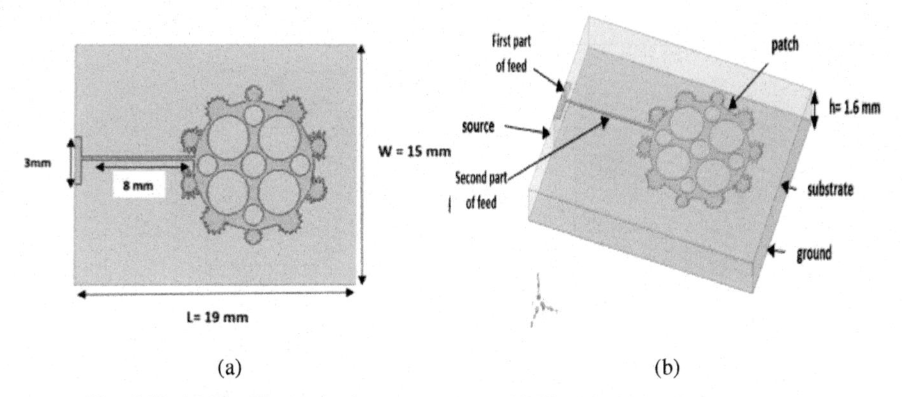

(a) (b)

Fig. 4.12: (a) The 2D single element structure. (b) The 3D single element structure.

The width W of thc feed of an impedance Z_0 of 50Ω, the following equations [27] was used:

$$W = \frac{2 * h}{\pi}\left\{B - 1 - ln(2B - 1) + \frac{\varepsilon_r - 1}{2\varepsilon_r} * \left[ln(B - 1) + 0.39 - \frac{0.61}{\varepsilon_r}\right]\right\} = 31mm \tag{4.4}$$

In the above equation,

$$B = \frac{377 \cdot \pi}{2 \cdot Z_0 \cdot \sqrt{\varepsilon_r}}$$

where Z_0 is the feeding line impedance.

When ε_r is 4.4 and $Z_{\circ}$ is 50Ω, the width is 3 mm and the length of the 50Ω resistor is optimized to be 0.5 mm. For the second part of the transmission line, and by using the same equations, Z_1 as indicated in Figure 4.12(a), is 100Ω. In addition, the width is found to be 0.2 mm. From the simulation, the length is 8 mm. Figure 4.13 shows different reflections coefficient curves for different feeding line length dimensions. The overall dimensions of the substrate for a single element miniaturized patch (L, W, h) are $(15\times19\times1.6)\text{mm}^3$. The 3D and the 2D radiation efficiency image are shown in Figure 4.14. It is clear from both figures that the reflection coefficient curve and the radiation pattern vary according to dimensions. Figure 4.14 shows on top the 2D and the 3D structure of the single element and the bottom shows the different reflection coefficient curves for different length values of the feeding lines.

4.6.2 Design of 2 × 1 Array

In this case, a parallel network feeding line connection was used to supply a uniform distribution of power to all the elements. The feeding network is constructed in two parts, the first part was connected to the patch which has an impedance of 100Ω. Then, another 100Ω feed line was used to connect the two patches to the 50Ω feeding line which was used to connect the array with the SMA input power connection. Next, the distance between the two connected elements was changed and the best results are found when the distance is 0.75λ from centre to centre. The geometry of the 2 × 1 array is shown in Figure 4.15.

Figure 4.16 shows the reflection coefficient curve when the spacing distance between the two connected elements varies from 0.35λ to 0.85λ. For a better understanding of the obtained results in Figure 4.15, Table 4.4 shows different values of the gain, the reflection coefficient, and the resonance frequency when the distance has been changed. As demonstrated in Table 4.4, the optimal results of this array are obtained when

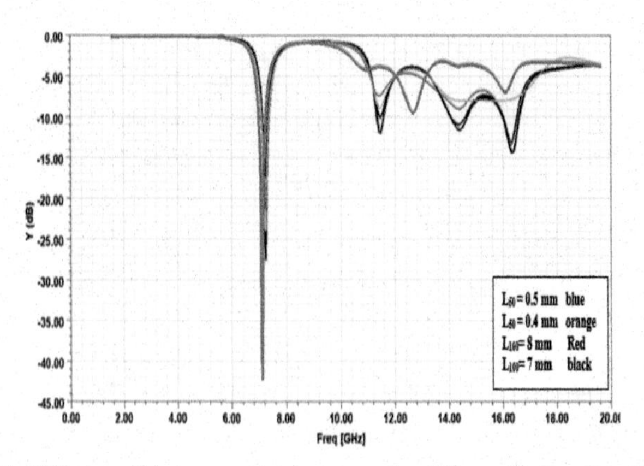

Fig. 4.13: Different reflection coefficient curves for different feeding line dimensions.

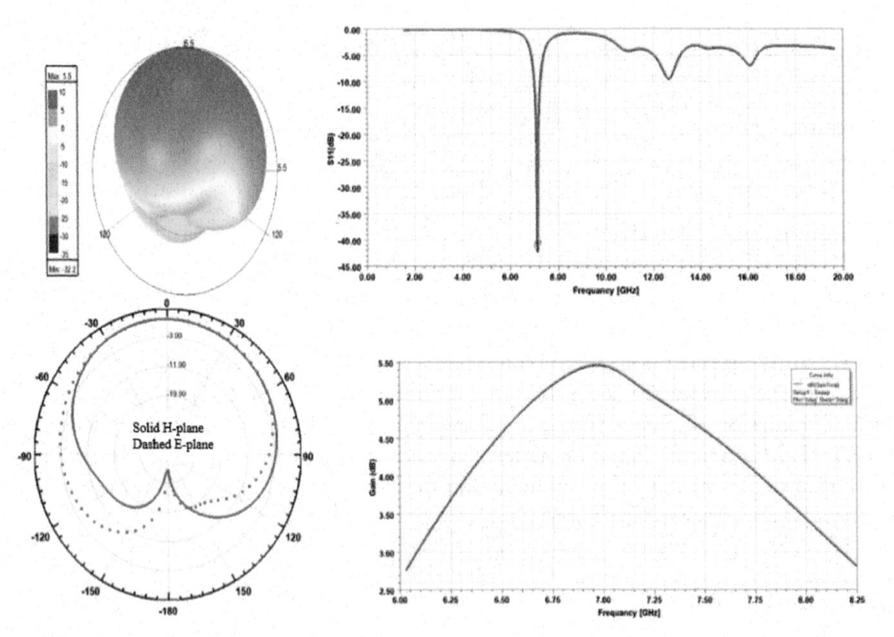

Fig. 4.14: Left: 3D and 2D radiation pattern. Right: reflection coefficient and gain curves versus frequency.

the spacing distance is 0.55λ from centre to centre. In this case, the 100Ω feed that connects directly to the patch has a length of 8.4 mm and a width of 0.2 mm which was calculated in the previous section. The 50Ω feeding line is (3mm × 1.35 mm). For the designated structure, the 2D 1 × 2 antenna structure and the 2D radiation efficiency are shown in Figure 4.16.

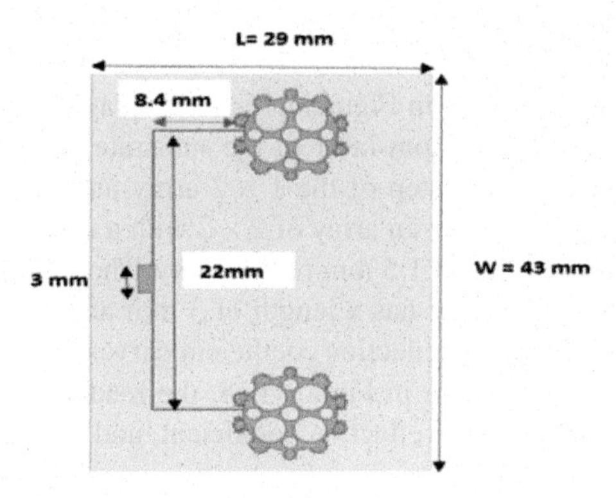

Fig. 4.15: Geometry and dimension of the 2 × 1 array.

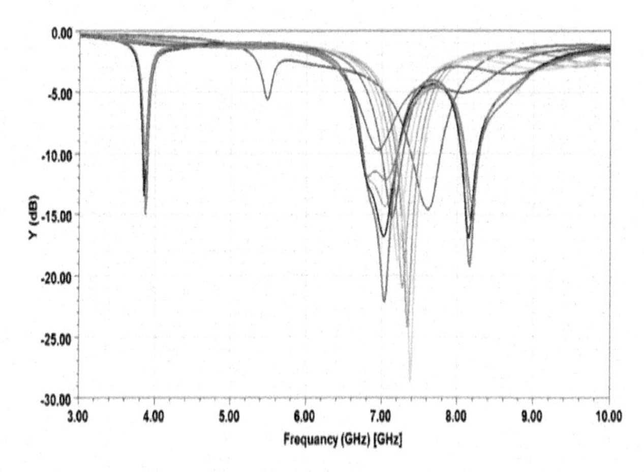

Fig. 4.16: Reflection coefficient curves for different spacing distance values.

Table 4.4: Results of 1 × 2 array concerning the spacing distance with resonance frequency 7.5 GHz.

Spacing distance with respect to λ	Line colour	Gain (dB)	Resonance frequency (GHz)	Reflection coefficient (dB)
0.35λ	Red	5.6	7.6	-14
0.45λ	Light blue	5.9	7.5	-19
0.5λ	Light green	6.5	7.3	-28
0.55λ	Dark blue	6.9	7.34	-24.25
0.6λ	Orange	6.85	7.2	-21
0.65λ	Gray	6.9	7.2	-18
0.7λ	Light brown	7	7.1	-15
0.75λ	Purple	-3, 6.8, 4.6	3.8, 7, 8.1	-15, -24, -18
0.8λ	Brown	6.7	7	-10
0.85λ	Pink	6.6	7.1	-14

4.6.3 Design of 2 × 2 Antenna Array

The 2 × 2 antenna array geometry is shown in Figure 4.17. As displayed in this figure, the patch is printed at the top layer of the substrate and the bottom layer of the substrate consists of a full ground plane. The considered configuration follows the same step of the 1 × 2 array and connected with a feeding network consisting form 70Ω, 100Ω, and 50Ω to have an array of 2 × 2 with a spacing distance of 0.55λ. The length and width of the 70Ω feeder are 9.2 mm and 1.5 mm respectively. The 50Ω feeder has a length of 1.35 mm and a width of 3 mm while the 100Ω feeder has a length of 3 mm and a width of 0.15 mm. The distance between the 2×2 array is optimized and the reflection coefficient curves for different distance values is shown in Figure 4.18. To explain the results shown in Figure 4.18, the reader is recommended to refer to Table 4.5 that shows the resonance frequency, the reflection coefficient, and the gain as a function of the spacing distance as a function of the wave length.

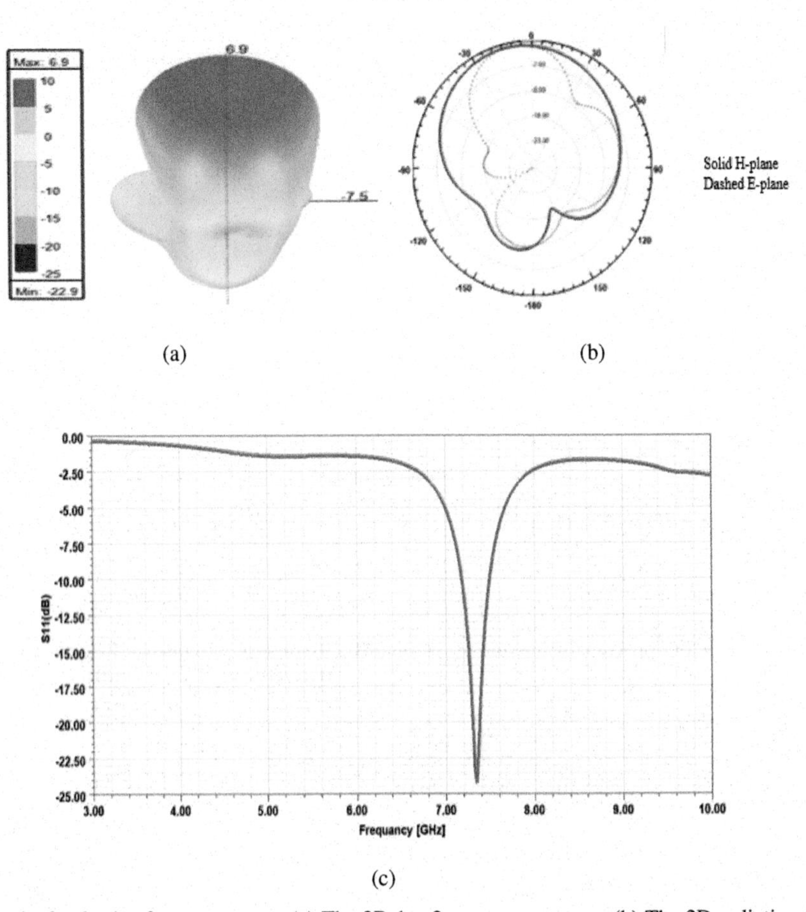

Fig. 4.17: Final results for the 1 × 2 antenna array. (a) The 2D 1 × 2 antenna structure. (b) The 2D radiation efficiency where the solid line is the H-plane and the dotted line is the E-plane. (c) The 3D radiation efficiency and on right is the S_{11} curve concerning frequency.

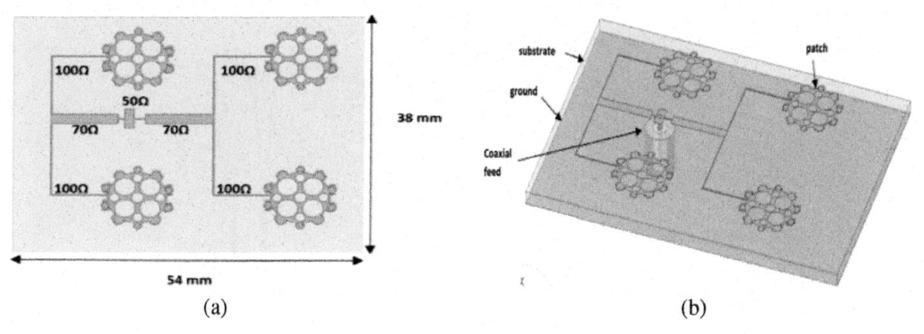

(a) (b)

Fig. 4.18: (a) Three-dimensional 2 × 2 COVID-19 patch antenna array. (b) Two-dimensional prototype of the simulated 2 × 2 COVID-19 patch antenna array.

Table 4.5: Results of 2 × 2 antenna array vs the spacing distance with resonance frequency 7.5 GHz.

Spacing distance with respect to λ	Line colour	Resonance frequency (GHz)	Reflection coefficient (dB)	Gain (dB)
0.35λ	Red	4.9, 10	-13.5, -26	1, 6
0.45λ	Blue	9.5	-9.4	7
0.55λ	Brown	7.15	-36.25	7.8
0.57λ	Green	6.97.8, 10.2	-18, 15	7.5
0.6λ	Light blue	7.2	-21	6.85
0.65λ	Gray	7.2	-18	6.9
0.7λ	Orange	7.1	-15	6

Based on the optimal results obtained, the reflection coefficient and the 3D Gains for both operating frequencies are shown in Figure 4.19. It is to note that the coaxial probe feeding method, used to excite this array and the dimensions of this probe, are identical to the coaxial used in building the single element. Moreover, the inner conductor of the coaxial is extended from the ground plane through the substrate to reach the topmost layer.

4.6.4 Design of 4 × 2 Array

The overall size of the proposed design is $(38 \times 100)\text{mm}^2$ as shown in Figure 4.20. The previous array was duplicated horizontally to build a 2 × 4 array. The coaxial probe feed is in the middle of the substrate connected to the main patch through the 50Ω feeder with (L, W) are (100 mm, 38 mm), the length of the 100Ω is 3 mm, and the width is 0.15 mm. The 70Ω line has a width of 1.5 mm, the length (L_{70}) is changed to have the best reflection coefficient as shown in Figure 4.21. As clear from this figure, the optimal value of L_{70} is 25 mm. The distance between every two patches is fixed at 22 mm which gives the optimal gain value at three frequency bands 5.63 GHz, 6.49 GHz, and 7.25 GHz. The results of this type of array are shown in Figures 4.22, 4.23 and 4.24 for S_{11} characteristic, 3D radiation patterns for different resonance frequencies, and 2D radiation patterns, respectively.

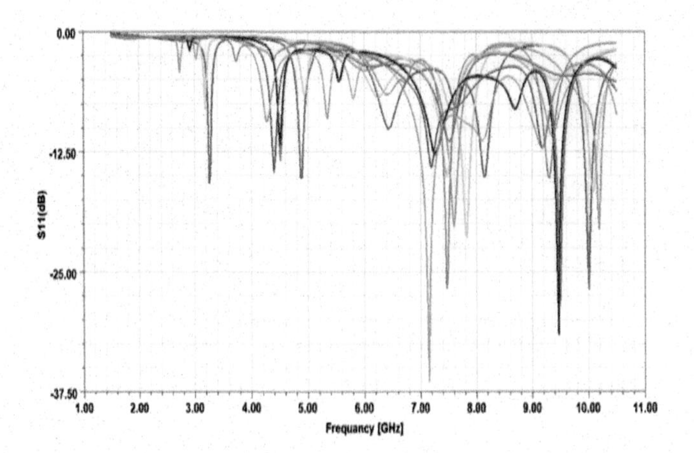

Fig. 4.19: Reflection coefficient curves concerning the spacing distance.

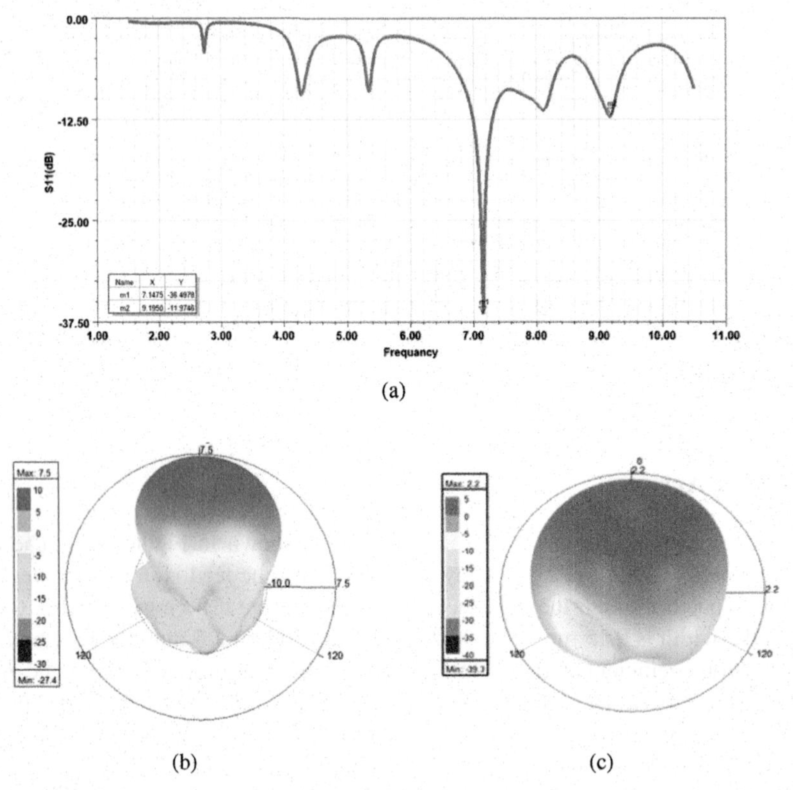

Fig. 4.20: (a) The reflection coefficient curve concerning the frequency. (b) 3D gain at a frequency of 7.28 GHz. (c) The 3D gain at 9.19 GHz.

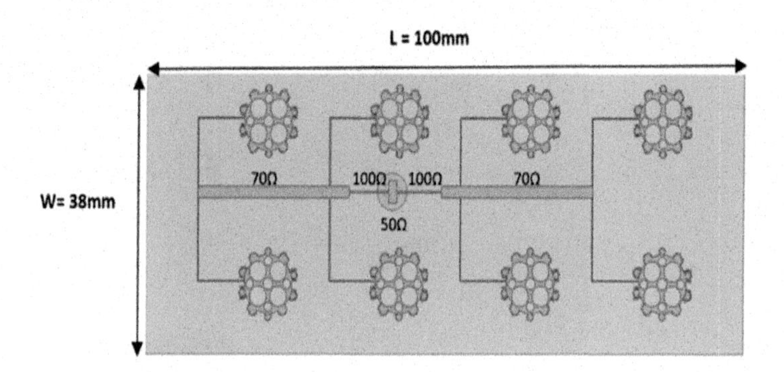

Fig. 4.21: The two-dimensional prototype of the simulated 2 × 4 COVID-19 antenna array.

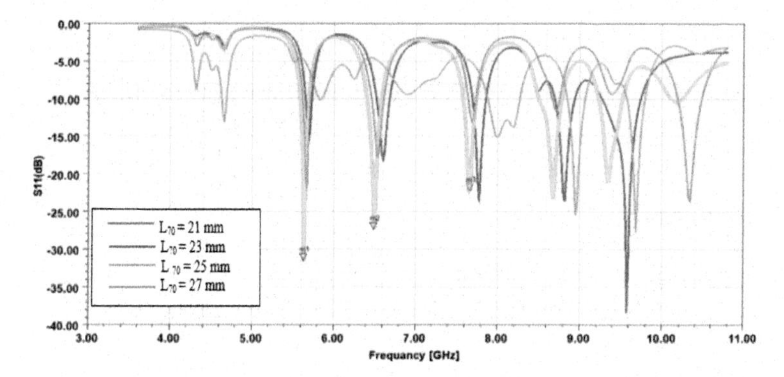

Fig. 4.22: Different reflection coefficient curves for different feeding line dimensions.

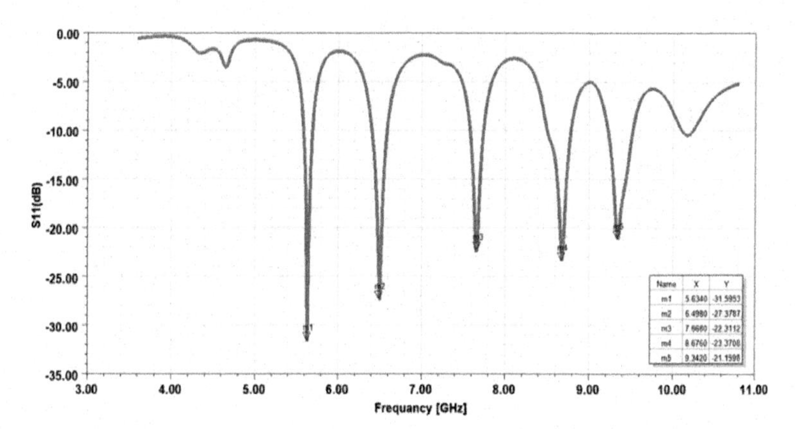

Fig. 4.23: S_{11} characteristic for the optimal case when L_{70} = 25mm.

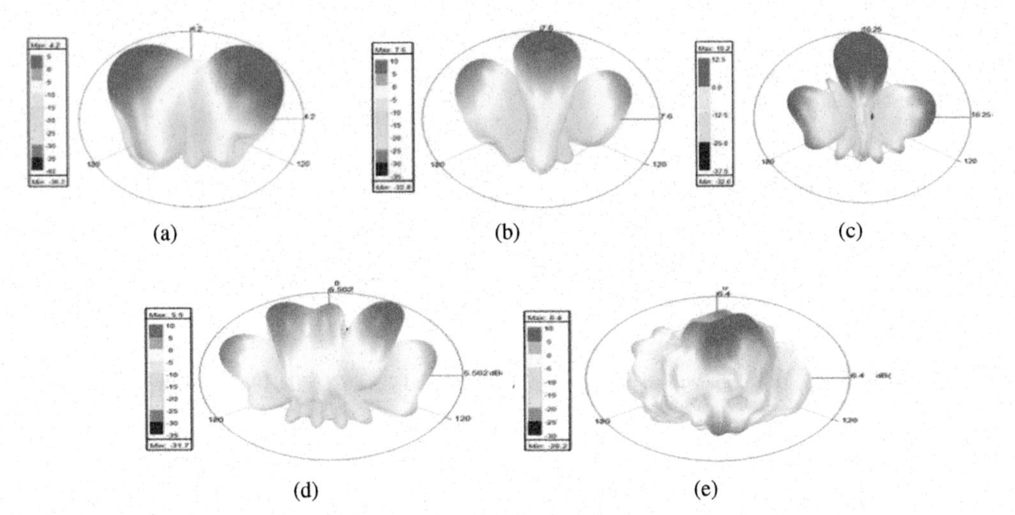

Fig. 4.24: 3D radiation patterns for frequencies (a) 5.634 GHz, (b) 6.498 GHz, (c) 7.668 GHz, (d) 8.676 GHz and (e) 9.342 GHz.

4.6.5 Design of 8 × 2 Array

The overall size of the proposed design is (40 mm×185 mm) as shown in Figure 4.25. The previous array 2 × 4 was duplicated horizontally to build a 2 × 8 array. The coaxial probe feed is in the middle of the substrate connected to the main patch through the 50Ω feeder with (L, W) are (100 mm, 38 mm), the length of the 100Ω is 3mm, and the width is 0.15 mm. The 70Ω line has a width of 1.5 mm, the length (L_{70}) is

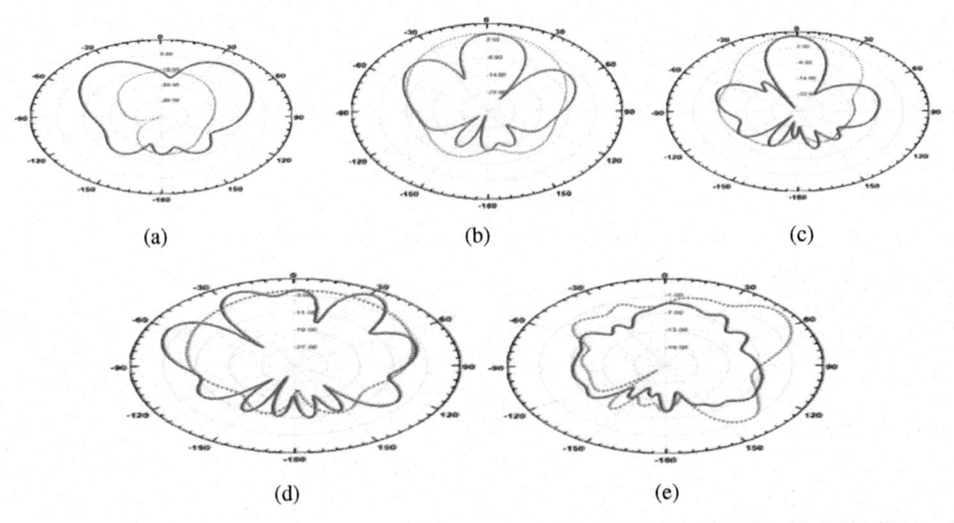

Fig. 4.25: 2D radiation patterns for (a) frequencies 5.634 GHz, (b) 6.498 GHz, (c) 7.668 GHz, (d) 8.676 GHz and (e) 9.342 GHz.

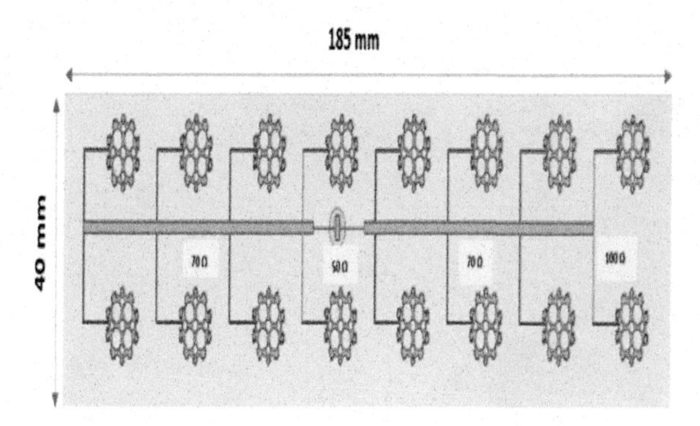

Fig. 4.26: The two-dimensional prototype of the simulated 2 × 8 COVID-19 antenna array.

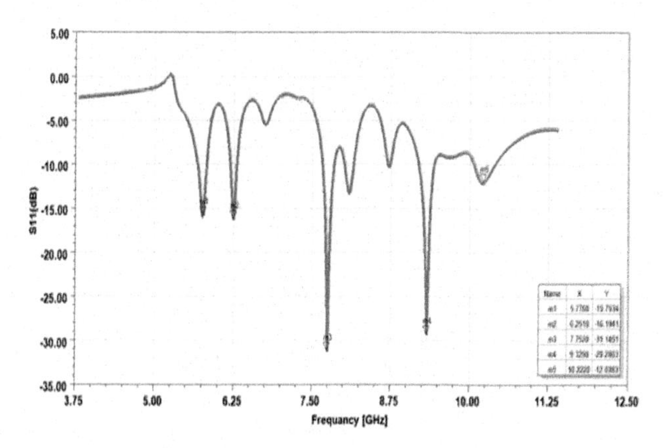

Fig. 4.27: S_{11} characteristic for the optimal case.

Table 4.6: Summary of the simulated COVID-19 miniaturized patch antenna.

Array type	Gain (dB)	S_{11}(dB)	Resonance frequency (GHz)
Single element	5.5	-43	7.1
1 × 2	6.9	-24	7.28
2 × 2	2.2,7.5	-12,-12.5	4.5,7.28
4 × 2	4.2,7.6,10.25,5.5,6.4	-31.5,-27.4,-22.3,-23.37,-21.15	5.63,6.49,7.66, 8.67,9.34
8 × 2	10,6.2,11.6,4.4,15.4	-15.7,-16.2,-31.15,-29.3,-12.03	5.77,6.25,7.75, 9.33,10.22

changed to have the best reflection coefficient and the optimal value of L_{70} is found to be 69.35 mm. The distance between every two patches is fixed at 22 mm which gives the optimal gain value at five resonance frequencies 5.776 GHz, 6.251 GHz, 7.752 GHz, 9.329 GHz and 10.222 GHz. The final results of this type of array are shown in Figures 4.26, 4.27 and 4.28 for S11 characteristic, 3D radiation patterns for different resonance frequencies, and 2D radiation patterns, respectively. To understand the results of the miniaturized antenna single patch and the array, a summary of the array results is presented in Table 4.6. This table shows the comparison of the previous antenna design in terms of gain resonance frequency and reflecting coefficient. From the performance of this type of array, the designed antenna array can be used in the

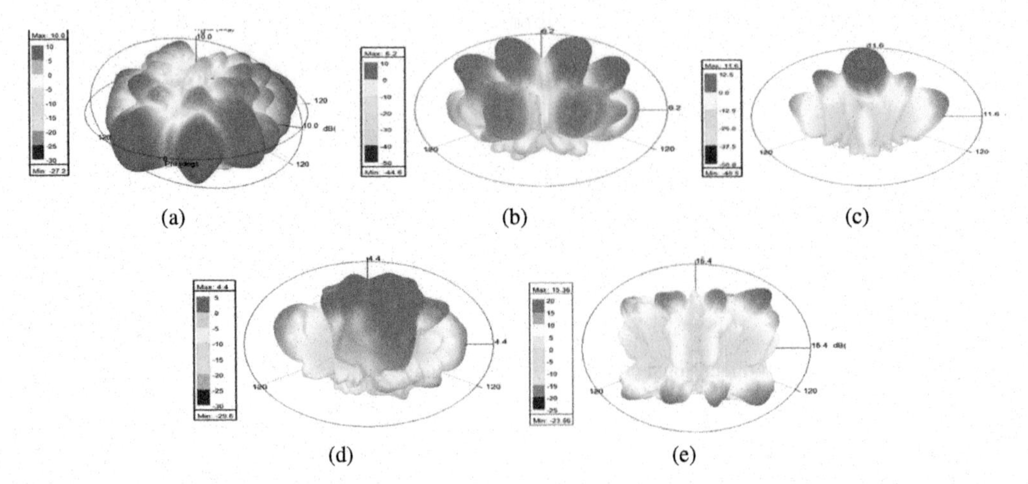

Fig. 4.28: 3D radiation patterns for frequencies (a) 5.776 GHz, (b) 6.251 GHz, (c) 7.752 GHz, (d) 9. 329 GHz and (e)10.222 GHz.

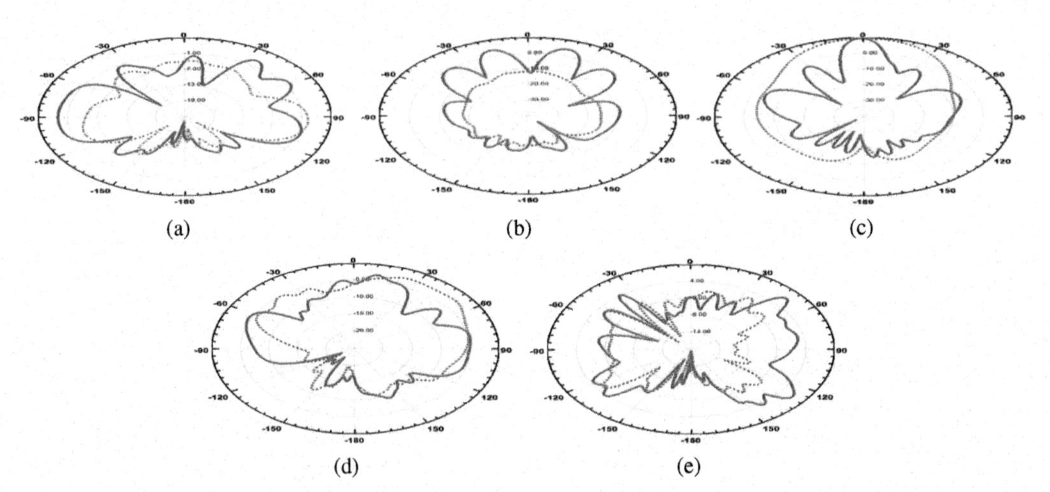

Fig. 4.29: 2D radiation patterns for frequencies (a) 5.776 GHz, (b) 6.251 GHz, (c) 7.752 GHz, (d) 9. 329 GHz and (e)10.222 GHz.

radiation of low radar cross-section characteristics [28]. The patch array is also suitable for the downlink of satellite communication systems, and the smart home concept (at 7.5 GHz) [24, 29]. Moreover, since 2002, the Federal Commission Comity in the United States has been authorized the frequency band from 3.1 to 10 GHz can be used in civil commercial services and the 5 G wireless applications. Because these arrays are resonating at the range of 7 GHz, they are suitable for this type of application.

4.7 Conclusion

The main goal of the current paper is to use the fractal geometry and the COVID-19 shape in order to create a miniature antenna for the implementation of dual-band wireless, satellite, and radar applications (when it is a part of an array) and civil commercial services. The proposed single patch with a low-weight antenna operates at two different frequency bands 7.5 GHz and 17 GHz with a maximum gain of 0.8 dB and 2.21 dB respectively for the simulated and 0.5 dB and 2 dB for the measured results. This innovative patch is suitably designed so that the current distribution density reaches the far edge of the crowns. The main purpose of these crown shapes is not only to give the patch its unique shape of the COVID-19 virus but also to improve the resonance frequency and reflection coefficient of the fractal circular patch. When the simulated results are finalized, the prototype is printed on a 1 cm $\times$1 cm substrate using chemical etching. There is an acceptable agreement between the simulated and measured results for both the input and output antenna characteristics. The discrepancy in the results is explained by errors in exact duplication of the design due to its miniature dimensions and mismatches or reflection in SMA and coaxial feed connection. When the simulated results are finalized, an antenna array of $1\times2, 2\times2, 4\times2$, and 8×2 are simulated from this miniaturized patch. The FR4-epoxy material of 0.16mm used as a substrate in the design of these arrays. The 8×2 array with size of $(18.5\times4)\text{cm}^2$ has the optimal number of antenna elements and it resonated at five frequency bands 5.77 GHz, 6.25 GHz, 7.75 GHz, 9.33 GHz, and 10.22 GHz with gain of 10 dB, 6.2 dB, 11.6 dB, 4.4 dB, and 15.4 dB. These resonated frequency bands make the array suitable for the commercial services in the 5G wireless network, downlink of the satellite communication systems, and smart home applications.

References

[1] Razi, Z.M., P. Rezaei and A. Valizade. 2015. A novel design of Fabry-Perot antenna using metamaterial superstrate for gain and bandwidth enhancement. International Journal of Electronics and Communications, 1525–1532.

[2] Jahani, S., J. Rashed-Mohassel and M. Shahabadi. 2013. Miniaturization of circular patch antennas using MNG metamaterials. IEEE Antennas Wirel. Propag. Lett., (9): 1194–1196.

[3] Aziz, C.H. and A.M. Al-Hindawiia. 2016. Electromagnetic effect of rectangular spiral metamaterial on microstrip patch antenna performance. Journal of Modeling and Simulation of Antennas and Propagation, 2(1): 24–29.

[4] Patel, A., R. Patel, A. Desai, T. Upadhaya and J. Patel. 2018. Design of Wideband Broccoli Fractal Antenna for WiMAX/WLAN Applications. 2018 Second International Conference on Inventive Communication and Computational Technologies (ICICCT), 958–961.

[5] Kula, J., D. Psychoudakis, W.J. Liao, C.C. Chen, J. Volakis and J. Halloran. 2006. Patch antenna miniaturization using recently available ceramic substrates. IEEE Antennas Propag. Mag., 48(6): 13–20.

[6] Musselman, R.L. and J.L. Vedral. 2019. Patch antenna size-reduction parametric study. ACES Journal, 34(2): 288–292.

[7] Nasimuddin, Z., N. Chen and X. Qing. 2010. Dual-band circularly polarized S-shaped slotted patch antenna with a small frequency-ratio. IEEE Transactions on Antennas and Propagation, 58(6): 2112–2115.

[8] Jang, H.A., D.O. Kim and C.Y. Kim. 2012. Size reduction of patch antenna array using CSRRs loaded ground plane. PIERS Proceedings, pp. 1487–1489, Kuala Lumpur, Malaysia, March 27–30.

[9] Goodwill, K., V.N. Saxena and M.V. Kartikeyan. 2013. Dual–band CSSRR inspired microstrip patch antenna for enhancing antenna performance and size reduction. 2013 International Conference on Signal Processing and Communication (ICSC), 495–497.

[10] He, M., X. Ye, P. Zhou, G. Zhao, C. Zhang and H. Sun. 2015. A small-size dual-feed broadband circularly polarized U-slot patch antenna. IEEE Antennas Wirel. Propag. Lett., 14: 898–901.

[11] Dwairi, M.O., M.S. Soliman, A.A. Alahmadi, I.M.A. Sulayman and S.H. Almalki. 2017. Design regular fractal slot-antennas for ultra-wideband applications. 2017 Progress In Electromagnetics Research Symposium – Spring (PIERS), 3875–3880, St. Petersburg, Russia, 22–25.

[12] Bakariya, P.S., P.S. Dwari and S. Sarkar. 2015. Triple band notch UWB printed monopole antenna with enhanced bandwidth. AEU Int. J. Electron. Commun.

[13] Jena, M.R., B.B. Mangaraj and R. Pathak. 2014. Design of a novel Sierpinski fractal antenna arrays based on circular shapes with low side lobes for 3G applications. American Journal of Electrical and Electronic Engineering, 2(4): 137–140.

[14] Chowdhury, B.B., R. De and M. Bhowmik. 2016. A novel design for circular patch fractal antenna for multiband applications. 2016 3rd International Conference on Signal Processing and Integrated Networks (SPIN), 449–453.

[15] Kumar, A. and A.P. Singh. 2019. Design of micro-machined modified Sierpinski gasket fractal antenna for satellite communications. International Journal of RF and Microwave Computer Aided Engineering, 29(8).

[16] Mandlebrot, B.B. 1983. The Fractal Geometry of Nature, New York: W.H. Freeman.

[17] Prajapati, P.R., G. Murthy, A. Patnaik and M. Kartikeyan. 2015. Design and testing of a compact circularly polarised microstrip antenna with the fractal defected ground structure for L-band application. IET Microw. Antennas Propag., 9: 1179–1185.

[18] Khanna, G. and P.N. Sharma. 2016. Fractal antenna geometries: A review. International Journal of Computer Applications, 153(7): 29–32.

[19] Madi, M.A., M. Al-Husseini, A.H. Ramadan, M. Mervat and A. El-Hajj. 2012. A reconfigurable cedar-shaped microstrip antenna for wireless applications. Progress in Electromagnetics Research C, 25: 209–221.

[20] Abraham, J., K.K. Aju John and T. Mathew. 2014. Microstrip antenna based on Durer pentagon fractal patch for multiband wireless applications. International Conference on Information Communication and Embedded Systems (ICICES2014), 1–5.

[21] Kaushal, D. and T. Shanmuganantham. 2018. Parametric enhancement of a novel microstrip patch antenna using circular SRR loaded fractal geometry. Alexandria Engineering Journal, 2551–2557.

[22] Gupta, M. and V. Mathur. 2017. Wheel shaped modified fractal antenna realization for wireless communications. International Journal of Electronics and Communications, 257–266.

[23] Bisht, N. and P. Kumar. 2011. A dual band fractal circular microstrip patch antenna for C-band applications. PIERS Proceedings, 852–855, Suzhou, China, September 12–16.

[24] Maria, N., M.A. Madi and K.Y. Kabalan. 2021. Miniaturized inward fractal antenna for breast cancer detection. Proc. of the International Conference on Electrical, Computer and Energy Technologies (ICECET), December 9–10.

[25] Deepak, G. and Sh. Mishr. 2016. Smart home networking. Jaipur International Journal of Converging Technologies and Management (IJCTM), 2(2).

[26] Balanis, C.A. 2005. Antenna Theory: Analysis and Design, 3rd Edition, John Wiley and Sons Inc., New York.

[27] Samsuzzaman, M., M.T. Islam, N. Misran and M.M. Ali. 2013. Dual band X shape microstrip patch antenna for satellite applications. Procedia Technology, 11: 1223–1228.

[28] Vijayvergiya, P.L. and R.K. Panigrahi. 2016. Single-layer single-patch dual band antenna for satellite applications. IET Microw., Antennas Propag., 11(5): 664–669.

[29] Saini, G.S. and R. Kumar. 2019. A low profile patch antenna for Ku-band applications. International Journal of Electronics Letters, 1–11.

Chapter 5

Fluctuation Analysis Through Multifractals for the Pathogenesis of SARS-CoV-2 aka nCoV-19 Community Spread in USA

Aashima Bangia[1] and *Rashmi Bhardwaj*[2,*]

5.1 Introduction

Corona-genomic viruses that are a member of the *Coronaviridae* species have viruses consisting of large strands of RNA sequences. RNA is sized about *27–32kb* engulfed with polyadenylated. In each cluster, viruses pigeon-hole their way into the host cells genomic sequence. This so-called *'Corona'* virus got first identified in animals like mice, horses and many reptiles as well as cows, bullocks, etc., that led to severe infections some of which were gastric and respiratory tract infections. Predominant infections associated with this virus are respiratory, gastric however, hepatic or neurological diseases have also been recorded. WHO reported the status of novel coronavirus in China on January 12, 2020. Figure 5.1 shows the viral-gene affecting host *RNA*-structure. Coronaviruses (Co-Vs) have been traced in the respiratory tract in addition to gastric-intestinal-tract. These have been studied under four genres namely, *Alpha*, *Beta*, *Gamma* and *Delta*. Basically, these structures have been described so far as non-segmented positively-sensed RNA genomic-viruses. As per existent trend analysis, a broad area of scaling of time series was required popularly known as Multi-fractal and then refined into Fractal. Multi-fractals were established as refined analysis techniques that included differentiation of pure fractal-based dynamics from the rest of the scaling variants, which had their own drawbacks as they could not detect and overcome the non-stationary occurrences in the corpora of datasets to be analyzed. The two major throwbacks noted from already existing conventional statistical processes that analyze time successions belonging to dynamics of various autonomous and non-autonomous systems are no. of series of data alongwith their durations been restricted which makes it difficult to extract significant information on system dynamics. Nonstationarities exist because external/internal effects result in continuous or sudden changes that are reflected averages, std. deviations and other such statistics. Thus, this important problem arising in the statistical characterization of dynamism, particularly for finding accurate conclusions related to the scaling properties of data considered.

[1] Assistant professor, ASMS, AAFT, Noida, Uttar Pradesh.
Email: aashima1408@gmail.com

[2] Professor Mathematics, Head, Non-Linear Dynamics Research Lab, University School of Basic and Applied Sciences (USBAS), G.G.S. Indraprastha University, Delhi.

* Corresponding author: rashmib@ipu.ac.in

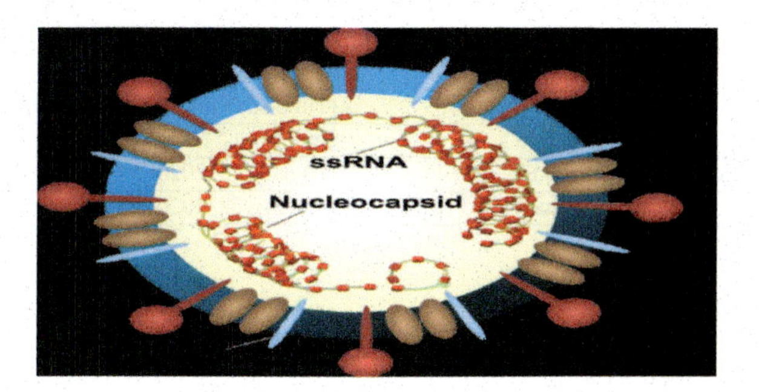

Fig. 5.1: Detailed diagram of COVID-19 affecting the host RNAs.

Various measures to discover drug mechanisms analogous to chloroquine by moving from malaria to multifarious diseases explored [1]. Studied meditating body complexity, HIV- dynamics, Neuro-fuzzy to study demonetization, Fuzzified-PID for the improvement of efficiency of battery devices, atmosphere pollutants' estimation, stock markets trends analyzed through soft-computing, malware spread in IoTs, stock prices variation, river water quality, COVID-19 pandemic spread through data driven system [2–11]. Deliberated reason coronaviruses in humans via spiked glycoprotein in receptor-binding areas [12]. Explained the timeseries transformations through different analysis [13]. Which modelled the spread of novel-coronavirus with the help of phases [14]. Modelled spread of novel-coronavirus via hand, foot and mouth [15]. Analyzed chloroquine medication towards SARS-CoV-2 2019 [16]. It further discussed global dynamical systems for acute/chronic HCV infections [17]. Studied the human-respiratory tract to isolate this virus [18]. Explained in details the coronavirus genomes. [19]. Concluded with the observations obtained from AIDS for the study of viral diseases [20]. Hazardness of coronaviruses present in acute lower respiratory tract of infants discussed [21]. Discussed the relation between coronavirus and pneumonia into infected living beings [22]. *Corona-theorem* in case of countably-many mappings explored [23]. Detailed form *corona theorem* with their applications in spectra have been studied [24].

WHO recorded the novel-coronavirus spread occurring in Japan. Surveies on updates of MERS-CoV disease were conducted [25, 26]. An analysis of molecules that target the SARS-human coronavirus has been studied [27]. The WHO reported new Coronavirus updates as recorded on *January 19, 2020* in detail discussed pneumonia outbreak within bats resulting in this virus. Discussed some important anti-biotics that could effectively hinder access in cases: *Ebolavirus*, *MERS CoV* and *SARS CoV* in host-cells [28–31].

None of the authors have studied Multi-fractal, including fractal, spectral, holder exponent, R/S algorithm, and further waveform signal analysis, denoising and decomposition towards the COVID-19 spread of the United States. In this article, the impact through scaling properties that vary for a stationarity and non-stationarity of time successions has been studied.

5.2 Dataset Collection

In this study, daily laboratory-confirmed records starting approximately from the last week of January through July with variations in time-periods. Daily *COVID-19* active and recovered cases data for the United States are taken for the time period January through July. The dataset for active and recovered cases contains a total of a little less than 200 days' observations as given in Table 5.1. A pragmatic approach assumes that the trend will continue indeterminately in the future, which is very different from various deterministic modeling methods that would perhaps tend towards convergence at future further on.

Table 5.1: Data sets for simulation for Fractal analysis.

Data	Cases	Time-span under consideration	
		From	Up to
Data type: United States	Active cases	January 22, 2020	July 25, 2020
	Recovered cases	January 22, 2020	July 25, 2020

5.3 Multi-fractal Analysis

Multifractality is better described as a self-affinity or particularly fractality is based on the fundamentals of scaling as:

Theorem 5.1 *Multifractals rescales the series values (y(t)) on rescaling the time, t by a constant factor such as γ^h resulting in a self- affine system, i.e., having statistical properties but on a completely different axis.*

Remark 5.1 Thus, the scaling relation as: $y(t) \rightarrow \gamma^h\ y(ht)$ holds for an arbitrary factor, h.

Multi-fractals are a general term to a fractal system, spectral system, and denoising procedures, eventually leading to waveform methods. Multi-fractals consist of a single exponent, which may not be enough to describe the complexity of the system requiring a continuous spectrum of exponents to be worked upon. This analysis helps investigate datasets in conjunction with fractal and lacunarity analysis techniques. This method requires distorting dataseries extracted (via patterns) which would generate multi-fractal spectrum demonstrating the applicability of scaling variations on corpora of data.

The capability of the description provided by signal regularity plays its part in handling situations with no characteristic scaling. For applying any kind of analyzation technique to raw data, an inbuilt invariability is assumed for the data. Hence, for translational invariance, autocorrelation or power spectral density are the best considered. It also directs that signal statistics such as mean, deviation, the variance shouldn't vary with time-period. Thus, signals without characteristic scaling known as scale-invariant, meaning signal statistics do not change on being stretched, shrinked over time.

Pointwise Holder exponent (PHE): Consider $\chi \in (0,1)$ & $y_0 \in \mathrm{K} \subset \mathrm{R}$. Then, function $h : \mathrm{K} \rightarrow \mathrm{R}$ lying in$C^{\chi}_{y_0}$ forall y in a neighborhood of y_0,

$$|h(y) - h(y_0)| \leq k|y - y_0|^{\chi}$$

having k as constant. Then, PHE(h) for y_0 represented through $\chi(y_0)$ is the sup.(χ) as per the definition above. Thus, this characterization is used by fractal analysis as it directly interprets the mathematics into applications.

5.3.0.1 Spectral Analysis

As it is known, time series are stationary and non-stationary.

Theorem 5.2 *For stationary time series analysis, commonly known Fourier transform, the spectral analysis leading to the simulation of the power spectrum, $\varsigma^n f_0$ of the time successions as a function of the frequency, f_i so that self-affined scaling fluctuations can be detected.*

Remark 5.2 For long-term correlated data associated via correlation exponent, ϖ is expressed as

$$\mathrm{P_s(f)} \sim f^{-\eta} \text{ where } \eta = 1 - \varpi$$

Clearly, η is the spectral exponent & ϖ is the correlation exponent to be computed through fitting the power-law observed via double logarithmic plot capturing power spectrum$P_s(f)$.

Logarithmic-Binning procedure is the core of $P_s(f)$ computation that makes it better and provides more precise results than the classical autocorrelation. It involves averaging the $log\, P_s(f)$ simulated as in the subsequently plus logarithmically wide-bands from $\varsigma^n f_0$to $\varsigma^{n+1} f_0, f_0$ denoting minimum frequency, $\varsigma > 1$- an arbitrary constant factor; n stands for counting these bins. The spectral analysis holds necessarily for the stationarity of the data considered.

5.4 Hurst Rescaled R/S Analysis

Technically known as Rescaled-range analysis (R/S analysis) proposed by H.E. Hurst meant to capture the long-term persistent behaviourism of time-series. It involves tracking ranges through max. as well as min. values alongwith computations of std. devs. considered denoted as:

$$
\begin{aligned}
&R_\phi(p) = \max_{i=1}^{p} X_\phi(i) - \min_{i=1}^{p} X_\phi(i),\\
&S_\phi(p) = \sqrt{\tfrac{1}{p}\textstyle\sum_{i=1}^{p} X_\phi^2(i)}\\
&p(k) = Ck^{-\alpha} \quad \text{where } C - \text{constant;}\\
&p(k) - \text{autocorrelation function with lag k}\\
&\mathrm{H} = 1-\tfrac{\alpha}{2}
\end{aligned}
$$

Hurst Exponent is basically, the slope of the regression-fitline of *'log-log curve'* of time-series in respect to time. It is defined through the rule of decay of power-law as:

$$p\,(k) = Ck^{-\alpha} \text{ where } \mathrm{C} - \text{const.; } \mathrm{p}\,(k) - \text{autocorrelation function having}'k'lag$$

It can be also calculated through: $H= 1-\frac{\alpha}{2}$. As and when $0 < \varpi < 1$, then $0.5<H_e <1$. In general, this may not be found true for all types of multifractals.

5.5 Discrete Waveform Signal Analysis (DWS)

The wavelet coeffs, $W_\varphi\,(\kappa, \mathrm{p})$ affect two features time-position, κas well as scaling, p. Thus, DWS transformation essential for data-signals, d_s is computed via following calculation of the time series, t_i, $i=1,\ldots,n$.

$$W_\varphi\,(\kappa, \mathrm{p}) = \frac{1}{p}\sum_{i=1}^{K} d_s(i)\varphi[(t-\kappa)/p].$$

5.6 Results and Discussions

For the stationarity of the data, multi-fractal and its associated components such as nonlinear pumping, L2 - norm (Least square) denoising, Bayesian form of denoising, power spectrum formulation through limsup dimensional analytics applied for the analysis. Waveform signal analysis applied to overcome the inbuilt non-stationarity in the datasets. This study is required as the outliers or inaccuracies may keep away the actual picture of the situation. Therefore, it became important to study this pandemic as it had been affecting people from all walks of life ever since its spread in case of the United States. Figure 5.2(a) and

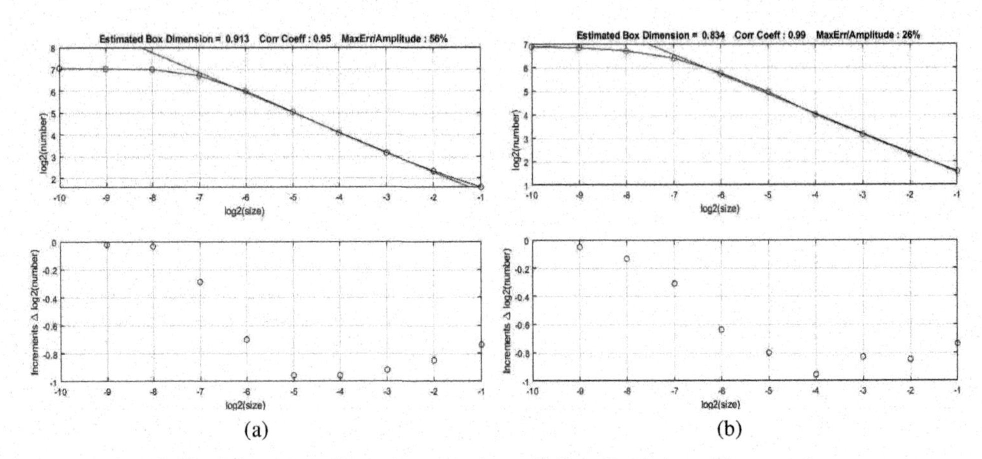

(a) (b)

Fig. 5.2: (a) Box dimension of Actives, (b) Box dimension of Recovereds.

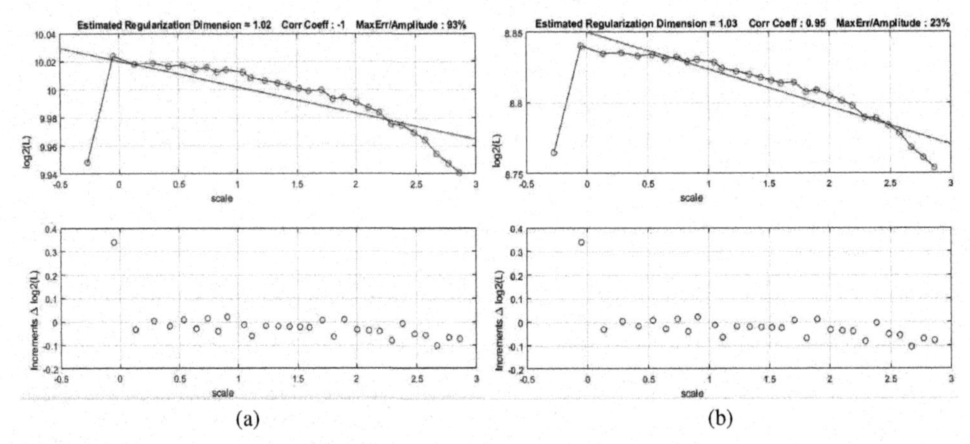

(a) (b)

Fig. 5.3: Regularization dimension of (a) Actives, (b) Recovereds.

5.2(b) shows the box dimension with its bounds and measure for active and recovered ones in the United States. Figure 5.3(a) and 5.3(b) depicts the regularization dimension with the bounds and numeric value. Figure 5.4(a) and 5.4(b) graphs the theoretical and empirical R-S algorithmic analysis for the Hurst of both the data sets. Figure 5.5(a) and 5.5(b) shows the local holder exponent and its measured numeric value for both cases. Figure 5.6(a) and 5.6(b) capture the Pointwise Holder Exponent and its value for both cases. Figure 5.7(a) and 5.7(b) depicts the discrete waveform signal analysis considering the cases as discrete time series.

Figure 5.8(a) and 5.8(b) encapsulate the Multi-fractal Bayesian denoising of both cases taken as signals for denoising. Figure 5.9(a) and 5.9(b) shows the multi-fractal L2-norm procedure denoising to trace the differences that may result. Figure 5.10(a) and 5.10(b) spectrum display through *limsupremum* of dimensions method that graphs the supremum reflecting the power spectrum of both the time data. Figure 5.11(a) and 5.11(b) shows multi-fractal nonlinear pumping of active and recovered. Figure 5.12(a) and 5.12(b) clearly shows the wavelet decomposition into coefficients of approx., and details through Daubechies (Db10) at four levels. Figure 5.13(a) and 5.13(b) depict wavelet denoising to overcome non-stationarities in the time

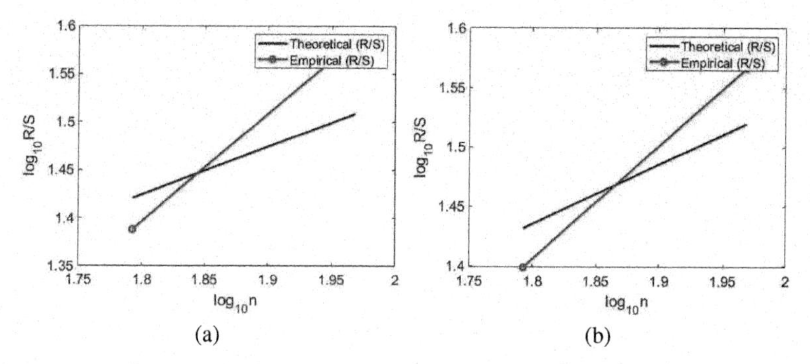

Fig. 5.4: R/S Analysis for (a) Active cases, (b) Recovered cases.

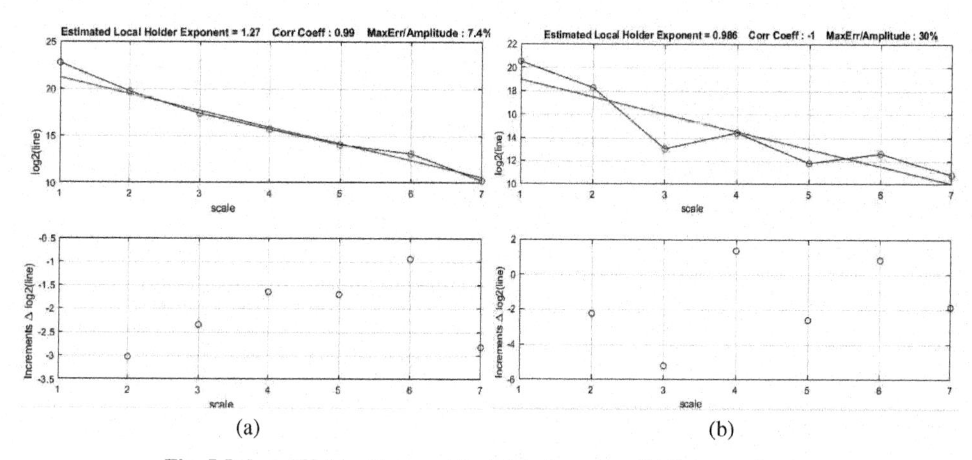

Fig. 5.5: Local Holder Exponent for (a) Active cases, (b) Recovered cases.

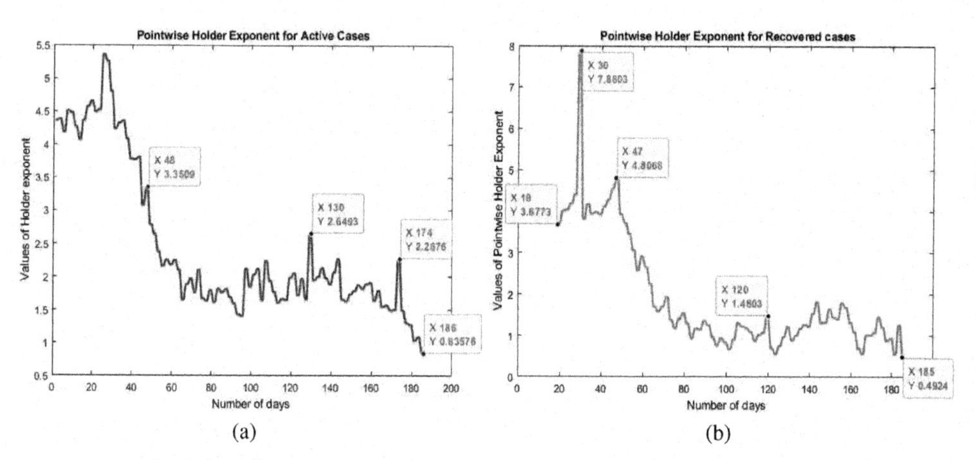

Fig. 5.6: Pointwise Holder Exponent for (a) Active cases, (b) Recovered cases.

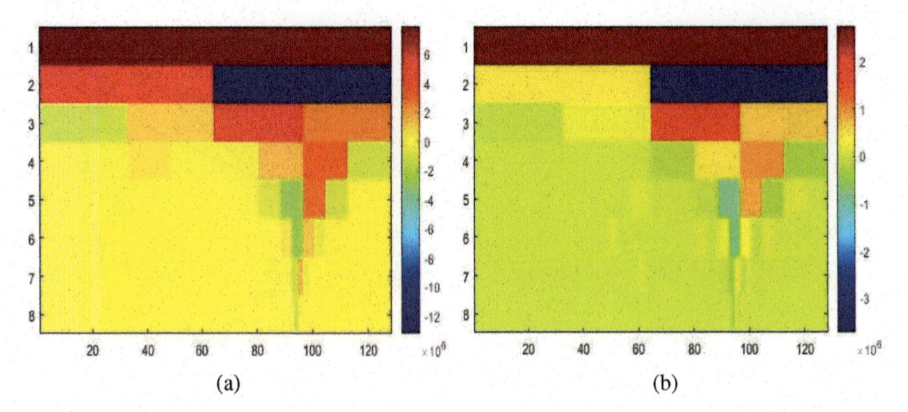

Fig. 5.7: Discrete Waveform Signal for (a) Active cases, (b) Recovered cases.

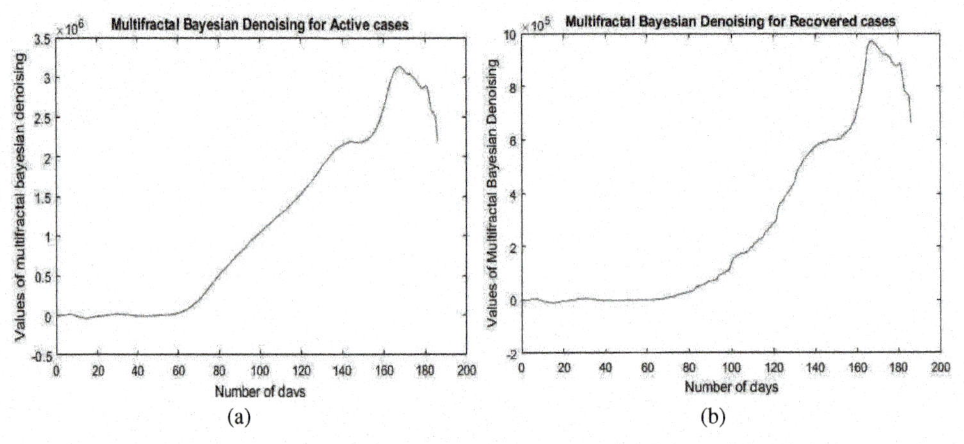

Fig. 5.8: Multi-fractal Bayesian Denoising for (a) Actives, (b) Recovered.

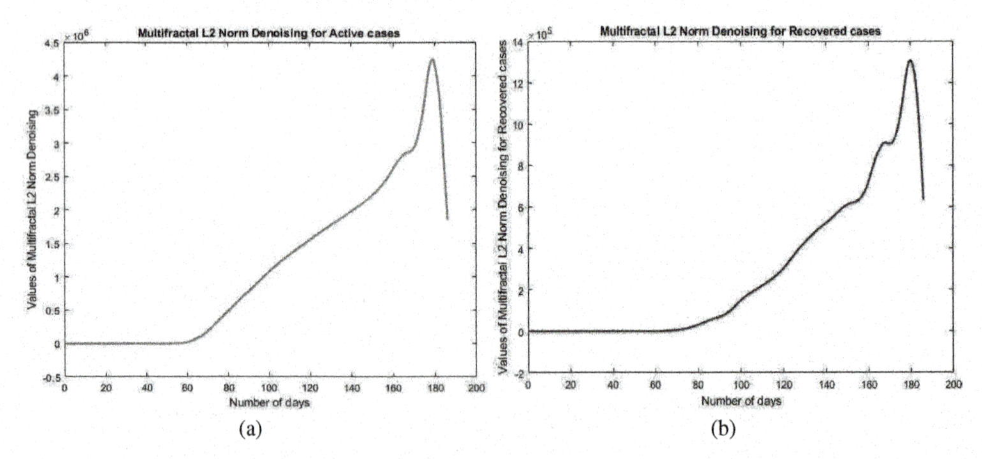

Fig. 5.9: Multi-fractal L2 Norm Denoising for (a) Actives, (b) Recovereds.

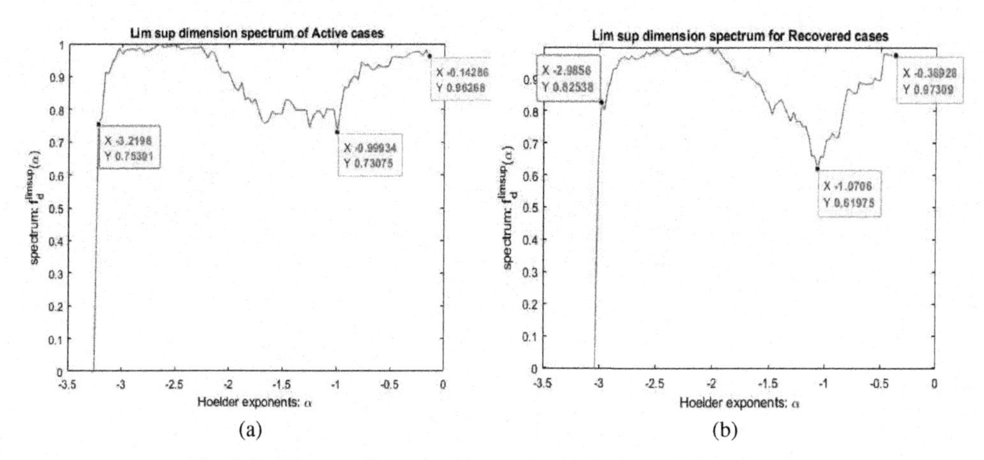

(a) (b)

Fig. 5.10: Lim sup dimension Spectra for (a) Actives, (b) Recovereds.

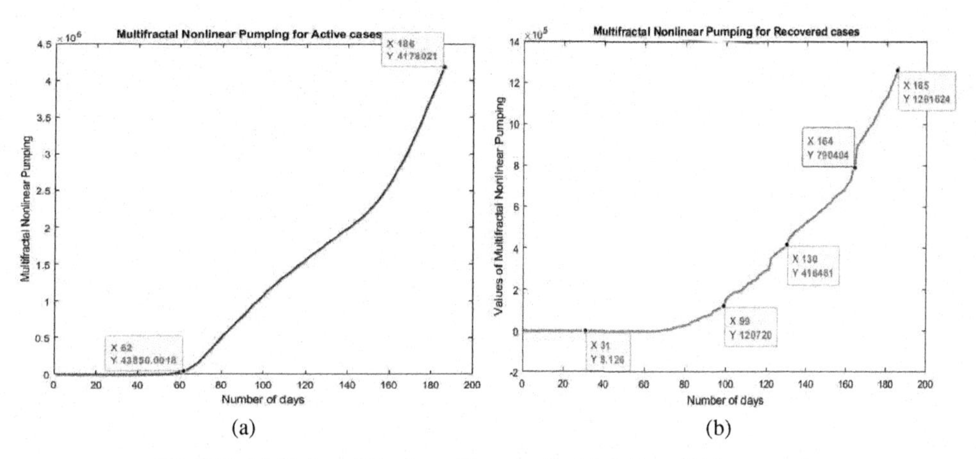

(a) (b)

Fig. 5.11: Multi-fractal Nonlinear Pumping for (a) Actives, (b) Recovereds.

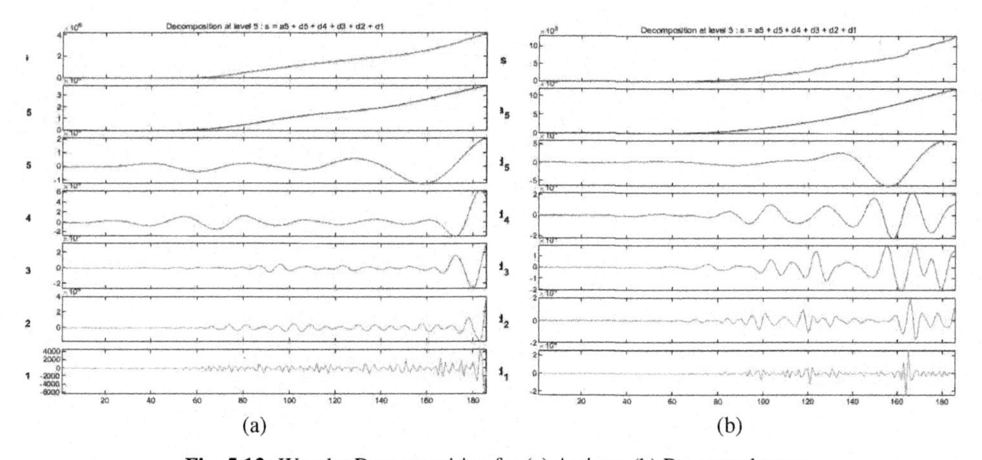

(a) (b)

Fig. 5.12: Wavelet Decomposition for (a) Actives, (b) Recovered cases.

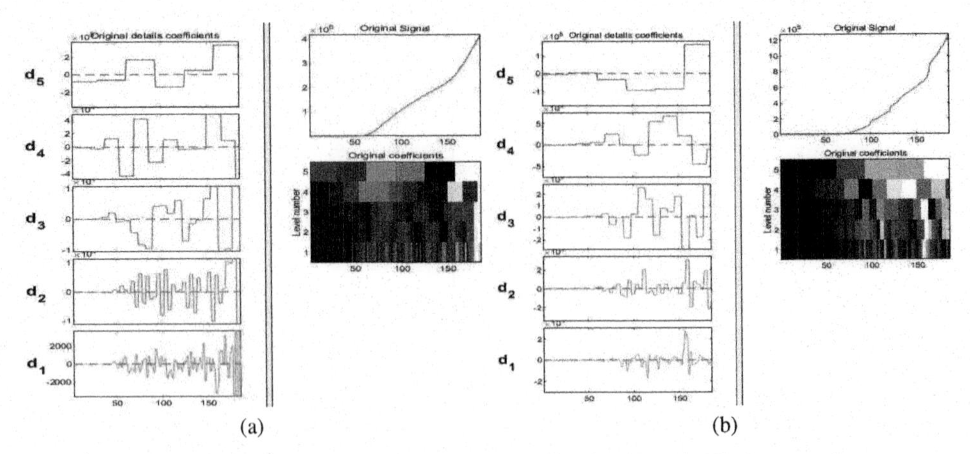

Fig. 5.13: (a) Wavelet Denoising Active cases, (b) Wavelet Denoising for Recovered cases.

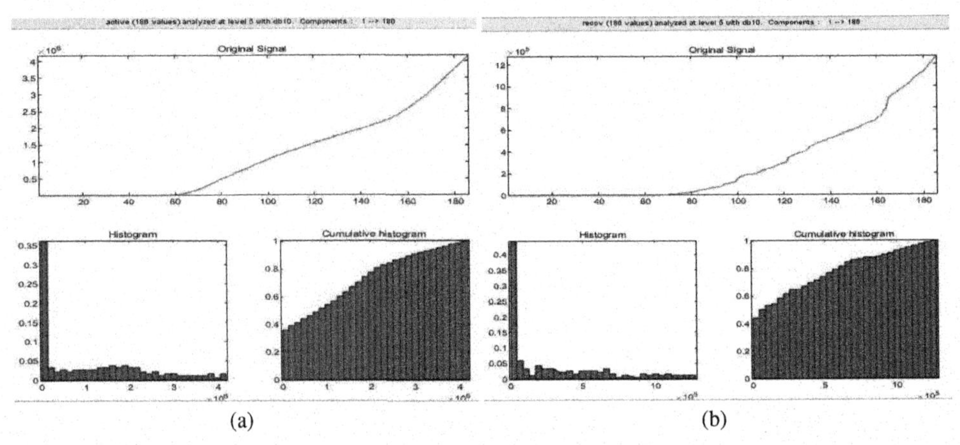

Fig. 5.14: (a) Wave-form signal analysis for Active cases, (b) Waveform signal analysis for Recovered cases.

successions data. Figure 5.14(a) and 5.14(b) conclude the waveform signal analysis of both the cases that eliminate the noises through filters and non-stationarities removed.

For Active and recovered cases, R/S-AL employs two divisors (62,...,93) for a sample of 186 values as considered for the computation of Hurst in Table 5.2. It holds the calculated Hurst exponent values, having corrected and computed theoretical and empirical values. Table 5.3 shows the confidence bounds and levels of R/S trajectories. Also, the algorithm utilizes (min(divisor)>50) two-sided for the empirical confidence intervals, as can be observed in Table 5.3. Table 5.4 tabulates the Holder exponent values recorded after the number of days passed and sudden changes observed to study the ongoing scenario of the pandemic. Table 5.5 represents various statistical characteristics for the two data types belonging to the United States. Table 5.6 and Table 5.7 give the valuation of Waveform signals via Daubechies 10 at level 4 for Active cases and recovered cases, respectively. It can be observed statistical properties vary for each synthesized signal recorded plus the coefficients of approximation and decomposition at four levels of Daubechies wavelet-type.

Table 5.2: Calculation of Hurst Exponent for both data types.

Calculation of Hurst	Active cases	Recovered cases
Corrected theoretical Hurst exponent	0.5	0.5
Corrected empirical Hurst exponent	1.119	0.952
Theoretical Hurst exponent	0.5566	0.5566
Empirical Hurst exponent	1.162	0.9886

Table 5.3: Calculation of two-sided empirical confidence intervals for both cases.

Confidence intervals bounds for both the data types for empirical confidence measures		
Lower bound	Higher bound	Confidence Level
0.1698	0.7949	0.9000
0.1110	0.8596	0.9500
0.0111	0.9963	0.9900

Table 5.4: Holder Exponent values for both cases.

Active Cases		Recovered Cases	
Days	Holder Exponent values	Days	Holder Exponent values
19	4.6508	19	3.6773
25	5.3564	30	7.8803
31	4.2422	31	3.8203
48	3.3509	47	4.8068
60	2.1803	60	2.9173
65	1.6541	101	0.68362
100	1.8498	120	1.4803
130	2.6493	123	0.55983
155	1.8224	155	1.8015
172	1.5025	165	0.57584
174	2.2676	173	0.4924
186	0.83576	185	1.4574

Table 5.5: Various statistical characteristics for the two data types belonging to the United States.

Data Types	Theoretical Hurst* (H_e)	R/S value	Entropy	Fractal Dimension (F_d=2-H_e)	Predictability Index (P_i=2| F_d - 1.5|)
Active cases	0.5566	37.3491	7.0815	1.4434	0.1132
Recovered cases	0.5566	35.7239	6.5559	1.4434	0.1132

Table 5.6: Evaluation of Waveform signals via Daubechies 10 at level 4 for Active cases.

	Active Cases data synthesized and decomposed as waveform signal at Db10 for four-level								
Statistical Properties	Synthesized signal	cA1	cA2	cA3	cA4	cD1	cD2	cD3	cD4
Mean	1.16×10^6	1.185×10^6	8.611×10^5	4.933×10^4	25.48	-27.83	242.2	-473.7	802.9
Median	8.898×10^5	5.682×10^5	372.7	25.39	24.91	0.2869	0.6592	0.699	-8.262
Maximum	4.178×10^6	4.333×10^6	3.857×10^6	8.744×10^5	44.41	3132	7709	6064	1.251×10^4
Minimum	1	1.316	-83.73	-1024	10.92	-3315	-1.021×10^4	-9586	-2383
Range	4.17×10^6	4.333×10^6	3.857×10^6	8.755×10^5	33.49	6447	1.792×10^4	1.565×10^4	1.489×10^4
Standard Deviation	1.202×10^6	1.344×10^6	1.285×10^6	1.848×10^5	12.95	937.6	3904	3667	3749
Median Absolute Deviation	1.027×10^6	5.682×10^5	456.4	18.41	11.55	405.2	693.2	292	16.68
Mean Absolute Deviation	8.897×10^5	1.185×10^6	1.086×10^6	8.791×10^4	12.13	610.3	2551	2330	1951
L1-norm	2.158×10^8	1.102×10^8	4.047×10^7	1.188×10^6	305.7	5.609×10^4	1.165×10^5	5.015×10^4	1.545×10^4
L2-norm	2.276×10^7	1.723×10^7	1.053×10^7	9.184×10^5	98.15	8997	2.653×10^4	1.774×10^4	1.274×10^4
Max norm	4.178×10^6	4.333×10^6	3.857×10^6	8.744×10^5	44.41	3315	1.021×10^4	9586	1.251×10^4

Table 5.7: Evaluation of Waveform signals via Daubechies 10 at level 4 for Recovered cases.

	Recovered Cases data synthesized and decomposed as waveform signal at Db10 for four levels								
Statistical Properties	Synthesized signal	cA1	cA2	cA3	cA4	cD1	cD2	cD3	cD4
Mean	2.889×10^5	2.695×10^5	1.525×10^5	1544	2.887×10^5	377.7	826.6	300.6	329
Median	8.964×10^4	3.049×10^4	10.96	0.007045	9.483×10^4	0.03436	-6.43×10^{-6}	0.0129	0.1026
Maximum	1.279×10^6	1.353×10^6	1.009×10^6	3.142×10^4	1.24×10^6	2.758×10^4	3.095×10^4	2.57×10^4	3171
Minimum	-4.491×10^{-7}	-0.1427	-3096	-2959	-1243	-1.648×10^4	-8580	-1.821×10^4	-0.09958
Range	1.279×10^6	1.353×10^6	1.009×10^6	3.438×10^4	1.24×10^6	4.406×10^4	3.953×10^4	4.391×10^4	3172
Standard Deviation	3.66×10^5	3.756×10^5	2.798×10^5	6588	3.654×10^5	5093	6369	8190	917.8
Median Absolute Deviation	8.964×10^4	3.049×10^4	12.07	0.1727	9.513×10^4	367.4	750.8	5.094	0.1781
Mean Absolute Deviation	3.052×10^5	3.113×10^5	2.103×10^5	2991	3.048×10^5	2484	3485	3851	537
L1-norm	5.373×10^7	2.507×10^7	7.167×10^6	4.399×10^4	5.374×10^7	2.168×10^5	1.462×10^5	8.905×10^4	3948
L2-norm	6.348×10^6	4.443×10^6	2.167×10^6	3.249×10^4	6.341×10^6	4.899×10^4	4.357×10^4	3.931×10^4	3250
Max norm	1.279×10^6	1.353×10^6	1.009×10^6	3.142×10^4	1.24×10^6	2.758×10^4	3.095×10^4	2.57×10^4	3171

5.7 Conclusion

It is the need of the hour to model the factors of COVID-19 transmission to minimize its spread and the extent to which it can be harmful. Thus, it is necessary to study the ongoing scenario of the pandemic. Also, this study concludes that in both the number of active and recovered people have seen a gradual dip, which indicates contrary to the perception of the pandemic, causing havoc in one of the most developed countries. Multifractal analysis is concerned with the study of the regularity structure of processes, both from a local and global point of view that included various methods such as nonlinear pumping, L2- norm denoising, Bayesian form of denoising, power spectrum formulation through limsup dimensional analytics. Box dimesion and regularization dimensions also played an important part. It is focusing on the concern of measuring the pointwise-regularity through Hölder exponents. In addition, Hurst exponent through R/S also clearly indicates the decay in the active cases and variations in recovered citizens. Secondly, providing a global description of the calculated regularity. This was done geometrically through Hausdorff dimension. The present investigation indicates the control in the numbers of affected and transmissions of the viral genome. Hence, the social distancing and subsequent preventive measures in the infected parts of different cities and countries might have been started to show substantial improvement in real and as well as the analytical front. No antiviral-genomic treatment for this pandemic has been proven to be effective to date. Herd immunity attains a level of 99%. In the long-range, it is observed that the pandemic will end between February 2021 to March 2021. The outcomes of this study can provide efficient learning and understanding of the pathogenesis of COVID-19. Also, it may aid in employing similar control strategies and various other measures taken by authorities and citizens against this pandemic.

Acknowledgment

Authors thank G.G.S.I.P. University for research facilities. No conflict of interest.

References

1. Al-Bari, M.A. 2015. Chloroquine analogues in drug discovery: new directions of uses, mechanisms of actions and toxic manifestations from malaria to multifarious diseases. Journal of Antimicrobial Chemotherapy, 70: 1608–1621.
2. Bhardwaj, R. and A. Bangia. 2016. Complexity dynamics of meditating body. Indian Journal of Industrial and Applied Mathematics, 7: 106–116.
3. Bhardwaj, R. and A. Bangia. 2018. Statistical time series analysis of dynamics of HIV. JNANABHA, Special Issue, 48: 22–27.
4. Bhardwaj, R. and A. Bangia. 2019. Neuro-fuzzy analysis of demonetization on NSE. pp. 853–861. *In*: Bansal, J.C., K.N. Das, A. Nagar, K. Deep and A.K. Ojha (eds.). AISC Springer Proceedings: Soft Computing for Problem Solving (SocPros-2017), Springer Singapore.
5. Bhardwaj, R. and A. Bangia. 2019. Hybrid Fuzzified-PID controller for non-linear control surfaces for DC motor to improve the efficiency of electric battery driven vehicles. International Journal of Recent Technology and Engineering™ (IJRTE), 8: 2561–2568.
6. Bhardwaj, R. and A. Bangia. 2019. Dynamic indicator for the prediction of atmospheric pollutants. Asian Journal of Water, Environment and Pollution, 16: 39–50.

7. Bhardwaj, R. and A. Bangia. 2019. Stock market trend analysis during demonetization using soft-computing techniques. 2018 International Conference on Computing, Power and Communication Technologies (GUCON-2018). IEEE Xplore, 696–701.
8. Bhardwaj, R. and A. Bangia. 2020. Dynamical forensic inference for Malware in IoT-based wireless transmissions. pp. 51–79. *In*: Sharma, K., M. Makino, G. Shrivastava and B. Agarwal (eds.). Forensic Investigations and Risk Management in Mobile and Wireless Communications.
9. Bhardwaj, R. and A. Bangia. 2020. Assessment of Stock prices variation using Intelligent Machine Learning Techniques for the prediction of BSE. Advances in Intelligent Systems and Computing (AISC) Volume 979. Numerical Optimization in Engineering and Sciences, Eds: Kacprzyk, J., Debashis Dutta and B. Mahanty, 107–123.
10. Bangia, A., R. Bhardwaj and K.V. Jayakumar. 2020. River water quality estimation through Artificial Intelligence conjuncted with Wavelet Decomposition. Advances in Intelligent Systems and Computing (AISC) Volume 979. Numerical Optimization in Engineering and Sciences, Eds: Kacprzyk, J., Debashis Dutta and B. Mahanty, 159–166.
11. Bhardwaj, R. and A. Bangia. 2020. Data driven estimation of novel COVID-19 transmission risks through hybrid soft-computing techniques. Chaos, Soliton and Fractals, 140: 110152.
12. Bonavia, A., B.D. Zelus, D.E. Wentworth, P.J. Talbot and K.V. Holmes. 2003. Identification of a receptor-binding domain of the spike glycoprotein of human coronavirus HCoV-229E. Journal of Virology, 77: 2530–2538.
13. Box, G.E.P. and D.R. Cox. 1964. An analysis of transformations. Journal of the Royal Statistical Society, Series B, 26: 211–252.
14. Chen, T.-M., J. Rui, Q.-P. Wang, Z.-Y. Zhao, J.-A. Cui and L. Yin. 2020. A mathematical model for simulating the phase-based transmissibility of a novel coronavirus. Infectious Diseases of Poverty, 9: 1–8.
15. Chen, S., D. Yang, R. Liu, J. Zhao, K. Yang and T. Chen. 2019. Estimating the transmissibility of hand, foot, and mouth disease by a dynamic model. Public Health, 174: 42-–48.
16. Colson, P., J.M. Rolain and D. Raoult. 2020. Chloroquine for the 2019 novel coronavirus SARS-CoV-2. International Journal of Antimicrobial Agents, 55: 105923.
17. Cui, J.-A., S. Zhao, S. Guo, Y. Bai, X. Wang and T. Chen. 2020. Global dynamics of an epidemiological model with acute and chronic HCV infections. Applied Math Letters, 103: 106–203.
18. Hamre, D. and J.J. Procknow. 1966. A new virus isolated from the human respiratory tract. Proc. Soc. Exp. Biol. Med., 121: 190–193.
19. Holmes, K.V. 2001. Coronaviruses. pp. 1187–1203. *In* Knipe, D.M. and P.M. Howley (ed.). Fields Virology, volume 1, 4th ed. Lippincott-Raven Publishers, New York.
20. Jubelt, B. and J.R. Berger. 2001. Does viral disease underlie ALS? Lessons from the AIDS pandemic. Neurology, 57: 945–946.
21. McIntosh, K., R.K. Chao, H.E. Krause, R. Wasil, H.E. Mocega and M.A. Mufson. 1974. Coronavirus infection in acute lower respiratory tract disease of infants. Journal of Infectious Diseases, 130: 502–507.
22. Frédéric Pene, Annabelle Merlat, Astrid Vabret, Flore Rozenberg, Agnès Buzyn, François Dreyfus, Alain Cariou, François Freymuth and Pierre Lebon. 2003. Coronavirus 229E-related pneumonia in immuno-compromised patients. Clinical Infectious Diseases, 37: 929–932.
23. Rosenblum, M.A. 1980. Corona theorem for countably many functions. Integral Equations Operator Theory, 3: 125–137.
24. Fuhrmann, P.A. 1968. On the corona theorem and its application to spectral problems in Hilbert space. Transactions of the American Mathematical Society, 132: 55–66.

25. World Health Organization (WHO). 2020. Novel Coronavirus – Japan (ex-China), World Health Organization, cited January 20, 2020.
Available: https://www.who.int/csr/don/17-january-2020-novel-coronavirus-japan-ex-china/en/.
26. World Health Organization (WHO). 2013. Middle East Respiratory Syndrome Coronavirus (MERS-CoV) - update:2 DECEMBER 2013.
Available: http://www.who.int/csr/don/2013_12_02/en/.
27. Chung-Yi Wu, Jia-Tsrong Jan, Shiou-Hwa Ma, Chih-Jung Kuo, Hsueh-Fen Juan, Yih-Shyun E. Cheng Hsien-Hua Hsu, Hsuan-Cheng Huang, Douglass Wu, Ashraf Brik, Fu-Sen Liang, Rai-Shung Liu, Jim-Min Fang, Shui-Tein Chen, Po-Huang Liang and Chi-Huey Wong. 2004. Small molecules targeting severe acute respiratory syndrome human coronavirus. Proceedings of National Academy of Sciences, 101: 10012–10017.
28. World Health Organization (WHO). 2020. Coronavirus. World Health Organization, cited January 19, 2020.
Available: https://www.who.int/health-topics/coronavirus.
29. Peng Zhou, Xing-Lou Yang, Xian-Guang Wang, Ben Hu, Lei Zhang, Wei Zhang, Hao-Rui Si, Yan Zhu, Bei Li, Chao-Lin Huang, Hui-Dong Chen, Jing Chen, Yun Luo, Hua Guo, Ren-Di Jiang, Mei-Qin Liu, Ying Chen, Xu-Rui Shen, Xi Wang, Xiao-Shuang Zheng, Kai Zhao, Quan-Jiao Chen, Fei Deng, Lin-Lin Liu, Bing Yan, Fa-Xian Zhan, Yan-Yi Wang, Geng-Fu Xiao and Zheng-Li Shi. 2020. A pneumonia outbreak associated with a new coronavirus of probable bat origin. Nature, 579: 270–273.
30. Nan Zhou, Ting Pan, Junsong Zhang, Qianwen Li, Xue Zhang, Chuan Bai, Feng Huang, Tao Peng, Jianhua Zhang, Chao Liu, Liang Tao and Hui Zhang. 2016. Glycopeptide antibiotics potently inhibit cathepsin L in the late endosome/lysosome and block the entry of Ebola virus, Middle East Respiratory Syndrome Coronavirus (MERS-CoV), and Severe Acute Respiratory Syndrome Coronavirus (SARS-CoV). Journal of Biological Chemistry, 291: 9218–9232.
31. World Health Organization (WHO). 2020. Novel coronavirus - China. Jan 12, 2020.
Available: http://www.who.int/csr/don/12-january-2020-novel-coronavirus-china/en/.

Chapter 6

Multifractal Detrended Fluctuation Analysis on COVID-19 Dynamics

M. Dhanzeem Ahmed,[1] *D. Easwaramoorthy,*[1,*] *Bilel Selmi*[2] and *Sara Darabi*[3]

6.1 Introduction

A "Fractal" is a rough or fragmented geometric shape that can be split into parts, and each of those is a reduced-size copy of the whole called self-similarity. Mathematically Mandelbrot defined a set with a Hausdorff dimension strictly greater than its topological dimension as Fractal [1]–[3].

The multifractal has a global reputation as one factor that describes non-trivial properties of observable data. Numerous researchers have investigated aspects of complex systems using fractals and multifractals. The research studies using the chaos theory have shown that biomedical signals have the property of fractality or self-similarity on various scales. The monofractality and multifractality are the two kinds of fractal theory. In comparison to monofractals, multifractals are inherently more complicated, non-homogeneous, with extremely irregular dynamics and high-frequency fluctuations [4]–[7].

With the development of technology, the multifractal theory can obtain the different fluctuation information of the market on different time scales and provide more analysis for the financial market. The multifractal theory is mostly utilized to analyze the return rates and the stock price indices [8]. In nature, the time series and its fractal representations are the most common ways to record observable quantities and the detailed investigations have been done on properties [2]. There is plenty of evidence to support this feature of empirical data coming from such a wide range of fields like geophysics [9], astrophysics [10], physiology [11], complex networks research [12] and econophysics [13], which are essential elements of systems that are considered to be complicated. Thus, multifractal concepts are important and the multifractal measures are applied in many medical and biological problems to estimate the complexity of the signals or images [14]–[24].

[1] Department of Mathematics, School of Advanced Sciences, Vellore Institute of Technology, Vellore, Tamil Nadu, India.
Email: dhanzeemahmed@gmail.com

[2] Department of Mathematics, Faculty of Sciences of Monastir, University of Monastir, Monastir 5000, Tunisia.
Email: bilel.selmi@fsm.rnu.tn;bilel.selmi@isetgb.rnu.tn

[3] Department of Mechanical Engineering, Science and Research Branch, Islamic Azad University, Tehran, Iran.
Email: sarah_darabi@ymail.com

* Corresponding author: easandk@gmail.com

A common tool to unveil the nature of the scaling and fractionality of a process, natural or computer-generated, is Multifractal Detrended Fluctuation Analysis (MFDFA) [6]. It was initially developed by Peng et al. [25] as a basic Detrended Fluctuation Analysis (DFA), and later extended to study multifractal processes. For different time scales, the multifractal detrended fluctuation analysis (MFDFA) method can determine the multifractal scale of time series and distinguish the generalized probability density function and the multifractality of long-range correlation. MFDFA is a numerical algorithm designed to determine the self-similarity of a stochastic process. Putting it simply, the algorithm examines the relationship between the diffusion of the process and its propagation in time or space.

In the medical field, COVID-19 is one of the major harmful diseases. The effects of COVID-19 have severely impacted the daily lives of the majority of people. The symptoms of COVID-19 are dry cough, sore throat, fever, headache, and shortness of breath. It is spread rapidly across the globe. The COVID-19 pandemic has caused the financial and health difficulties for people all over the world [26]. Numerous researches have been done on COVID-19 by fractal and multifractal perspective [27]–[30].

The MFDFA (Multifractal Detrended Fluctuation Analysis) approach has the advantages of easy implementation, high precision, and low computational time. It has been widely used to investigate the fractal behavior of time series [31]–[34]. The multifractal spectrum offers pertinent information regarding the proportion of the time series under the multifractality qualities. The degree of multifractality is defined and determined by the width of multifractal spectrum. A wider spectrum corresponds to a stronger multifractal system. We analyze the daily infected cases, death cases, and vaccinated cases of COVID-19 for the highly impacted countries like United States of America (USA), France, Germany, Brazil, India, and Tunisia by using Multifractal Detrended Fluctuation Analysis (MFDFA).

6.2 Mathematical Methods

6.2.1 Multifractal Detrended Fluctuation Analysis

Multifractal detrended fluctuation analysis (MFDFA), which examines the multifractal characteristics of time series using various time scales, is a common technique for studying multifractality in time series. With increasing segments of a time series, a multifractal detrended fluctuation study analyzes the variances of the fluctuations of a particular process. There are five steps in the generalized MFDFA method.

Step 1

Establish the Profile

$$Y(i) = \sum_{k=1}^{i} x_k - < x >, \quad i = 1, 2, \ldots, N. \tag{6.1}$$

where x_k is the data of length N and $< x >$ is the mean.

Step 2

The profile $Y(i)$ divided into

$$N_s = int(N/s)$$

where N_s is non overlapping segments of equal length s, s is scale.

Step 3

Use a least-squares fit of the series to calculate the local trend for each segment. After that, determine the variance.

$$F^2(v,s) = \frac{1}{s}\sum_{i=1}^{s}\{y[(v-1)s+i] - y_v(i)\}^2 \tag{6.2}$$

where $y_v(i)$ is fitting polynomial in segment v; $v = 1, \ldots, N_s$.

Step 4

To obtain the qth order fluctuation function, averaging over all segments is used.

$$F_q(s) = \left\{\frac{1}{N_s}\sum_{v=1}^{N_s}[F^2(v,s)]^{q/2}\right\}^{1/q} \tag{6.3}$$

where $F_q(s)$ depends on scale s for different values of q. $F_q(s)$ will increase with increasing s.

Step 5

Examine log-log plots to determine the scaling properties of the fluctuation functions. $F_q(s)$ versus s for each value of q. If there is a long-range power-law correlation between the series x_i, $F_q(s)$ increases as a power law for high values of s.

$$F_q(s) \sim s^{h(q)}. \tag{6.4}$$

For very high scales, $s > N/4$, $F_q(s)$ becomes statistically unreliable because the length of segments N_s because the Eq. (6.3) average became very small. Therefore, we often do not include scales $s > N/4$ in the fitting process to determine $h(q)$. Generally, the exponent may depend on $h(q)$. For stationary time series, the exponent $h(2)$ is identical to the Hurst exponent. The exponents $h(q)$ are called the generalized Hurst exponents.

For monofractal time series, which are characterized by a single exponent over all scales, $h(q)$ is independent of q, whereas for a multifractal time series, $h(q)$ varies with q. This dependence is considered to be a characteristic property of multifractal processes [6].

When the exponent $h(q)$ depends on q, the multifractal scaling exponent is given by

$$\tau(q) = qh(q) - 1. \tag{6.5}$$

By Eq. (6.4) $h(q)$ is defined and it is related to multifractal scaling exponent $\tau(q)$.

An alternative measure to analyze the multifractal characteristics of a series is to calculate the singularity spectrum, also called multifractal spectrum $f(\alpha)$. The multifractal spectrum may be related to $\tau(q)$ through the Legendre transform.

$$\alpha = \tau'(q) \quad \textit{and} \quad f(\alpha) = q\alpha - \tau(q) \tag{6.6}$$

where $\tau'(q)$ stands for the derivative of $\tau(q)$ with respect to q.

By Eq. (6.5), we can directly relate α and $f(\alpha)$ to $h(q)$.

$$\alpha = h(q) + qh'(q) \quad \textit{and} \quad f(\alpha) = q[\alpha - h(q)] + 1 \tag{6.7}$$

where $h'(q)$ represents the derivative of $h(q)$ with respect to q and α is singularity strength and $f(\alpha)$ is dimension of the subset of series characterized by α.

6.2.2 Strength of Multifractality

According to the generalized multifractal model, the difference between the maximum and minimum values of α can be used to measure the strength of multifractality in a time-series. The larger multifractal spectrum represents how much larger the multifractality of the time series will be.

$$\Delta\alpha = \alpha_{max} - \alpha_{min} \tag{6.8}$$

Algorithm 1 Multifractal Detrended Fluctuation Analysis

Step 1 Integrate the time series to generate a profile.
Step 2 Divide the time series into nonoverlapping segments.
Step 3 Calculate a local trend for each segment.
Step 4 Define a qth-order fluctuation function.
Step 5 Calculate the multifractal spectrum.
Step 6 Calculating the multifractality measure by the width of its spectrum.

6.3 Data Description

The daily data of COVID-19 from 01 January 2022 to 30 June 2022 from USA, France, Germany, Brazil, India and Tunisia are taken from Our World in Data [35] and utilized in the research study.

Table 6.1: Daily Infected Cases, Death Cases, and Vaccinated Cases.

Countries	Infected Cases	Death Cases	Vaccinated Cases
World	258040776	879320	2867036068
USA	32829824	191552	77263587
France	21156205	25797	21852440
Germany	21143594	29277	28983194
Brazil	10066179	52165	110713331
India	8607655	43653	516016107
Tunisia	316229	3126	682211

6.4 Results and Discussion

The simulations are carried out in MATLAB software by using the multifractal detrended fluctuation analysis algorithm to analyze the highest multifractality for COVID-19 infected cases, death cases, and vaccinated cases.

6.4.1 Daily Infected Cases of COVID-19

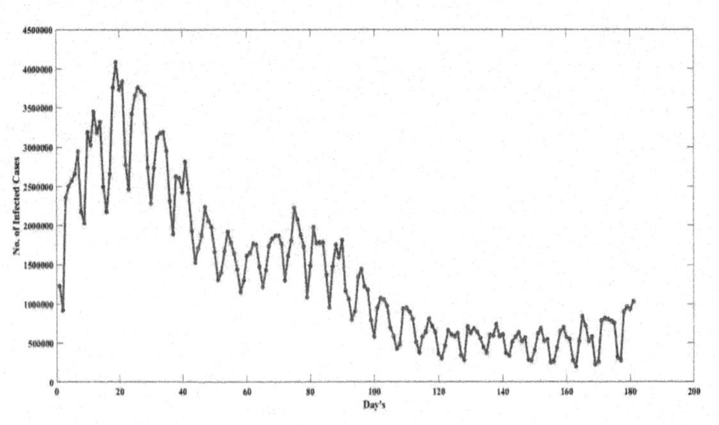

Fig. 6.1: Daily Infected Cases of World.

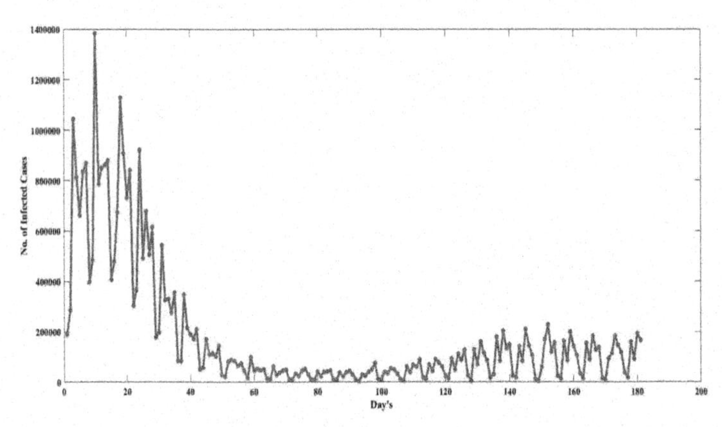

Fig. 6.2: Daily Infected Cases of USA.

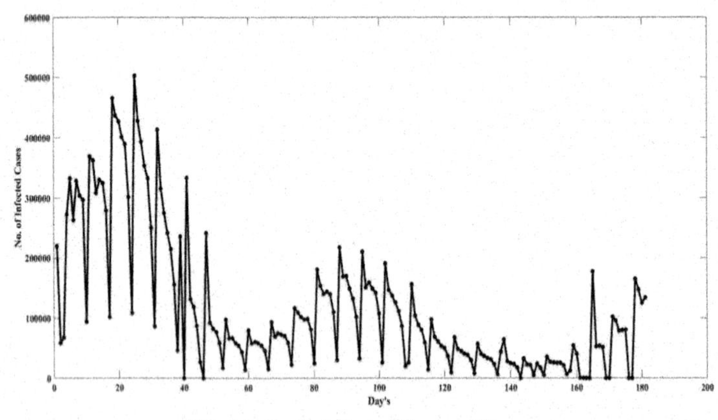

Fig. 6.3: Daily Infected Cases of France.

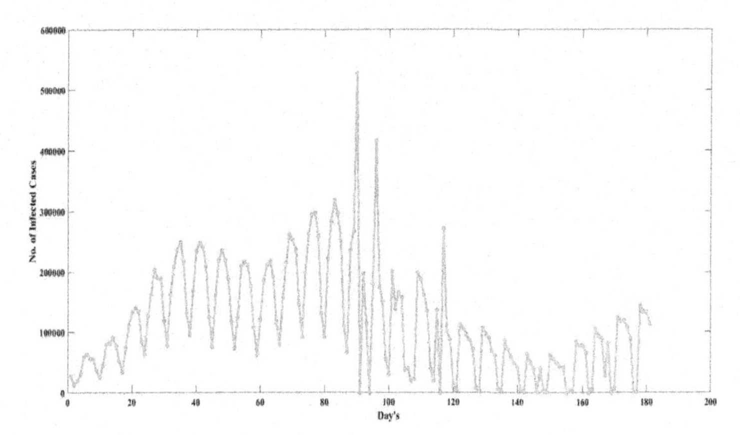

Fig. 6.4: Daily Infected Cases of Germany.

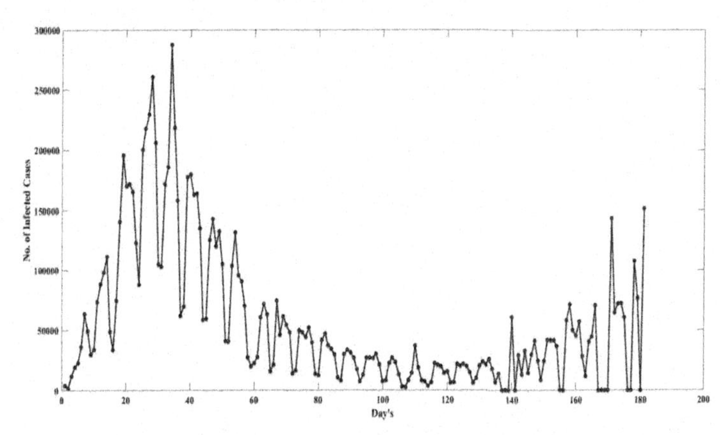

Fig. 6.5: Daily Infected Cases of Brazil.

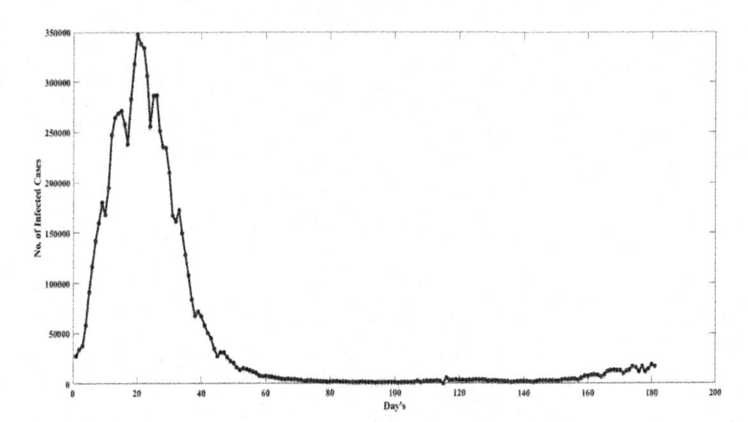

Fig. 6.6: Daily Infected Cases of India.

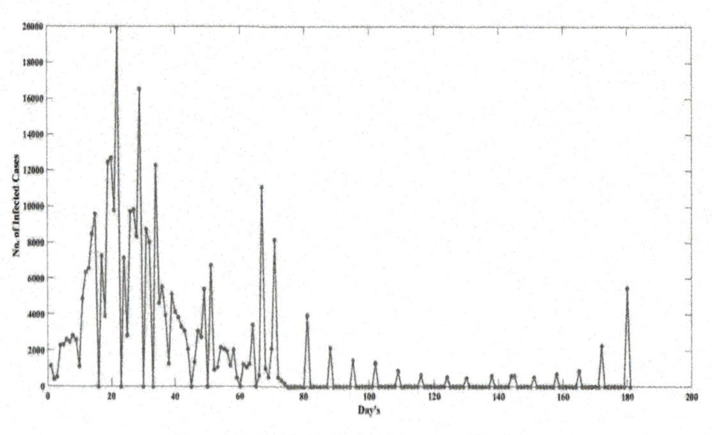

Fig. 6.7: Daily Infected Cases of Tunisia.

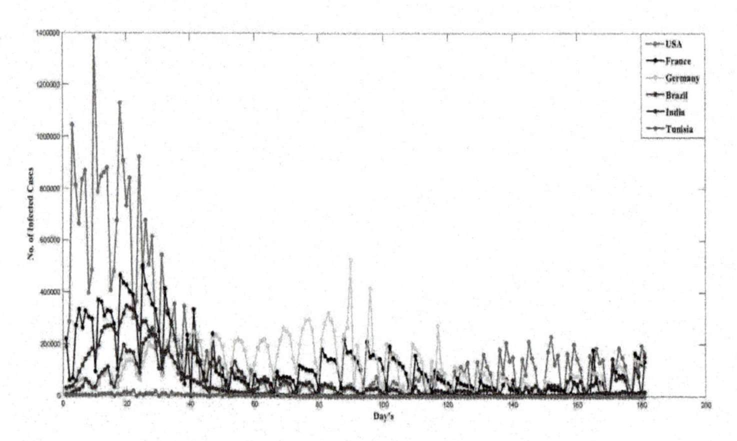

Fig. 6.8: Daily Infected Cases of USA, India, Brazil, France, Germany and Tunisia.

6.4.2 Multifractal Spectrum of COVID19 Infected Cases

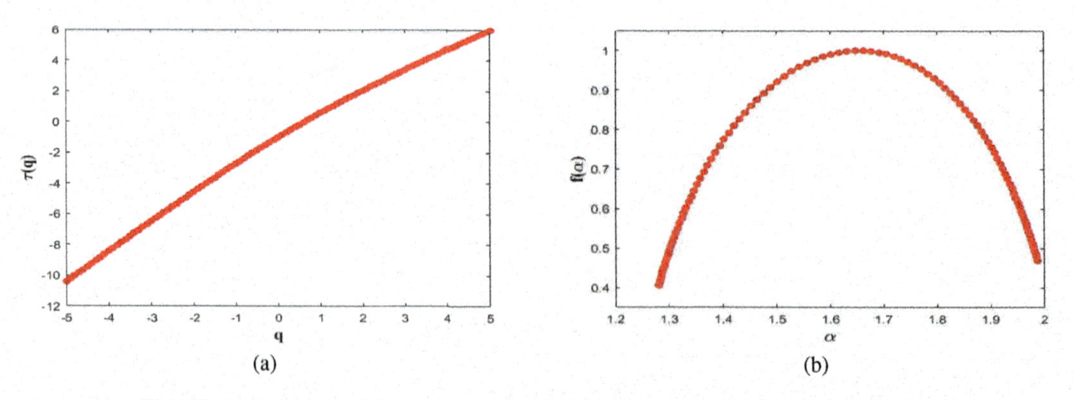

Fig. 6.9: Multifractal scaling exponent and multifractal spectrum of Infected Cases in World.

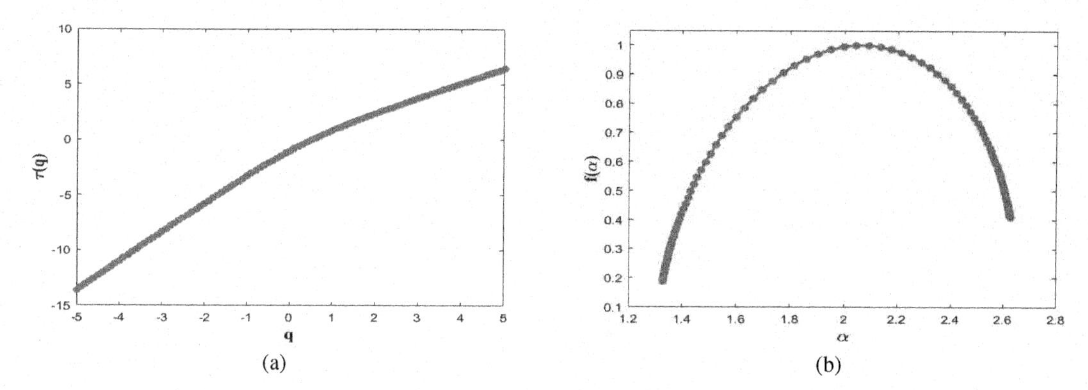

Fig. 6.10: Multifractal scaling exponent and multifractal spectrum of Infected Cases in USA.

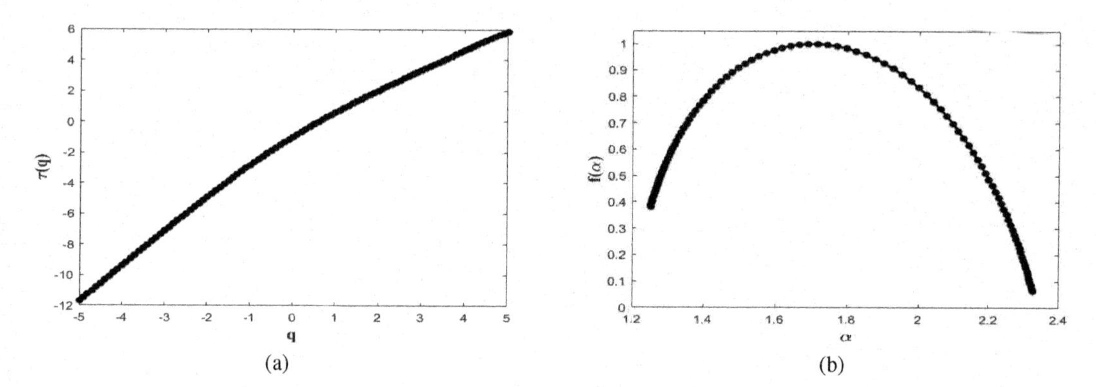

Fig. 6.11: Multifractal scaling exponent and multifractal spectrum of Infected Cases in France.

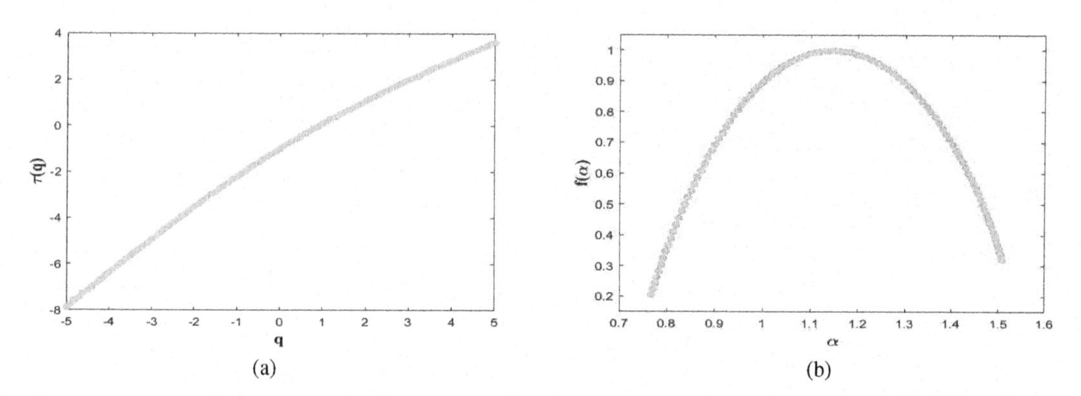

Fig. 6.12: Multifractal scaling exponent and multifractal spectrum of Infected Cases in Germany.

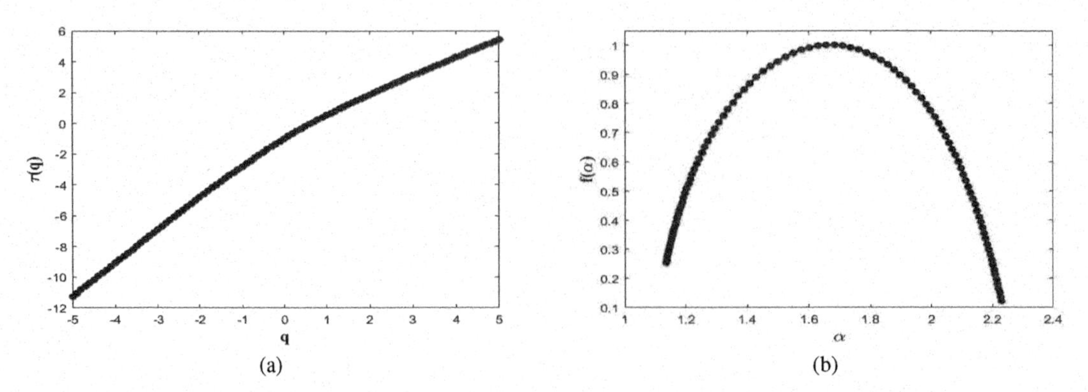

Fig. 6.13: Multifractal scaling exponent and multifractal spectrum of Infected Cases in Brazil.

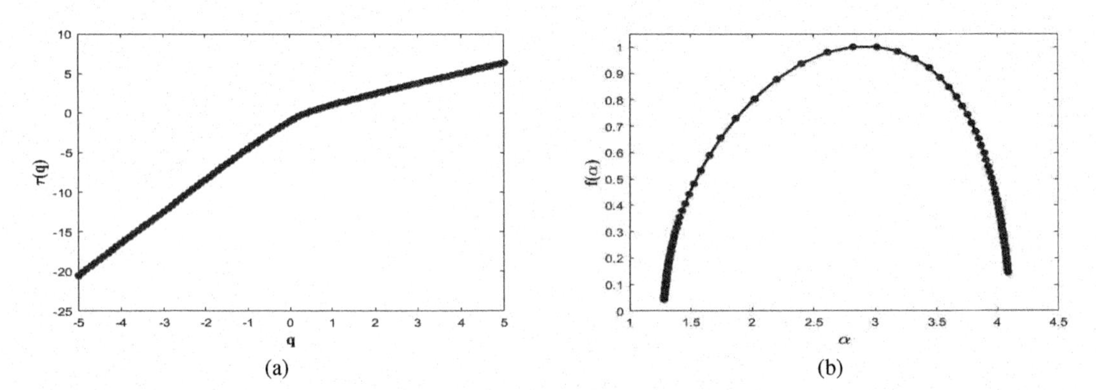

Fig. 6.14: Multifractal scaling exponent and multifractal spectrum of Infected Cases in India.

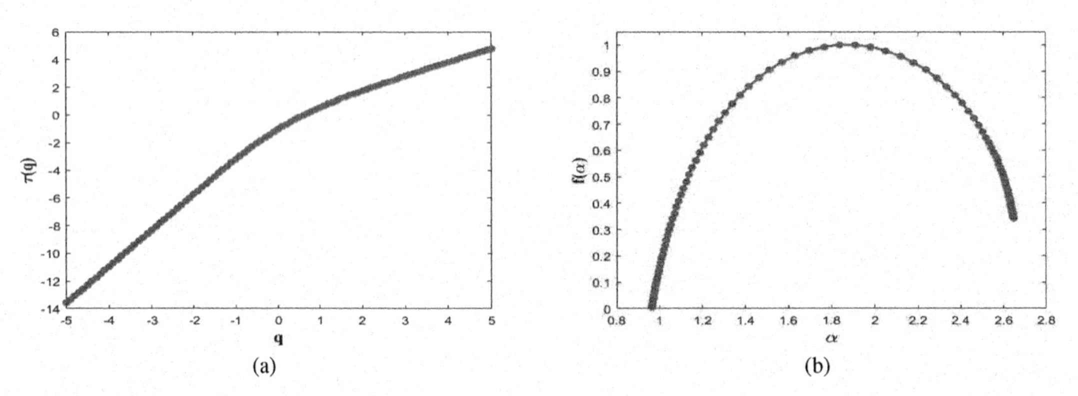

Fig. 6.15: Multifractal scaling exponent and multifractal spectrum of Infected Cases in Tunisia.

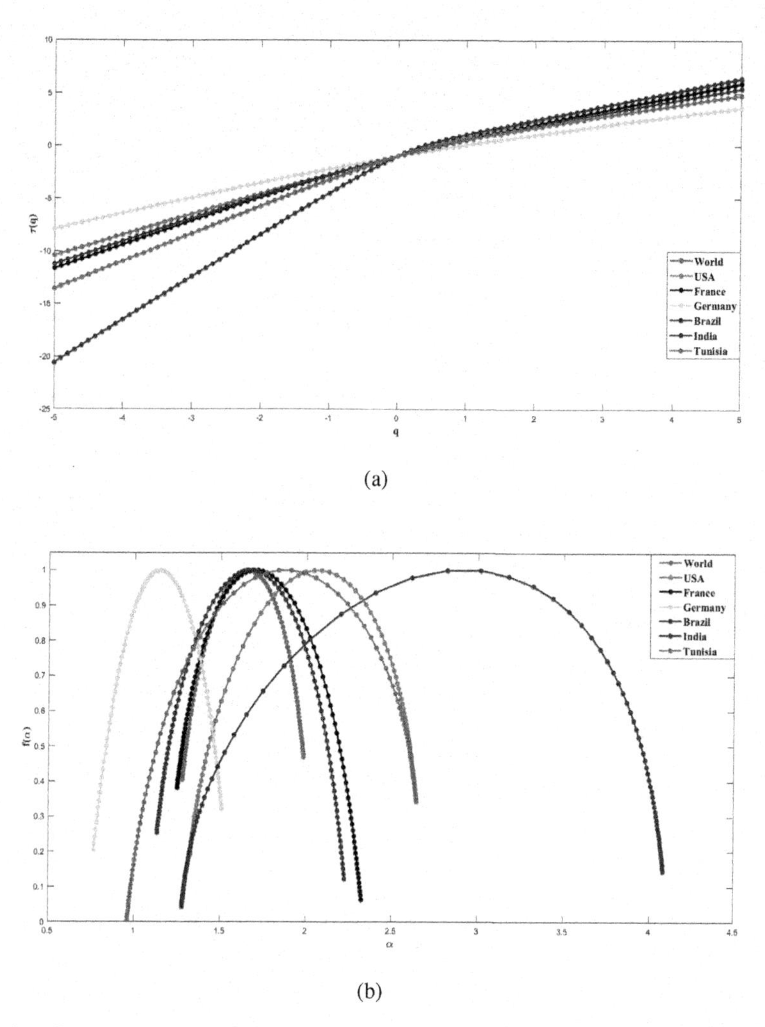

Fig. 6.16: Multifractal scaling exponent and multifractal spectrum of Infected Cases in World, USA, France, Germany, Brazil, India and Tunisia.

Table 6.2: Multifractality strength of Infected Cases in World, USA, France, Germany, Brazil, India, and Tunisia.

Country	α_{min}	α_{max}	$\triangle\alpha = \alpha_{max} - \alpha_{min}$
World	1.2796	1.9860	0.7064
USA	1.3270	2.6266	1.2996
France	1.2509	2.3255	1.0746
Germany	0.7668	1.5085	0.7417
Brazil	1.1349	2.2283	1.0934
India	1.2799	4.0826	2.8026
Tunisia	0.9631	2.6459	1.6828

The multifractal scaling exponent $\tau(q)$ is not linear indicating the time-series is multifractal. We see that India has the highest Multifractality compared to other countries and Germany has the lowest Multifractality. There are high fluctuations of COVID-19 infected cases in India. We strongly suggest that taking COVID-19 safety precautions, attempting to avoid social gatherings, maintaining social distance, and implementing more awareness campaigns to inform people about COVID-19 safety precautions to decrease the number of infected cases in the future.

6.4.3 Multifractal Spectrum of COVID-19 Death Cases

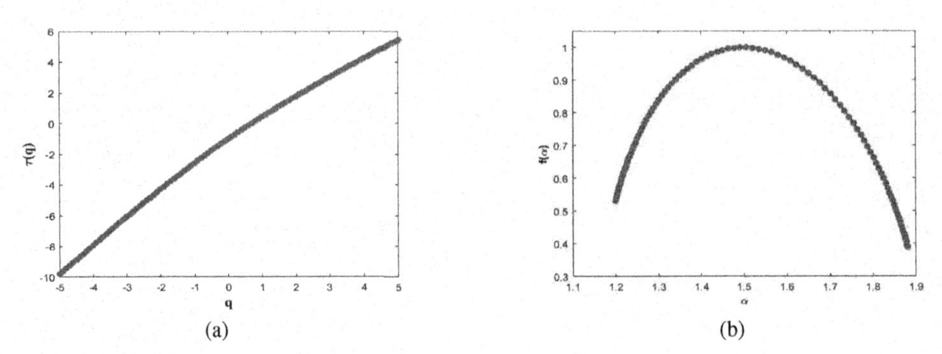

Fig. 6.17: Multifractal scaling exponent and multifractal spectrum of Death Cases in World.

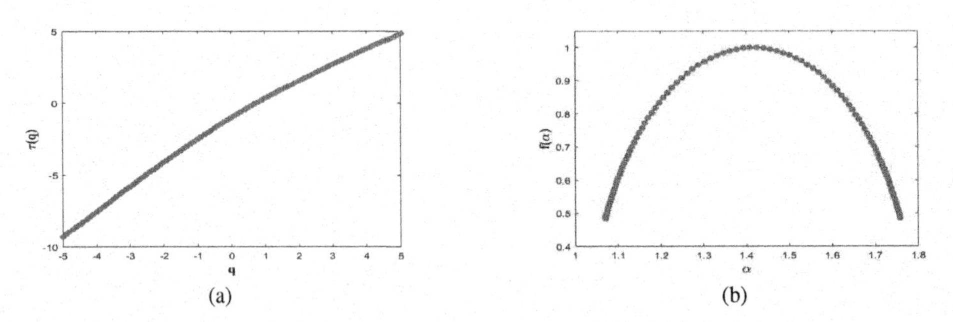

Fig. 6.18: Multifractal scaling exponent and multifractal spectrum of Death Cases in USA.

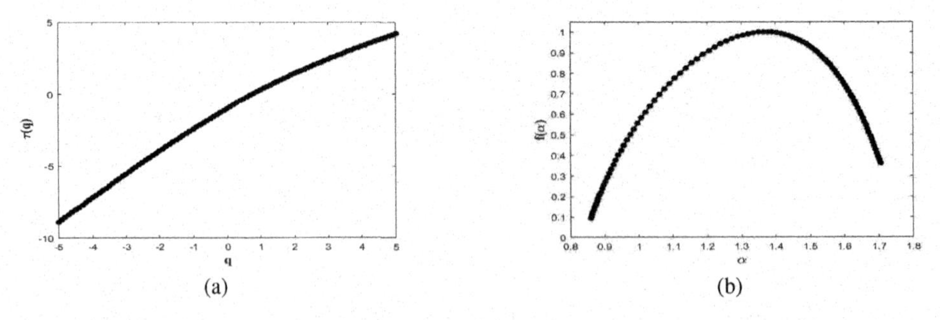

Fig. 6.19: Multifractal scaling exponent and multifractal spectrum of Death Cases in France.

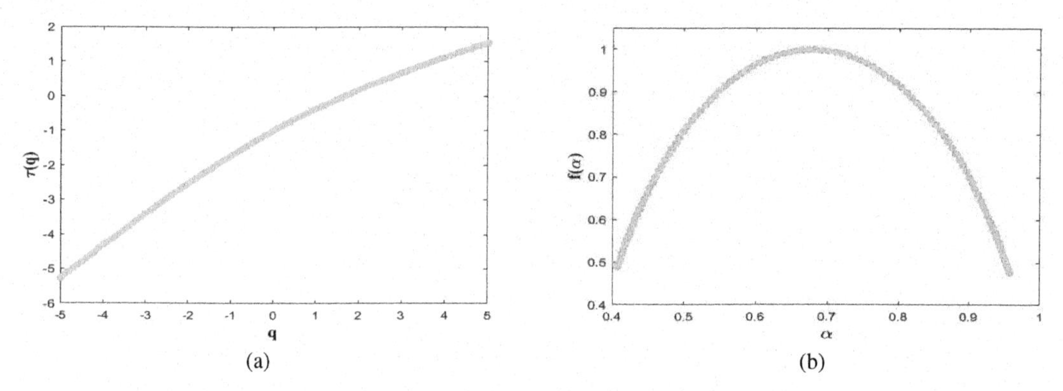

(a) (b)

Fig. 6.20: Multifractal scaling exponent and multifractal spectrum of Death Cases in Germany.

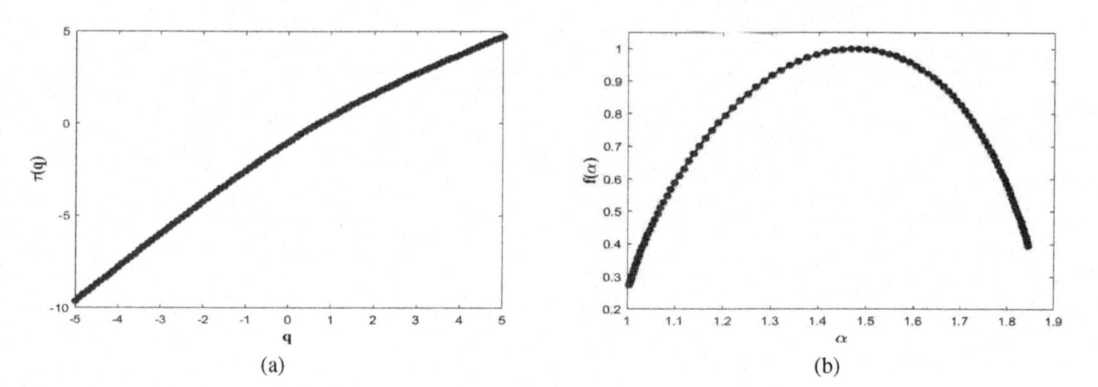

(a) (b)

Fig. 6.21: Multifractal scaling exponent and multifractal spectrum of Death Cases in Brazil.

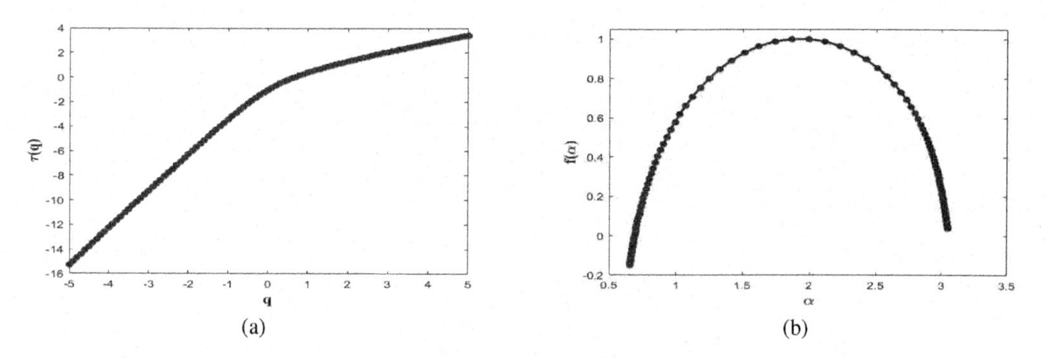

(a) (b)

Fig. 6.22: Multifractal scaling exponent and multifractal spectrum of Death Cases in India.

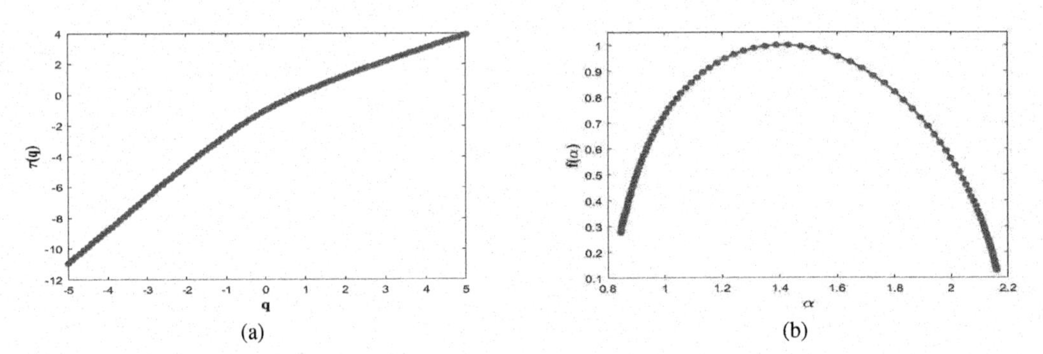

(a) (b)

Fig. 6.23: Multifractal scaling exponent and multifractal spectrum of Death Cases in Tunisia.

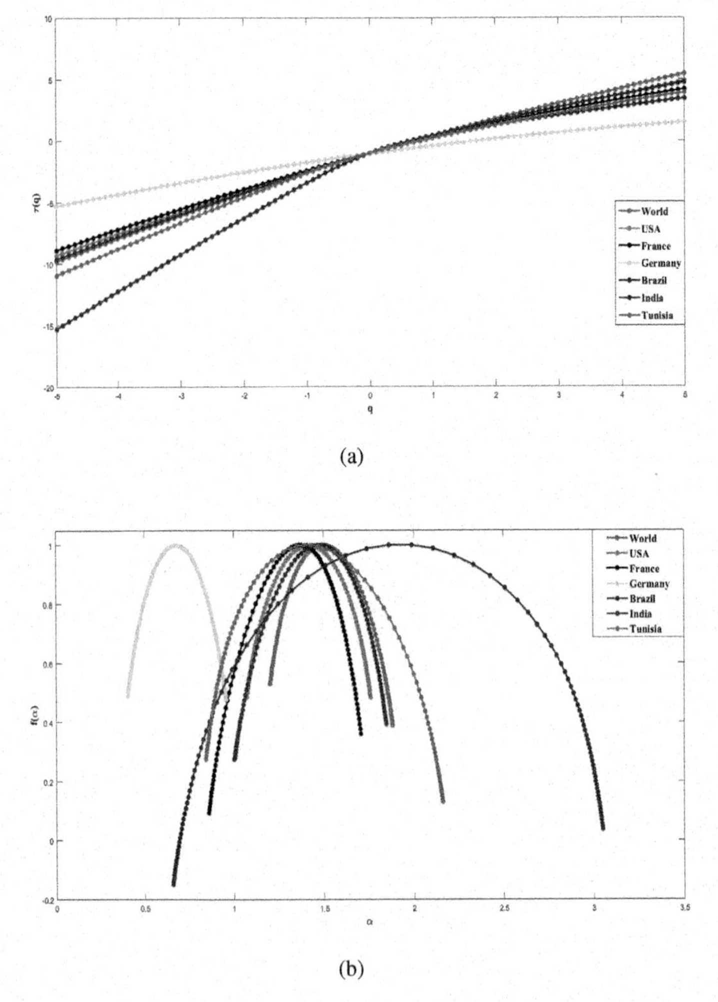

(b)

Fig. 6.24: Multifractal scaling exponent and multifractal spectrum of Death Cases in World, USA, France, Germany, Brazil, India, and Tunisia.

Table 6.3: Multifractality strength of Death Cases in World, USA, France, Germany, Brazil, India, and Tunisia.

Country	α_{min}	α_{max}	$\Delta\alpha = \alpha_{max} - \alpha_{min}$
World	1.1990	1.8803	0.6813
USA	1.0695	1.7576	0.6881
France	0.8594	1.7044	0.8449
Germany	0.4069	0.9575	0.5505
Brazil	1.0043	1.8450	0.8407
India	0.6566	3.0495	2.3929
Tunisia	0.8442	2.1596	1.3155

The multifractal scaling exponent $\tau(q)$ is not linear indicating the time-series is multifractal. We see that India has the highest Multifractality compared to other countries and Germany has the lowest Multifractality. There are high fluctuations of COVID-19 death cases in India. We strongly advise getting vaccinated against COVID-19 as early as possible for older adults, children, and individuals with low immunity as they have the lowest survival rates and are more susceptible to serious sickness from the virus. This will help to reduce the number of Covid-19 Death Cases.

6.4.4 Multifractal Spectrum of COVID-19 Vaccinated Cases

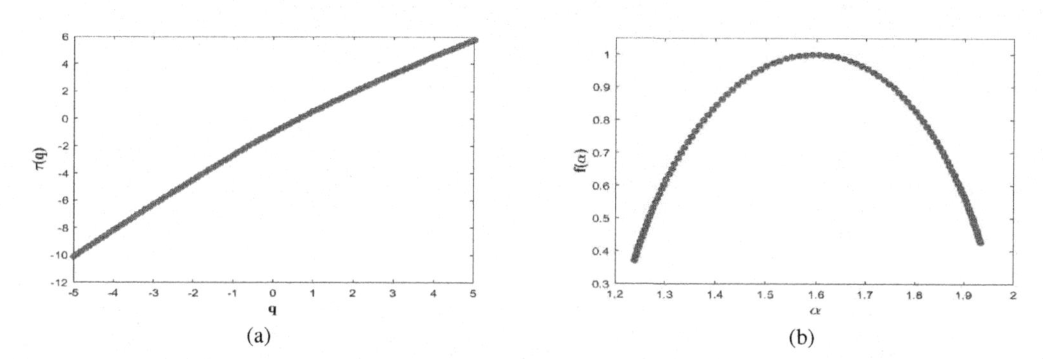

Fig. 6.25: Multifractal scaling exponent and multifractal spectrum of Vaccinated Cases in World.

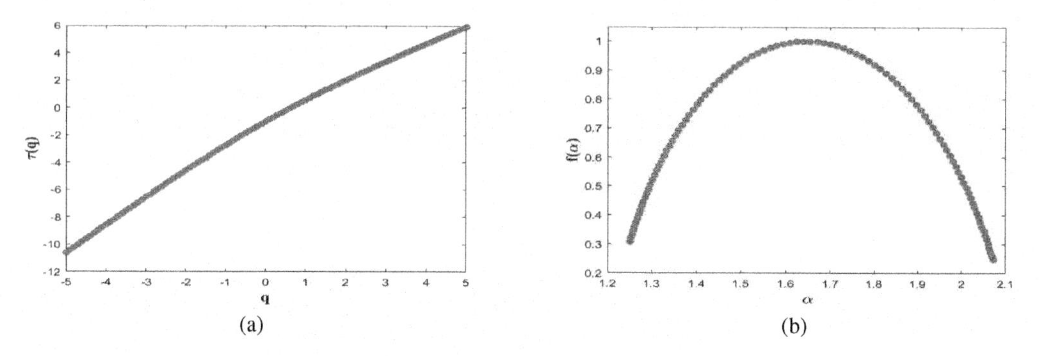

Fig. 6.26: Multifractal scaling exponent and multifractal spectrum of Vaccinated Cases in USA.

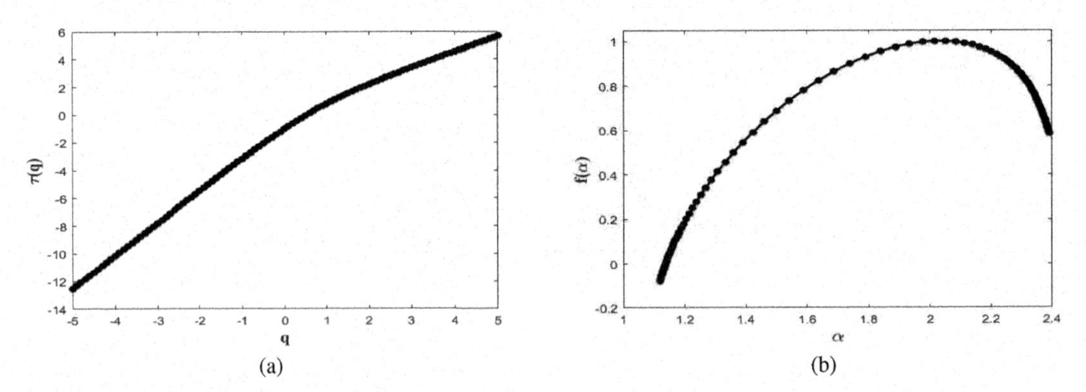

Fig. 6.27: Multifractal scaling exponent and multifractal spectrum of Vaccinated Cases in France.

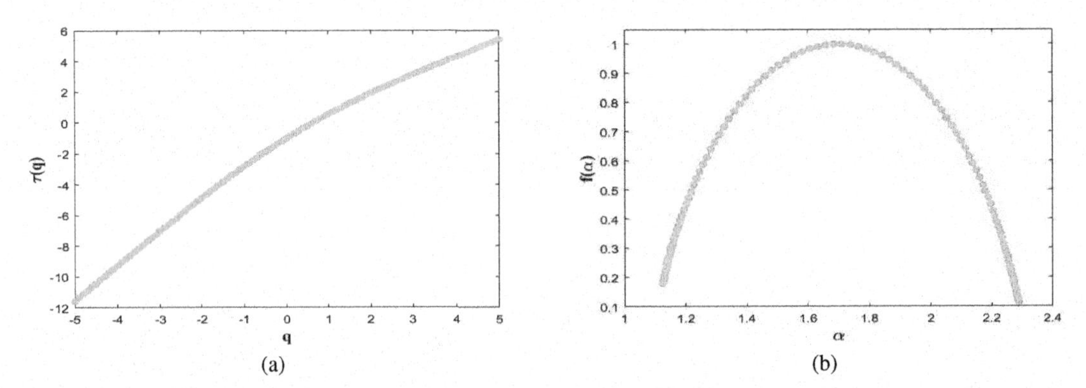

Fig. 6.28: Multifractal scaling exponent and multifractal spectrum of Vaccinated Cases in Germany.

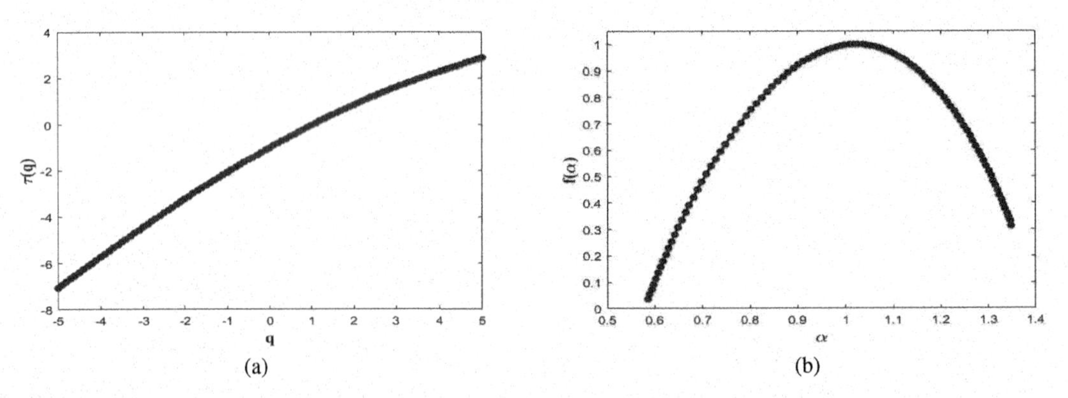

Fig. 6.29: Multifractal scaling exponent and multifractal spectrum of Vaccinated Cases in Brazil.

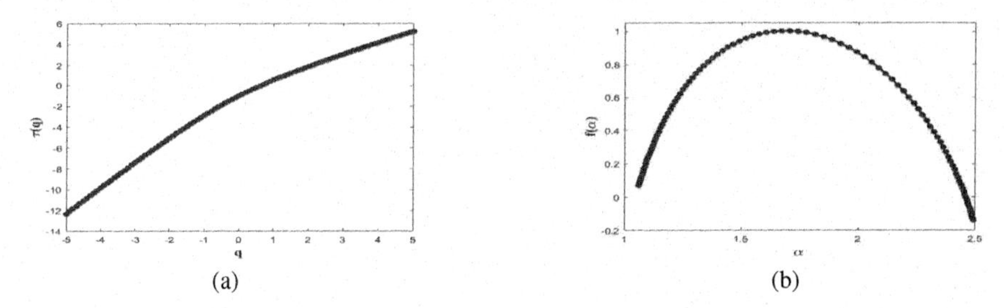

(a) (b)

Fig. 6.30: Multifractal scaling exponent and multifractal spectrum of Vaccinated Cases in India.

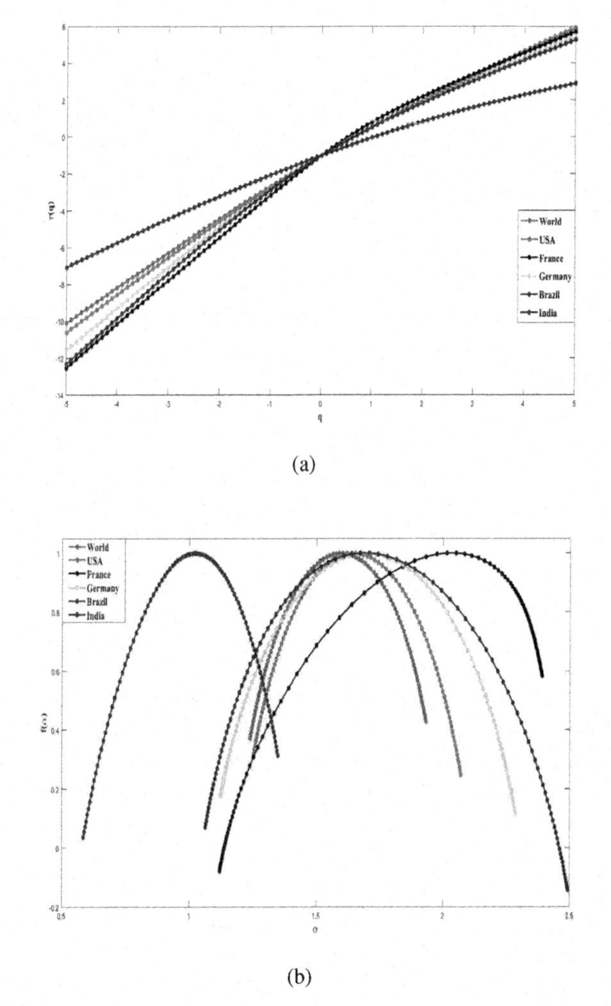

(a)

(b)

Fig. 6.31: Multifractal scaling exponent and multifractal spectrum of Vaccinated Cases in World, USA, France, Germany, Brazil, India and Tunisia.

Table 6.4: Multifractality strength of Vaccinated Cases in World, USA, France, Germany, Brazil, India and Tunisia.

Country	α_{min}	α_{max}	$\Delta\alpha = \alpha_{max} - \alpha_{min}$
World	1.2389	1.9330	0.6941
USA	1.2503	2.0720	0.8217
France	1.1197	2.3902	1.2705
Germany	1.1244	2.2867	1.1623
Brazil	0.5855	1.3485	0.7630
India	1.0633	2.4923	1.4290

The multifractal scaling exponent $\tau(q)$ is not linear indicating the time-series is multifractal. We clearly see that India has the highest Multifractality compared to other countries and Brazil has the lowest Multifractality. There are high fluctuations of COVID-19 Vaccinated cases in India, suggest that a lot of vaccinations are done in the past compared to other countries.

From the infected cases and death cases, India has the highest multifractality and the lowest is Germany in the vaccinated cases, India has the highest multifractality and the lowest of Brazil. It is advised that by taking the COVID-19 vaccine, we can reduce our risk of passing on COVID-19 infections and may reduce the infected cases and death cases in the world.

6.5 Conclusion

This study evaluated the multifractality of the top affected countries of COVID-19 in the first half of 2022. We apply the multifractal detrended fluctuation analysis to investigate the multifractal properties of COVID-19 Infected Cases, Death Cases, and Vaccinated Cases in the World, USA, France, Germany, Brazil, India, and Tunisia. This chapter provides an methodology of analyzing COVID-19 from multifractal perspectives. The obtained results play a crucial role and give an idea that there might be some risk for the countries involved and the need to understand the current situations compared to other countries. Based on the results on the top multifractality countries, it is suggested that we need to increase vaccinations to reduce the rate of infections and deaths.

References

[1] Falconer, K. 2003. Fractal Geometry: Mathematical Foundations and Applications, John Wiley and Sons Ltd.

[2] Mandelbrot, B.B. 1983. The Fractal Geometry of Nature, W.H. Freeman and Company, New York.

[3] Santo Banerjee, D. Easwaramoorthy and A. Gowrisankar. 2021. Fractal Functions, Dimensions and Signal Analysis, Understanding Complex Systems, Springer: Complexity, Springer, Cham.

[4] Yu, S., D. Meifeng, S. Yanqiu and S. Shuxiang. 2016. Scaling of the average receiving time on a family of weighted hierarchical networks. Fractals, 24(3): 1650038.

[5] Meifeng, D., H. Jie, G. Jianyu et al. 2016. Mixed multifractal analysis of China and US stock index series. Chaos, Solitons and Fractals, 87: 268–275.

[6] Kantelhardt, J.W., S.A. Zschiegner, E. Koscielny-Bunde, S. Havlin, A. Bunde and H.E. Stanley. 2002. Multifractal detrended fluctuation analysis of nonstationary time series. Physica A, 316(1): 87–114.

[7] Davis, A., A. Marshak, W. Wiscombe and R. Cahalan. 1994. Multifractal characterizations of non stationarity and intermittency in geophysical fields: Observed, retrieved, or simulated. Journal of Geophysical Research, 99(4): 8055–8072.
[8] Li, W. and X. Zhao. 2018. Multiscale horizontal-visibility-graph correlation analysis of stock time series. Europhysics Letters, 122(4): 40007.
[9] Dimitriu, P.P., E.M. Scordilis and V.G. Karacostas. 2000. Multifractal analysis of the Arnea, Greece Seismicity with potential implications for earthquake prediction. Natural Hazards, 21: 277–295.
[10] Chappel, D. and J. Scalo. 2001. Multifractal scaling, geometrical diversity and hierarchical structure in the cool interstellar medium. Astrophysical Journal 551: 712–729.
[11] Ivanov, P.C., L.A.N. Amaral, A.L. Goldberger, S. Havlin, M.G. Rosenblum, Z.R. Struzik and H.E. Stanley. 1999. Multifractality in human heartbeat dynamics. Nature, 399: 461–465.
[12] Bianconi, G. and A.L. Barabasi. 2001. Competition and multiscaling in evolving networks. Europhysics Letters, 54(4): 436–442.
[13] Fisher, A., L. Calvet and B.B. Mandelbrot. 1997. Multifractality of Deutschemark/US Dollar Exchange Rates, Cowles Foundation Discussion Papers, 1166.
[14] Easwaramoorthy, D. and R. Uthayakumar. 2010. Estimating the complexity of biomedical signals by multifractal analysis. Proceedings of the IEEE Students' Technology Symposium, IEEE Xplore Digital Library, IEEE, USA, 6–11.
[15] Easwaramoorthy, D. and R. Uthayakumar. 2010. Analysis of EEG Signals using Advanced Generalized Fractal Dimensions. Proceedings of the Second International Conference on Computing, Communication and Networking Technologies, IEEE Xplore Digital Library, IEEE, USA, 1–6.
[16] Easwaramoorthy, D. and R. Uthayakumar. 2010. Analysis of biomedical EEG signals using wavelet transforms and multifractal analysis. Proceedings of the IEEE International Conference on Communication Control and Computing Technologies, IEEE Xplore Digital Library, IEEE, USA, 544–549.
[17] Easwaramoorthy, D. and R. Uthayakumar. 2011. Improved generalized fractal dimensions in the discrimination between healthy and epileptic EEG signals. Journal of Computational Science, 2(1): 31–38.
[18] Uthayakumar, R. and D. Easwaramoorthy. 2012. Multifractal-wavelet based denoising in the classification of healthy and epileptic EEG signals. Fluctuation and Noise Letters, 11(4): 1250034.
[19] Uthayakumar, R. and D. Easwaramoorthy. 2012. Generalized fractal dimensions in the recognition of noise free images. Proceedings of the International Conference on Computing, Communication and Networking Technologies, IEEE Xplore Digital Library, IEEE, USA, 1–5.
[20] Uthayakumar, R. and D. Easwaramoorthy. 2012. Multifractal analysis in denoising of color images. Proceedings of the International Conference on Emerging Trends in Science, Engineering and Technology, IEEE Xplore Digital Library, IEEE, USA, 228–234.
[21] Uthayakumar, R. and D. Easwaramoorthy. 2013. Epileptic seizure detection in EEG signals using multifractal analysis and wavelet transform. Fractals, 21(2): 1350011.
[22] Uthayakumar, R. and D. Easwaramoorthy. 2014. Fuzzy generalized fractal dimensions for chaotic waveforms. Chaos, Complexity and Leadership 2012, Springer Proceedings in Complexity, 411–422.
[23] Easwaramoorthy, D., P.S. Eliahim Jeevaraj, A. Gowrisankar, A. Manimaran and S. Nandhini. 2018. Fuzzy generalized fractal dimensions using inter-heartbeat interval dynamics in ECG signals for age related discrimination. International Journal of Engineering and Technology (UAE), 7(4.10): 900–903.
[24] Nandhini, S., D. Easwaramoorthy and R. Abinands. 2020. An extensive review on recent evolutions in object detection algorithms. International Journal of Emerging Trends in Engineering Research, 8(7): 3766–3776.
[25] Peng, C.K., S.V. Buldyrev, S. Havlin, M. Simons, H.E. Stanley and A.L. Goldberger. 1994. Mosaic organization of DNA nucleotides. Phys. Rev. E, 49: 1685–1689.

[26] Ding, Q., P. Lu, Y. Fan, Y. Xia and M. Liu. 2020. The clinical characteristics of pneumonia patients coinfected with 2019 novel coronavirus and influenza virus in Wuhan, China. Journal of Medical Virology, 92(9): 1549–1555.

[27] Easwaramoorthy, D., A. Gowrisankar, A. Manimaran, S. Nandhini, Lamberto Rondoni and Santo Banerjee. 2021. An exploration of fractal-based prognostic model and comparative analysis for second wave of COVID-19 diffusion. Nonlinear Dynamics, 2021.

[28] Qiusheng Rong, C. Thangaraj, D. Easwaramoorthy and Shaobo He. 2021. Multifractal based image processing for estimating the complexity of COVID-19 dynamics. The European Physical Journal Special Topics, 230(21-22): 3947–3954.

[29] Shaobo He, C. Thangaraj, D. Easwaramoorthy and G. Muhiuddin. 2022. Multifractal analysis on age-based discrimination in X-ray images for sensing the severity of COVID-19 disease. The European Physical Journal Special Topics.

[30] Thangaraj, C. and D. Easwaramoorthy. 2022. Generalized fractal dimensions based comparison analysis of edge detection methods in CT images for estimating the infection of COVID-19 disease. The European Physical Journal Special Topics.

[31] Gu, G.F. and W.X. Zhou. 2006. Detrended fluctuation analysis for fractals and multifractals in higher dimensions. Phys. Rev. E, 74: 061104.

[32] Silva, L.B.M., M.V.D. Vermelho, M.L. Lyra and G.M. Viswanathan. 2009. Multifractal detrended fluctuation analysis of analog random multiplicative processes. Chaos Solitons Fractals, 41: 2806.

[33] Bolgorian, M. and R. Raei. 2011. A multifractal detrended fluctuation analysis of trading behavior of individual and institutional traders in Tehran stock market. Physica A, 390: 3815.

[34] Wang, F., G.P. Liao, J.H. Li, X.C. Li and T.J. Zhou. 2013. Multifractal detrended fluctuation analysis for clustering structures of electricity price periods. Physica A: Statistical Mechanics and its Applications, 392: 5723.

[35] Mathieu, E., H. Ritchie, L. Rodés-Guirao, C. Appel, C. Giattino, J. Hasell, B. Macdonald, S. Dattani, D. Beltekian, E. Ortiz-Ospina and M. Roser. 2020. "Coronavirus Pandemic (COVID-19)", https://ourworldindata.org/coronavirus.

Chapter 7

An Integrated Perspective of Fractal Time Series Analysis for Infected Cases of COVID-19

A. Gowrisankar,[1] *D. Easwaramoorthy,*[1,*] *R. Valarmathi,*[1] P.*S. Eliahim Jeevaraj,*[2] *Christo Ananth*[3] and *Ilie Vasiliev*[4]

7.1 Introduction

An unidentified pneumonia outbreak is reported in December 2019 in Wuhan, Hubei Province, China. It was then discovered that cases of pneumonia were related to the Huanan Seafood Wholesale Market. As a result of the inoculation of respiratory materials into human airway epithelial cells, Vero E6 and Huh7 cell lines, an unidentified pneumonia outbreak in Wuhan was identified as a novel coronavirus (SARS-CoV-2) related to SARS-CoV after genetic analysis. The disease caused by SARS-CoV-2 was named COVID-19. Although there are many similarities between the new COVID-19 and the virus that caused the SARS infection, there are differences due to the mutations in their genes which include the way of transmission and the symptomatic behaviors. Preliminary reports indicate that the new corona virus infection is more likely to be caused by SARS but less likely to cause serious illness. Approximately 80% of patients recover completely from the illness without needing any more care. About 1 in 6 people infected with COVID-19 experience severe illness and respiratory problems. Older adults and those with underlying medical conditions such as high blood pressure, heart problems or diabetes are more likely to develop severe disease. Additionally, more people died as a result of lack of ventilator facilities, even though they were plagued by this type of respiratory issue. This was because one of the largest factors was not realizing how severe the illness was at the appropriate moment. As a result, the polymerase chain reaction (RT-PCR) instrument is regarded as a superb tool for detecting this disease. Despite this it serves a very useful purpose, this technology is not used

[1] Department of Mathematics, School of Advanced Sciences, Vellore Institute of Technology, Vellore, Tamil Nadu, India.
Emails: gowrisankargri@gmail.com; valarmathi.2142@gmail.com
[2] Department of Computer Science, Bishop Heber College, Tiruchirappalli, Tamil Nadu, India.
Email: eliahimps@gmail.com
[3] Samarkand State University, Uzbekistan.
Email: dr.christoananth@gmail.com
[4] The World Academy of Medical Sciences, Netherlands.
Email: ilievasiliev@gmail.com
* Corresponding author: easandk@gmail.com

to predict the effects of the disease or to identify issues with the human lungs. Therefore, imaging the human lung and its effects using medical imaging technology like computed tomography (CT)-Scan and X-ray is highly helpful. In fact, X-ray is more effective and more affordable than CT scan for identifying respiratory issues caused on by COVID-19.

All viruses, including the SARS-CoV-2 virus that causes COVID-19, change over time. However, certain changes might affect the virus characteristics, such as how quickly it spreads, the severity of the illness it causes, or the efficacy of vaccines, therapeutic medications, diagnostic devices, or other public health and societal interventions. The identification of particular Variants of Interest (VOIs) and Variants of Concern (VOCs) was triggered by the appearance of variants that, by the end of 2020, posed a greater risk to the world's public health. In order to prioritise worldwide surveillance and investigation and, eventually, to inform the current response to the COVID-19 virus, this has been done. The nomenclature systems now in use by GISAID, Nextstrain, and Pango are used by scientists to name and track SARS-CoV-2 genetic lineages. WHO brought together researchers from the Technological Advisory Committee on Virus Evolution, the WHO COVID-19 reference research lab system, representatives from GISAID, Nextstrain, and Pango, as well as other experts in virology, microbial nomenclature, and interaction from various nations and organizations to discuss simple and non-stigmatizing labels for VOI and VOC. Later, the WHO-convened expert committee advised utilizing the Greek letters Alpha, Beta, Gamma, and Delta since they are simpler and more useful for discussions with non-scientific audiences. These working definitions may occasionally be modified due to the ongoing development of such that causes SARS-CoV-2 as well as ongoing advancements in our knowledge of the effects of variations. In discussion with the Technical Advisory Committee on Virus Development, variants may need to be reclassified when necessary, and those offering a reduced risk compared to other existing variants may be identified as VOCs/VOIs/VUMs. The circulating variants of concern and variants of interest are respectively provided in Tables 7.1 and 7.2. Updates on SARS-CoV-2 classifications, geographic VOC distribution, and overviews of their phenotypic characteristics based on published studies are regularly provided by the WHO weekly epidemiological updates.

The prevailing consequences of coronavirus disease has undoubtedly lead to the global threat of the public health, healthcare benefactors, social systems and finance. Developed countries have been fighting to control this present outbreak and trying to develop a vaccine, whereas the developing countries have been battling against COVID-19 with lack of social-distancing, economic impacts caused by the pandemic, inadequate health infrastructure due to the higher population. Therefore, there is a need for prompt investigation to

Table 7.1: Circulating Variants of Concern (VOCs).

WHO label	Pango lineage	Earliest documented samples	Date of designation
Alpha	B.1.1.7	United Kingdom, Sep-2020	VOC: 18-Dec-2020 Previous VOC: 09-Mar-2022
Beta	B.1.351	South Africa, May-2020	VOC: 18-Dec-2020 Previous VOC: 09-Mar-2020
Gamma	P.1	Brazil, Nov-2020	VOC: 11-Jan-2021 Previous VOC: 09-Mar-2022
Delta	B.1.617.2	India, Oct-2020	VOI: 4-Apr-2021 VOC: 11-May-2021 Previous VOC: 7-Jun-2022
Omicron	B.1.1.529	Multiple countries, Nov-2021	VUM 24-Nov-2021 VOC 26-Nov-2021

Table 7.2: Circulating Variants of Interest (VOIs).

WHO label	Pango lineage	Earliest documented samples	Date of designation
Epsilon	B.1.427 B.1.429	United States of America, Mar-2020	VOI: 5-Mar-2021 Previous VOI: 06-Jul-2021
Zeta	P.2	Brazil, Apr-2020	VOI: 17-Mar-2021 Previous VOI: 06-Jul-2021
Eta	B.1.525	Multiple countries, Dec-2020	VOI: 17-Mar-2021 Previous VOI: 20-sep-2021
Theta	P.3	Philippines, Jan-2021	VOI: 24-Mar-2021 Previous VOI: 06-Jul-2021
Iota	B.1.526	United States of America, Nov-2020	VOI: 24-Mar-2021 Previous VOI: 20-sep-2021
Kappa	B.1.617.1	India, Oct-2020	VOI: 4-Aprl-2021 Previous VOI: 20-Sep-2021
Lambda	C.37	Peru, Dec-2020	VOI: 14-Jun-2021 Previous VOI:09-Mar-2022
Mu	B.1.621	Colombia, Jan-2021	VOI: 30-Aug-2021 Previous VOI: 09-Mar-2022

understand the outbreak so that the most affected countries can take the appropriate strategies in their healthcare system as well as in their economic crisis. In recent days, researchers are analyzing SARS-CoV-2 to achieve the sustainable promotion of public health care services and systems in terms of forecasting, comparison, post-challenges and vaccination in which there is a large amount of speedy researches functioning through the prediction pipeline at extraordinary levels [1]–[6].

The public health system is demarcated as the construction of scheme for precluding infectious disease, protracting lifespan and stimulating healthiness through the systematized endeavours of the society. The global vision is to endorse greater health and well-being in sustainable practices, while establishing the unified public health services and dropping disparities. In order to achieve this goal, the public health methodology comprises the strategies employed with other firms to overcome the broader factors of health, and engaged with the health authorities. The primary health care specialists can play a main part in stopping the deadly infections and stimulating the public health care services [7]. The prediction analysis on diseased and death cases for the viewpoint of our future is the key factor in the route for reaching the goal and it could definitely create the expedient strategies and long term polices to attain the environmentally sustainable public health care systems. So the scientific community is functioning earnestly on the forecasting schemes by using mathematical and statistical methods.

Methodical planning and techniques are needed to control the COVID-19 virus outbreak, in that case the researchers' study on the COVID-19 data can make use of mathematical modelling. Mathematical analysis can be used to identify some of the fundamental components that govern eruptions and epidemics and to identify patterns and general principles that underpin the development of the disease. Recently, a lot of academics have concentrated on making predictions about the precise amount of COVID-19 cases using some mathematical analysis. In [8], a simple econometric model is proposed to predict the spread of Covid-19, and an ARIMA model is used to predict the prevalence and incidence of the virus in the Covid-19 dataset. In [9], the authors have proposed three quarantine models to deal with the pandemic disease by considering a number of compartments including the easily affected population, immigrant population, home seclusion population, contagious population, medical quarantine population, and recovered population. The prediction on corona virus epidemics in Brazil, Turkey, and South Africa has been presented in [10]. In this respect, the fractal dimension and fractal interpolation functions have been used effectively in clinical image analysis and COVID-19 data approximation in recent years. The modern mathematician, Mandelbrot mathematically characterized a Fractal as a set with the Hausdorff dimension strictly greater than its topological dimension [11–13]. In order to deal the objects with chaotic nature, a geometry with non-integer dimension called the fractal geometry, has been introduced. Such a non-integer dimension is known as the fractal dimension and it is defined as a non-linear measure for describing fractal patterns or quantifying the complexity of the set. The fractal dimensions are employed to inspect a broad spectrum of applications ranging from the abstract to practical phenomena, comprising turbulence structures, medical disorders, public health care systems, market fluctuations, economic trends and environmental sustainability. Generally, the biomedical waveforms with more complexity resemble the Weierstrass function (a continuous nowhere differentiable function), hence the most of the real time data are very irregular and so they are represented as Fractal Time Series for the detailed study on prediction [18].

In the literature of approximation theory, the interpolation is a process of fabricating new data from known data. The fractal interpolation technique can be considered as an advancement of the classical interpolation methods and the same is based on the iterated function systems of contractions. As an application of fractal interpolation function technique, the interpolated or predicted data can be generated accurately for the given set of realistic data [11–13]. Consequently, a FIF of a specific type can be implicated in the infectious data to interpolate the predicted data so that the forecasted information may help the society to upstream the environmentally sustainable health system. In the view of investigative schemes, the fractal dimension measurement is one of the most achievable amid all types of non-linear approaches. However, the single valued fractal dimension is insufficient to reveal the intricacy nature of the disordered systems. Such a non-homogeneous system with uncertain nature is called a multifractal and is studied by the multi-level fractal dimensions called the Generalized Fractal Dimensions (GFD) [19]. As the multifractal formalism have been applied to real time data and experimental signals, the improved version of GFD measures have predominantly been utilized to study the variations in the disordered features in various physical environments and to explore the complexity in forecasting practices [14]–[55]. Among all the non-linear systems, the Improved Generalized Fractal Dimensions (IGFD) method [44] has more feasible factors in analyzing the real time based transmission data with more difficulty in the way for medical prognostication. Hence, these scientific impressions motivate us to step into the predictive analysis on the current deadly coronavirus dispersion by using the proposed fractal features. Based on the forecasting results in this integrated research study, the control measures can be taken up by the public health care sectors in order to attain the sustainable environment by controlling the fatal virus diffusion.

The main task of constructing the executable model to forecast this destructive infectious disease is very essential at this moment as the real time data is highly noisy and not always compatible. In [22], the authors have realized that the uncertainty in COVID-19 data present a fractal like pattern. Therefore, the epidemic representation curves have been evaluated as a fractal function and scanned for a new data that can be reflected for comparing various outbreaks or forecasts. In order to develop the public health care sectors, the fatal coronavirus growth rate and transitivity nature have been modelled and analyzed by the scientific executives through the emerging mathematical, statistical and technological methods such as fractals, modified SEIR model, random forest machine learning model, effective reproduction number, component analysis, Poisson regression, negative Binomial regression analysis and IoT frameworks [23]–[32].

The fundamental qualities of the transmissibility and the natural behaviour of the pathogen of COVID-19 are observed as obscure in this crisis period. In the current medical emergency, it is perceived that there is an uncertainty in coronavirus transmission and its crucial transmission can be interpreted as a fractal structure facilitating the scientific community in a superfluous comprehension to significantly aid in further surveying of different outbreaks and their progress. This study focus to provide feasible reconstruction of the epidemic curves based on the fractal interpolation function with variable scaling parameter to construct the predicted data. As a sample data, the daily positive and death cases of COVID-19 are taken for 100 days till 1st September 2020, in this similar approach, data can be taken during any time interval for the reconstruction process using the fractal interpolation functions. Consequently, the improvised generalized fractal dimensions spectra is computed for the predicted data, derived through the fractal interpolation function with the variable and constant scaling factors which estimate the accuracy of the prediction.

The rest of the chapter is sketched as follows: Section 7.2 elaborates the mathematical background of the fractal interpolation function with variable scaling factor and the procedure of improved generalized fractal dimensions. In Section 7.3, the clinical data information is explored briefly. The scientific results obtained for forecasting the transmission of COVID-19 is illustrated and the key inferences of the attained results are discussed intensely in Section 7.4. Finally, the concluding remarks with findings, contributions, future study and limitations are provided in Section 7.5.

7.2 Methods

This section describes the mathematical contextual of fractal interpolation function with the constant and variable scaling factors; and the improved generalized fractal dimensions to propose a combined fractal based prognostic model for examining the infectious nature of COVID-19.

7.2.1 Fractal Interpolation Function with Variable Scaling

The method of fractal interpolation with the variable scaling is presented in this section concisely. For more detailed discussions, the readers may see [33]–[43].

The COVID-19 data can be considered as a time series (t_n, y_n), where y_n denotes the number of confirmed positive cases or the number of confirmed death cases at the time t_n (in days). Thus, the present model investigates the prediction of y_n value corresponding to t_n. Since positive cases are commonly are encountered day by day in epidemic analysis, here time is regarded as in days. The fractal interpolation function (FIF) with the variable scaling factor is constructed as follows: $\{[t_0, t_N] \times \mathbb{R}; f_n : n \in \{0, 1, 2, \dots, N\}\}$, where

$$f_n \begin{pmatrix} t \\ y \end{pmatrix} = \begin{pmatrix} a_n & 0 \\ c_n & s_n(t) \end{pmatrix} \begin{pmatrix} t \\ y \end{pmatrix} + \begin{pmatrix} b_n \\ d_n \end{pmatrix} \tag{7.1}$$

and $s_n(t)$ is a continuous function from $[t_0, t_N]$ to $(-1, 1)$ for all $n \in \{1, 2, \dots, N\}$ such that $\|s_n\|_\infty = \sup\{|s_n(t)| : t \in [t_0, t_N]\} < 1$, $s_n(t)$ is known as variable scaling factor. In the given set of data points $\{(t_n, y_n) : n \in \{0, 1, 2, \dots, N\}\}$, f_n maps the endpoints to the endpoints. Thence, f_n maps (t_0, y_0) to (t_{n-1}, y_{n-1}) and image of (t_N, y_N) under the mapping f_n is (t_n, y_n) for each n. Hence, the mapping f_n obey the conditions.

$$f_n \begin{pmatrix} t_0 \\ y_0 \end{pmatrix} = \begin{pmatrix} t_{n-1} \\ y_{n-1} \end{pmatrix} \text{ and } f_n \begin{pmatrix} t_N \\ y_N \end{pmatrix} = \begin{pmatrix} t_n \\ y_n \end{pmatrix} \tag{7.2}$$

for all $n \in \{1, 2, \dots, N\}$. If s_n is predefined in the system of equations (12.1) with the condition (12.2), then the system (12.1) has a unique solution. Therefore, the constants a_n, b_n, c_n, d_n are estimated as follows

$$\begin{aligned} a_n &= \frac{t_n - t_{n-1}}{t_N - t_0}, \\ b_n &= \frac{t_N t_{n-1} - t_0 t_n}{t_N - t_0}, \\ c_n &= \frac{(y_n - y_{n-1}) - s_n(t_n)(y_N - y_0)}{t_N - t_0}, \\ d_n &= \frac{(t_N y_{n-1} - t_0 y_n) - s_n(t_n)(t_N y_0 - t_0 y_N)}{t_N - t_0}. \end{aligned} \tag{7.3}$$

If $s_n(t) = k$ for all $n \in \{1, 2, \ldots, N\}$, then the above construction gives the fractal interpolation function with the constant scaling factor. Here, the variable scaling factor $s_n(t)$ decides the flexibility and smoothness of the fractal curve more properly than the constant scaling factor s_n.

7.2.2 Improved Generalized Fractal Dimensions

The Improved Generalized Fractal Dimensions (IGFD) method is presented mathematically in this Section.

The probability distribution of a given Fractal Time Series is constructed to define IGFD as follows.

The total range of the Signal Time Series is divided into $N_V \times N_t$ bins (boxes) such that

$$N_V = \frac{V_{max} - V_{min}}{r} \quad \text{and} \quad N_t = \frac{t_{max} - t_{min}}{r}$$

where V_{max} & V_{min} are the maximum & the minimum values of the experimentally obtained data and t_{max} & t_{min} are the maximum & minimum time of the experimental period, respectively; and r is the uncertainty factor.

Now the probability that the signal passes through the ij^{th} bin (box) of size r is given by

$$p_{I_{ij}} = \lim_{N_V, N_t \to \infty} \frac{N_{ij}}{N_V \times N_t}, \tag{7.4}$$

$$i = 1, 2, ..., N_V \quad \text{and} \quad j = 1, 2, ..., N_t$$

where N_{ij} is the number of times the signal passes through the ij^{th} bin of size r.

Then, the *Improved Rényi Fractal Dimensions or Improved Generalized Fractal Dimensions (IGFD)* of order $q \in (-\infty, \infty)$ for the known probability distribution, denoted by ID_q, can be defined as

$$ID_q = \lim_{r \to 0} \frac{1}{q-1} \frac{log_2 \sum_{i=1}^{N_V} \sum_{j=1}^{N_t} p_{I_{ij}}^q}{log_2 r}. \tag{7.5}$$

Here ID_q is also defined in terms of generalized Rényi Entropy with the probability given in Eqn. (7.4). Eqn. (7.5) is called the Improved form of the Generalized Fractal Dimensions.

7.3 Clinical Data

The World Health Organization has reported that the total number of confirmed positive cases is 2,57,19,569 and the total number of confirmed death cases is 8,56,275 globally as of 1st September 2020; and a total of 216 countries are affected by COVID-19 [7]. In this present study, we have considered the time series of confirmed positive and death cases for the countries the USA, Brazil and India to analyze the COVID-19 diffusion process. Meanwhile, the USA recorded 62,17,573 infected cases, Brazil registered 39,08,272 infected cases and the disease has since affected 37,33,936 people in India. The infectious disease has killed 1,87,891 people in the USA, 1,21,381 people enlisted in Brazil and 65,922 individuals in India [7, 56, 57]. The total number of confirmed infected cases, death cases, recovered cases are given in "Our World in Data"[57]. Since the USA, Brazil and India are the most affected nations among 216 countries; hence we have considered USA, Brazil and India for prediction analysis.

The datasets used in this study are obtained from the Center for Systems Science and Engineering (CSSE) at Johns Hopkins University [56] and "Our World in Data"[57]. It comprises of 2 separate time series data of daily confirmed positive and death cases of COVID-19 in each of the three representative countries and world during the above mentioned period. All the datasets are processed in MATLAB software with the recent version for predicting the data with future scope. The graphical representation of the epidemic curves with the daily infected and daily death cases are plotted against the number of days. The daily confirmed positive cases and the daily confirmed death cases of COVID-19 are graphically illustrated in Figure 7.1(a) and Figure 7.1(b) respectively. The uncertainty of the data occurred in COVID-19 infected and death are observed in Figure 7.1.

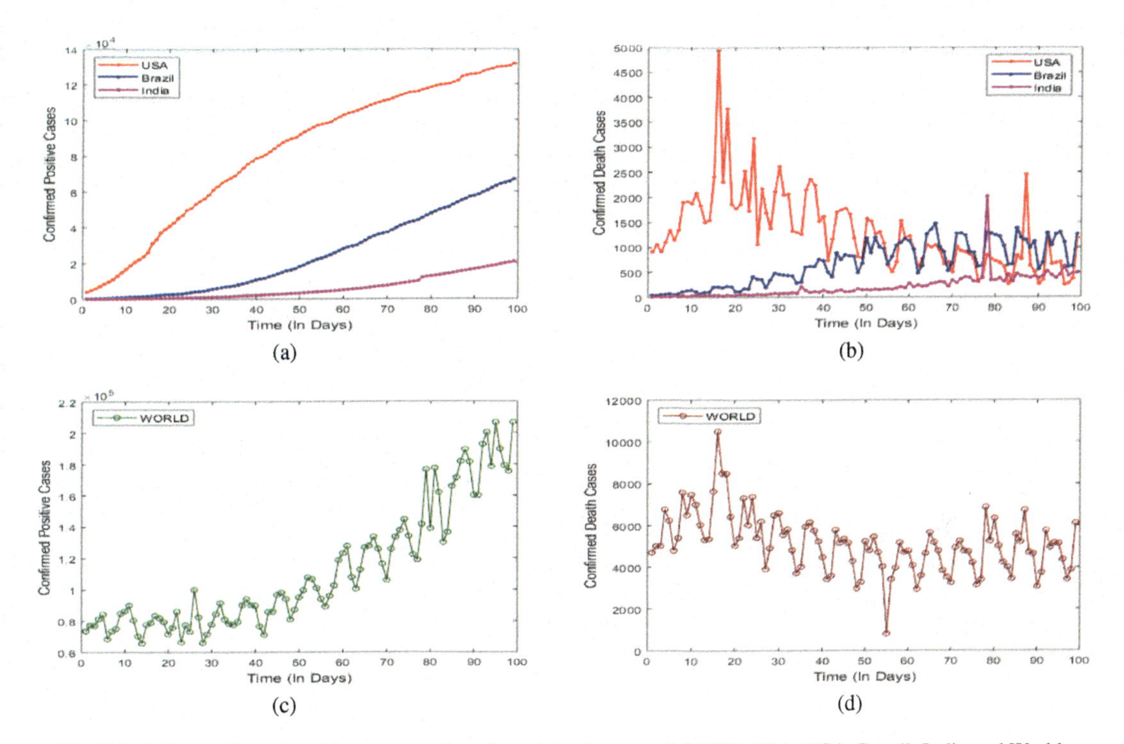

Fig. 7.1: Daily confirmed positive cases and confirmed death cases of COVID-19 in USA, Brazil, India and World.

7.4 Results and Discussion

The proposed research work focused on the combined method of fractal functions and multifractal dimensions to precisely analyze the uncertainty and to predict the infected and death rates for the near future. Figure 7.2 portrays the predicted values interpolated by the fractal interpolation method with the variable scaling versus the original values of the daily confirmed positive cases of USA, Brazil, India and the world. Whereas, Figure 7.3 depicts the result of the predicted values through the fractal interpolation with the constant scaling versus the original values of the daily infected cases of the specified countries and the worldwide cases. By comparing the graphs represented in Figure 7.2 and Figure 7.3, some noteworthy qualitative inferences can be taken up. In the predicted curve for each of the countries, there are some degree of self-similarity and smoothness in variable scaling, however the sharp peaks are available more in the case of constant scaling factor. Similarly, Figure 7.3 describes the forecasted data interpolated by the fractal interpolation with the variable scaling versus the original data of the daily confirmed death cases of USA, Brazil, India and the overall global cases. Additionally, Figure 7.5 outlines the expected data by the fractal interpolation with the constant scaling versus the original data of the death cases for the representative countries and the global deaths per day. Aside, from that the assessment between Figure 7.3 and Figure 7.5 narrates that the predicted death curve through the fractal interpolation function with the variable scaling factor has more smoothness than the constant scaling factor. Accordingly, the variable scaling factor controls the noisy peaks and precisely predicts the transmission of the outbreak of this harmful virus.

In Figure 7.5, the IGFD spectra between the predicted daily confirmed positive cases through the fractal interpolation function with the variable and the constant scaling factors are demonstrated as well. Also, the graphical depiction of the improved generalized fractal spectra of the predicted data obtained by the fractal interpolation function with the variable scaling and the constant scaling for daily infected cases against the order of the exponent are elucidated in Figure 7.7. The comparative analysis between the graphs in Figure 7.5 as well as Figure 7.7 conspicuously shows that the improved generalized fractal spectra (ID_q)

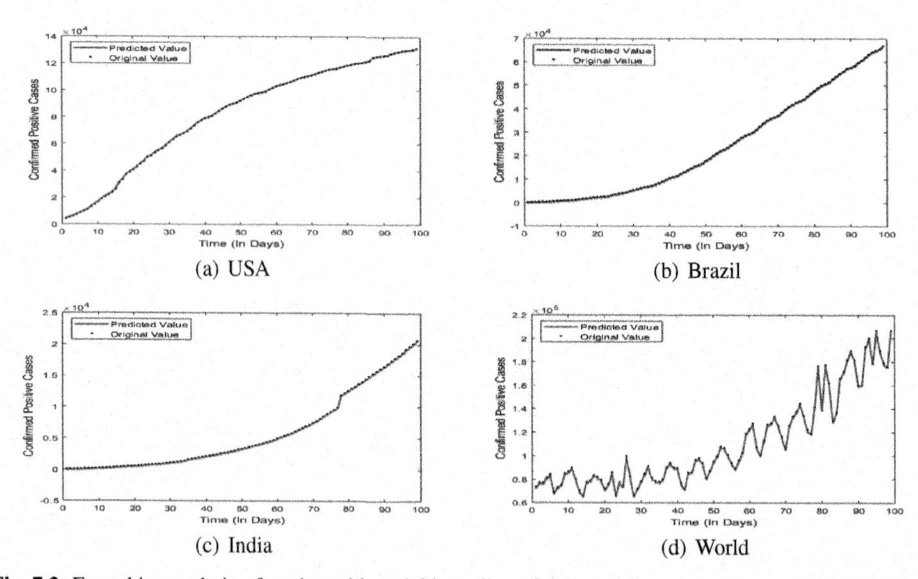

Fig. 7.2: Fractal interpolation function with variable scaling of daily confirmed positive cases of COVID-19.

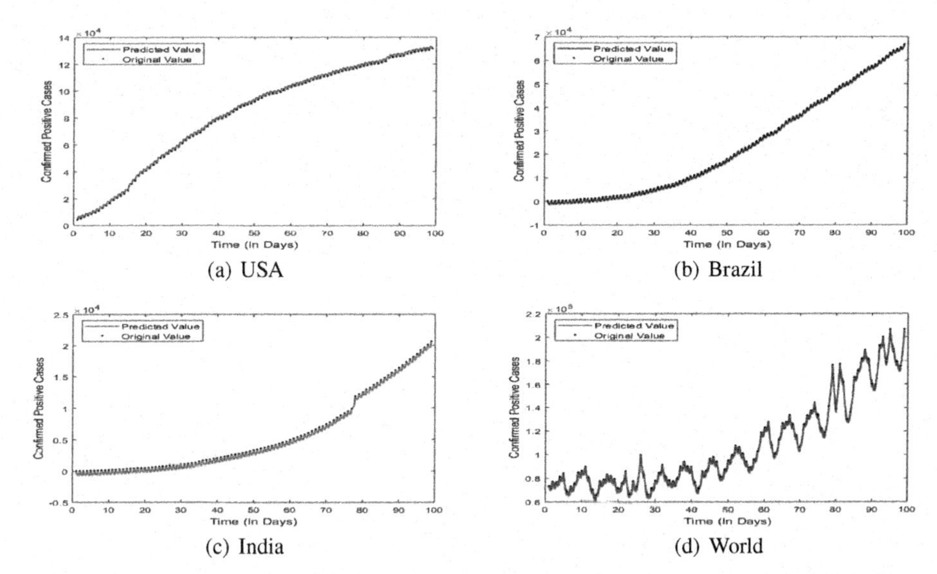

(a) USA (b) Brazil

(c) India (d) World

Fig. 7.3: Fractal interpolation function with constant scaling of daily confirmed positive cases of COVID-19.

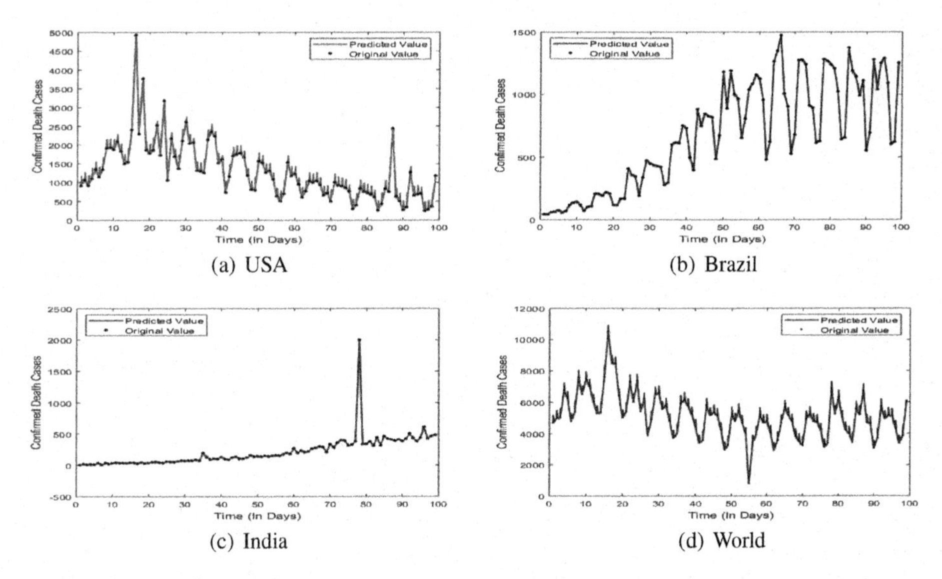

(a) USA (b) Brazil

(c) India (d) World

Fig. 7.4: Fractal interpolation function with variable scaling of daily confirmed death cases of COVID-19.

for predicted values corresponding to the variable scaling of both the infected and the death cases are higher than the predicted values with respect to the constant scaling factor for all orders of the exponent q. This demonstrates that the fractal interpolation function with the variable scaling factors has significantly predicted the irregularity of the COVID-19 data and it is more flexible than the constant scaling factor category.

A few key characteristics of the pandemic spread and the natural behavior of the coronavirus are currently unclear. For instance; How many secondary infections are possible from the infected person? How long will the infectious stage last? As the number of positive cases keeps increasing daily and is quite irregular,

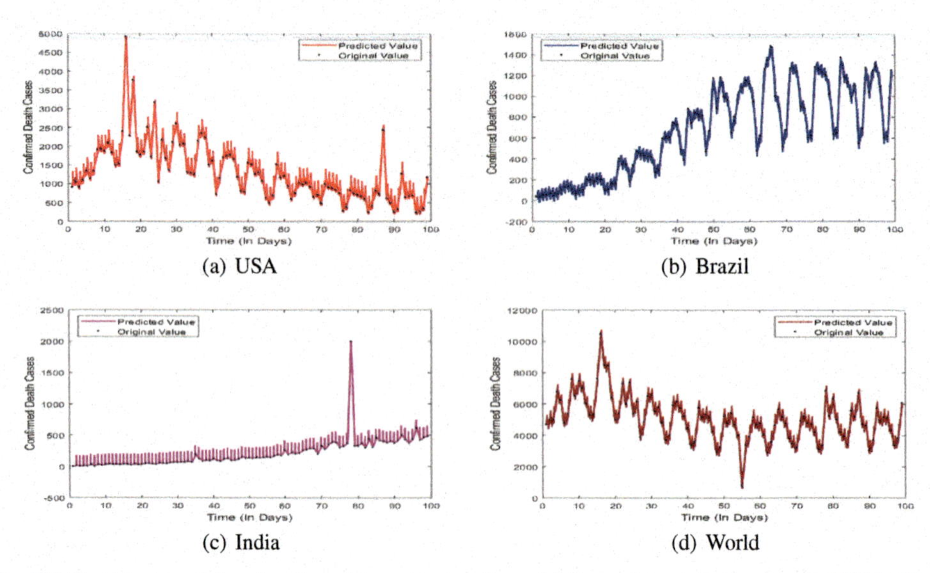

Fig. 7.5: Fractal interpolation function with constant scaling of daily confirmed death cases of COVID-19.

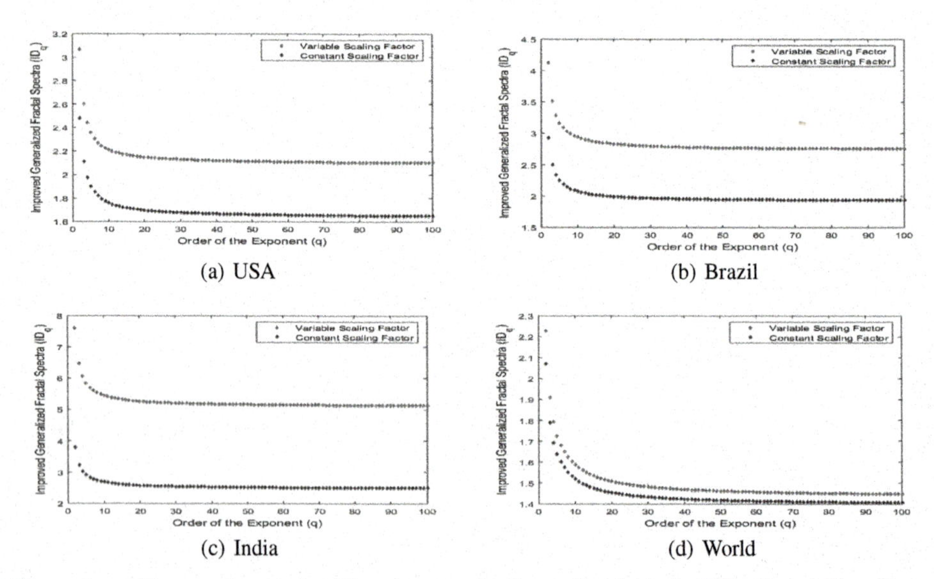

Fig. 7.6: Comparison of improved generalized fractal spectra for the predicted data by FIF with variable and constant scaling factors of daily confirmed positive cases.

there is an uncertainty in the COVID-19 transmission rate. Henceforth, the spread of the epidemic can be considered as a fractal like time series. The proposed fractal perspective on the transmission of the pandemic may uncover the significant method for foretelling the progress of the disease. The epidemic curves presented in Figure 7.1 noticeably possess roughness and some kind of self-similar pattern, which substantiate the

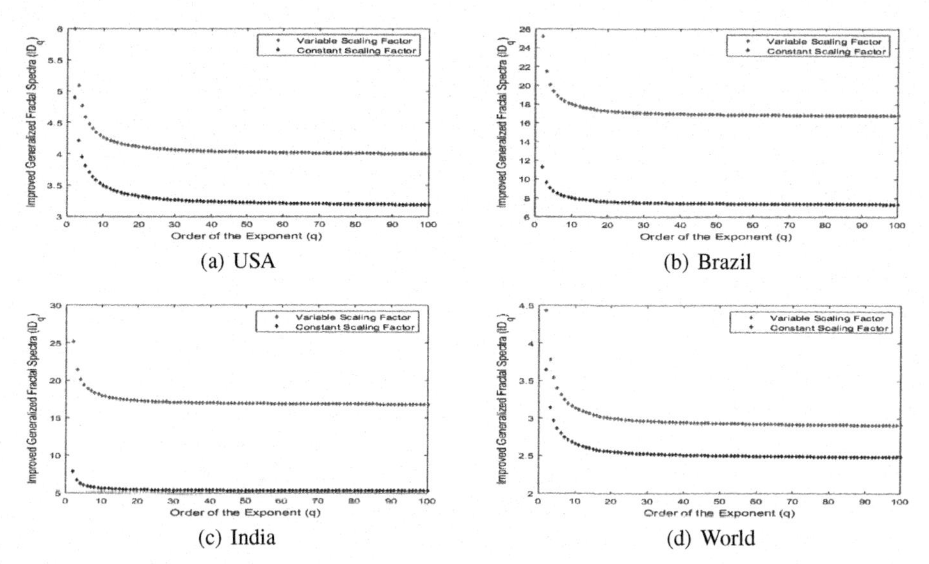

Fig. 7.7: Comparison of improved generalized fractal spectra for the predicted data by FIF with variable and constant scaling factors of daily confirmed death cases.

interpretation of this study. Also, this kind of similarity plays a vital role in measuring the present situation and predicting the upcoming progressions in the epidemic curves.

Though, the epidemiological curve is viewed as a fractal and figured it as the aftereffect of fractal interpolation, the powerful methods for reproducing or predicting bits of information have not been reported concretely. In this regard, we have to underline that the number of cases reported is exceptionally reliant on the quantity of tests performed by every nation on a specific day. Investigating the information utilized from the fractal interpolation; a few bits of the daily increasing information might be missing to show the signs of improvement in the pandemic [24]. It is clearly noticed that this study is differed in terms of choosing the scale factor. The comparison between the obtained results represented in Figure 7.2–Figure 7.5 indicate that the flexibility and versatility gained by extending the usual fractal interpolation function with the constant scaling to the fractal interpolation with the variable scaling parameter.

Moreover, the epidemic curves are predicted by assuming the variable scaling factor as $s_n(t) = \sin(1/t)$ and fixing the constant scaling factor as $s_n = 0.1$ for all n. Hence, if the comparison is made by means of IGFD spectra of the epidemic curves, then the similar results are acquired because of the scaling parameter. Here, COVID-19 data has been considered as a fractal time series during the prescribed period. Moreover, the improved generalized fractal dimensions of COVID-19 time series are computed and we have done the comparative study between two types of scaling factors. Further, the comparative results in Figure 7.5 and Figure 7.7 demonstrates that the fractal interpolation function with the variable scaling parameter predicted the number of infected cases and the number of daily deaths significantly more than the constant scaling factor.

7.5 Conclusion

The fundamental qualities of the transmissibility and the natural behaviour of the pathogen of COVID-19 are observed as obscure in this crisis period. Since it is perceived as an uncertainty in coronavirus transmission; the current diffusion process can be a considered as a fractal. Hence, the proposed research work focuses on the combined method of fractal functions and multifractal dimensions to precisely analyze the uncertainty and to predict the infected and the death rates of COVID-19. Based on the predicted results in this study, the control measures can be taken up by the public health care services and systems to control the deadly virus diffusion in order to attain the sustainable environment in the world.

The increasing number of infected cases and deaths of the pandemic demands a continuous data analysis, so that the dynamical behavior of the pathogen can be understandable and it leads us towards the controllability of the epidemic growth. Hence, this research explored the integrated fractal based prognostic model for COVID-19 pandemic by dealing the currently available data. However, the prediction of the confirmed cases of the infectious disease is liable to change in general, if an extensive amount of data is available and in such a scenario, the rudiments of outbreak prevention, testing, tracking and treating must be concentrated. This study demonstrated the combined fractal based framework for the epidemic curves prediction or reproduction and illustrated the roughness and statistical self-similar patterns behind the epidemic curves. One can understand that the present situation requires the forecasting techniques to estimate the upcoming progress of the epidemic data with respect to the fractal self-similar designs. Also, the forthcoming trends of the epidemic curve can be easily anticipated when the future value in a particular day is estimated by applying statistical measures on the currently available data. Along these pipelines, future directions can explore forecasting techniques to access the infection rate of the epidemic, based on the fractals with fuzzy and probabilistic measures.

References

[1] Palayew, A., O. Norgaard, K. Safreed-Harmon, T.H. Andersen, L.N. Rasmussen and J.V. Lazarus. 2020. Pandemic publishing poses a new COVID-19 challenge. Nature Human Behaviour. https://doi.org/10.1038/s41562-020-0911-0

[2] Zhao, S., Q. Lin, J. Ran, S.S. Musa, G. Yang, W. Wang, Y. Lou, D. Gao, L. Yang, D. He and M.H. Wang. 2020. Preliminary estimation of the basic reproduction number of novel coronavirus (2019-nCoV) in China, from 2019 to 2020: A data-driven analysis in the early phase of the outbreak. International Journal of Infectious Diseases 92: 214–217.

[3] Yuana, J., M. Lib, L. Gang and Z.K. Lu. 2020. Monitoring transmissibility and mortality of COVID-19 in Europe. International Journal of Infectious Diseases, 95: 311–315.

[4] Marimuthu, S., M. Joy, B. Malavika, A. Nadaraj, E.S. Asirvatham and L. Jeyaseelan. 2020. Modelling of reproduction number for COVID-19 in India and high incidence states. Clinical Epidemiology and Global Health. https://doi.org/10.1016/j.cegh.2020.06.012.

[5] Hellewell, J., S. Abbott, A. Gimma, N.I. Bosse, C.I. Jarvis, T.E. Russell, J.D. Munday, A.J. Kucharski, W.J. Edmunds, F. Sun and S. Flasche. 2020. Feasibility of controlling COVID-19 outbreaks by isolation of cases and contacts. The Lancet Global Health, 8(4): 488–496.

[6] Arino, J. and S. Portet. 2020. A simple model for COVID-19. Infectious Disease Modelling 5: 309–315.

[7] World Health Organization. https://covid19.who.int/.

[8] Benvenuto, D., M. Giovanetti, L. Vassallo, S. Angeletti and M. Ciccozzi. 2020. Application of the ARIMA model on the COVID-2019 epidemic dataset. Data in Brief, 29: 105340.

[9] Mishra, B.K., A.K. Keshri, Y.S. Rao, B.K. Mishra, B. Mahato, S. Ayesha and A.K. Singh. 2020. COVID-19 created chaos across the globe: Three novel quarantine epidemic models. Chaos, Solitons & Fractals, 138: 109928.
[10] Djilali, S. and B. Ghanbari. 2020. Coronavirus pandemic: A predictive analysis of the peak outbreak epidemic in South Africa, Turkey, and Brazil. Chaos, Solitons & Fractals, 138: 109971.
[11] Mandelbrot, B.B. 1983. The Fractal Geometry of Nature. W.H. Freeman and Company, New York.
[12] Barnsley, M. 1993. Fractals Everywhere. Second ed., Academic Press, USA.
[13] Santo, B., M.K. Hassan, M. Sayan and A. Gowrisankar. 2019. Fractal Patterns in Nonlinear Dynamics and Applications, CRC Press.
[14] Sharma, M., R.B. Pachori and U. Rajendra Acharya. 2017. A new approach to characterize epileptic seizures using analytic time-frequency flexible wavelet transform and fractal dimension. Pattern Recognition Letters, 94: 172–179.
[15] Sharma, M. and R.B. Pachori. 2017. A novel approach to detect epileptic seizures using a combination of tunable-Q wavelet transform and fractal dimension. Journal of Mechanics in Medicine and Biology, 17(7): 1740003.
[16] Gupta, V. and R.B. Pachori. 2019. Epileptic seizure identification using entropy of FBSE based EEG rhythms. Biomedical Signal Processing and Control, 53: 101569.
[17] Fatimah, B., P. Singh, A. Singhal and R.B. Pachori. 2020. Detection of apnea events from ECG segments using Fourier decomposition method. Biomedical Signal Processing and Control, 61: 102005.
[18] Gupta, V. and R.B. Pachori. 2020. Classification of focal EEG signals using FBSE based flexible time-frequency coverage wavelet transform. Biomedical Signal Processing and Control, 62: 102124.
[19] Grassberger, P. 1983. Generalized dimensions of strange attractors. Physics Letters A, 97: 227–320.
[20] Hentschel, H.G.E. and I. Procaccia. 1983. The infinite number of generalized dimensions of fractals and strange attractors. Physica 8D, 8(3):435–444.
[21] Uthayakumar, R. and A. Gowrisankar. 2016. Mid-sagittal plane detection in magnetic resonance image based on multifractal techniques. IET Image Processing, 10(10): 751–762.
[22] Cristina-Maria, P. and N. Bogdan-Radu. 2020. An analysis of COVID-19 spread based on fractal interpolation and fractal dimension. Chaos, Solitons and Fractals, 139: 110073.
[23] Liu, M., J. Ning, Y. Du, J. Cao, D. Zhang, J. Wang and M. Chen. 2020. Modelling the evolution trajectory of COVID-19 in Wuhan, China: Experience and suggestions. Public Health, 183: 76–80.
[24] Massimo Materassi. 2020. Some fractal thoughts about the COVID-19 infection outbreak. Chaos, Solitons and Fractals: X, 4: 100032.
[25] Abdon Atangana. 2020. Modelling the spread of COVID-19 with new fractal-fractional operators: Can the lockdown save mankind before vaccination? Chaos, Solitons and Fractals, 136: 109860.
[26] Gowrisankar, A., R. Lamberto and B. Santo. 2020. Can India develop herd immunity against COVID-19? The European Physical Journal Plus, 135: 526.
[27] Cobb, J.S. and M.A. Seale. 2020. Examining the effect of social distancing on the compound growth rate of COVID-19 at the county level (United States) using statistical analyses and a random forest machine learning model. Public Health, 185: 27–29.
[28] Das, A. 2020. An approximation-based approach for periodic estimation of effective reproduction number: A tool for decision-making in the context of coronavirus disease 2019 (COVID-19) outbreak. Public Health, 185: 199–201.
[29] Youa, C., Y. Dengb, W. Hub, J. Sunb, Q. Linb, F. Zhouc, C.H. Pangd, Y. Zhange, Z. Chenf and X.H. Zhoua. 2020. Estimation of the time-varying reproduction number of COVID-19 outbreak in China. International Journal of Hygiene and Environmental Health, 228: 113555.

[30] Das, A., S. Ghosh, K. Das, T. Basu, M. Das and I. Dutta. 2020. Modeling the effect of area deprivation on COVID-19 incidences: A study of Chennai megacity, India. Public Health, 185: 266–269.
[31] Oztig, L.I. and O.E. Askin. 2020. Human mobility and COVID-19: A negative binomial regression. Public Health. https://doi.org/10.1016/j.puhe.2020.07.002.
[32] Otoom, M., N. Otoum, M.A. Alzubaidi, Y. Etoom and R. Banihani. 2020. An IoT-based framework for early identification and monitoring of COVID-19 cases. Biomedical Signal Processing and Control, 62: 102149.
[33] Barnsley, M.F. 1986. Fractal functions and interpolation. Constructive Approximation, 2(1): 303–329.
[34] Wang, H.Y. and J.S. Yu. 2013. Fractal interpolation functions with variable parameters and their analytical properties. Journal of Approximation Theory, 175: 1–8.
[35] Yong-Shun Liang. 2019. Progress on estimation of fractal dimensions of fractional calculus of continuous functions. Fractals, 27(5): 1950084.
[36] Maria Vasilieva, Ilie Vasiliev, Irina Vasilieva and Stanislav Groppa. 2022. Recurrence of COVID-19 infection with meningitis without pulmonary involvement. Clin. Neurophysiol., 141: 53.
[37] Vasilieva, M., Vasiliev, Vasilieva and S. Groppa. 2022. TU-237. Recurrence of COVID-19 infection with meningitis without pulmonary involvement. Clinical Neurophysiology: Official Journal of the International Federation of Clinical Neurophysiology, 41: S53–S53.
[38] Raghavendra Rao, M.M. Karindas, Ilie Vasiliev, Chennamchetty Vijay Kumar, Hitesh Lakshmi Billa, Dilip Mathai, Manick Dass and Mahendra Kumar Verma. International Journal of Current Medical and Pharmaceutical Research, 8: 294–300.
[39] Punam Kumari, P., A. Gowrisankar, A. Saha and Santo Banerjee. 2020. Dynamical properties and fractal patterns of nonlinear waves in solar wind plasma. Physica Scripta, 95(6): 065603.
[40] Fataf, N.A.A., A. Gowrisankar and B. Santo. 2020. In search of self-similar chaotic attractors based on fractal function with variable scaling. Physica Scripta, 95(7): 075206.
[41] Gowrisankar, A. and R. Uthayakumar. 2016. Fractional calculus on fractal interpolation function for a sequence of data with countable iterated function system. Mediterranean Journal of Mathematics, 13(6): 3887–3906.
[42] Katiyar, S.K., A.K.B. Chand and G. Saravana Kumar. 2019. A new class of rational cubic spline fractal interpolation function and its constrained aspects. Applied Mathematics and Computation, 346: 319–335.
[43] Gowrisankar, A. and M.G.P. Prasad. 2019. Riemann-Liouville calculus on quadratic fractal interpolation function with variable scaling factors. The Journal of Analysis, 27(2): 347–363.
[44] Easwaramoorthy, D. and R. Uthayakumar. 2011. Improved generalized fractal dimensions in the discrimination between healthy and epileptic EEG signals. Journal of Computational Science, 2(1): 31–38.
[45] Uthayakumar, R. and D. Easwaramoorthy. 2012. Multifractal-wavelet based denoising in the classification of healthy and epileptic EEG signals. Fluctuation and Noise Letters, 11(4): 1250034.
[46] Uthayakumar, R. and D. Easwaramoorthy. 2012. Multifractal analysis in denoising of color images. Proceedings of the International Conference on Emerging Trends in Science, Engineering and Technology, IEEE Xplore Digital Library, IEEE, USA, 228–234.
[47] Uthayakumar, R. and D. Easwaramoorthy. 2013. Epileptic seizure detection in EEG signals using multifractal analysis and wavelet transform. Fractals, 21(2): 1350011.
[48] Uthayakumar, R. and D. Easwaramoorthy. 2014. Fuzzy generalized fractal dimensions for chaotic waveforms, chaos, complexity and leadership 2012. Springer Proceedings in Complexity, 411–422.

[49] Easwaramoorthy, D., P.S. Eliahim Jeevaraj, A. Gowrisankar, A. Manimaran and S. Nandhini. 2018. Fuzzy generalized fractal dimensions using inter-heartbeat interval dynamics in ECG signals for age related discrimination. International Journal of Engineering and Technology (UAE), 7(4.10): 900–903.

[50] Nandhini, S., D. Easwaramoorthy and R. Abinands. 2020. An extensive review on recent evolutions in object detection algorithms. International Journal of Emerging Trends in Engineering Research, 8(7): 3766–3776.

[51] Santo Banerjee, D. Easwaramoorthy and A. Gowrisankar. 2021. Fractal Functions, Dimensions and Signal Analysis. Understanding Complex Systems, Springer: Complexity, Springer, Cham.

[52] Easwaramoorthy, D., A. Gowrisankar, A. Manimaran, S. Nandhini, Lamberto Rondoni and Santo Banerjee. 2021. An exploration of fractal-based prognostic model and comparative analysis for second wave of COVID-19 diffusion. Nonlinear Dynamics.

[53] Qiusheng Rong, C. Thangaraj, D. Easwaramoorthy and Shaobo He. 2021. Multifractal based image processing for estimating the complexity of COVID-19 dynamics. The European Physical Journal Special Topics, 230(21-22): 3947–3954.

[54] Shaobo He, C. Thangaraj, D. Easwaramoorthy and G. Muhiuddin. 2022. Multifractal analysis on age-based discrimination in X-Ray images for sensing the severity of COVID-19 disease. The European Physical Journal Special Topics.

[55] Thangaraj, C. and D. Easwaramoorthy. 2022. Generalized fractal dimensions based comparison analysis of edge detection methods in CT images for estimating the infection of COVID-19 disease. The European Physical Journal Special Topics.

[56] Center for Systems Science and Engineering (CSSE) at Johns Hopkins University. https://systems.jhu.edu/research/public-health/ncov-model-2/.

[57] Our World in Data. https://ourworldindata.org/coronavirus.

Chapter 8

A Mathematical Model for COVID-19 Pandemic with the Impact of Economic Development

Jayanta Mondal,[1] *Subhas Khajanchi*[2,*] and *Md Nasim Akhtar*[2]

8.1 Introduction

Coronavirus disease 2019 (COVID-19) emerged in Wuhan, China as global healthcare concern. Due to its high transmission ability via aerosol, and due to lack of a specific treatment in the early stage of the COVID-19 Alpha variant pandemic a significant number of people have been infected. Upon recognition of the coronavirus (SARS-CoV-2) in 2019, laboratories throughout the world started to perform research on the pathogen and the disease to investigate its transmissibility, pathogen survivability and transport. In the year 2020, a Nature review delineated the exponential increase in research articles associated to COVID-19, as well as the trends in topics [1]. The review report showed that the research on epidemic modeling and its control the spread of the disease initially outpaced research on diagnostics and testing, public health. At the beginning, highly cited articles exhibited the proof of person-to-person transmission, medical characteristics of infected individuals, and transmission stemming from asymptomatic individuals [2–5]. The transmission became increasingly well-known as the dominant mechanism of contagion, modeling efforts pivoted towards better understanding incubation periods, aerosol survivability, and reproduction numbers; these observations were geared towards comprehending the outbreak of novel coronavirus and mechanisms for reduction casualties [6–9]. Due to the variable characteristics of COVID-19 in these early days and no modern pandemic to act as a foundational case study, model parameters and considerations were missing and not well defined, which could have resulted in additional uncertainties around results.

These problems have become additionally pronounced in the context of the present coronavirus pandemic, which, since being unprecedented in many aspects, underlines the necessity to expand the commonly used epidemiological models. Progress has been made in various directions, for example, by considering the effects of quarantine [10], temporary immunity [11], vaccination or medication [12], different levels of population susceptibility [13], stratification by age [14], competitive virus strains of various severity and transmissibility [15, 16] and media-related awareness [17] and so on. Particularly, the attempts to fight the disease led to the incorporation of contact-tracing, social distancing quantifies the scales hardly imaginable. While it is clear

[1] Department of Mathematics, Diamond Harbour Women's University, Sarisha, West Bengal 743368, India.
[2] Department of Mathematics, Presidency University, 86/1 College Street, Kolkata 700073, India.
* Corresponding author: subhas.maths@presiuniv.ac.in

that they have an impact on the epidemiological dynamic, their affects are not yet well defined [18], despite a lot of undergoing effort to introduction the impact of these measures into the existing epidemiological models [19, 20]. Common for all these extensions of epidemiological models are depending on numerical illustrations to determine the relations among independent variables and some epidemiological outputs.

While the superiority of the theoretical methods are clear, all of the investigated models in epidemiology, incorporating the basic ones such as SIR (Susceptible-Infected-Removed) [21] are nonlinear and the associated ordinary differential equations cannot be solved in an easy method. Over the last two decades, there was a substantial improvement in the field. To the best of our knowledge, the earliest progresses in this direction appeared with the turn of the century and were related to the SIR model, on network approach [22] and its stochasticity [23], followed by solutions given in the forms of convergent series, for SIR [21] and then also for SIR and SIS (Susceptible-Infected-Susceptible) models. Further development was made by Harko et al. [24], by providing the SIR model analytical solutions, albeit in parametric form and up to an integral inexpressible by elementary functions. Recently, there has been also some progress even with compartmental models more complex than the basic SIR variant.

A significant amount of research, clinical and analytical investigations have been done to better comprehend the dynamics of novel coronavirus and its consequences, and investigate more effective intervention policies [25, 26]. In particular, various mathematical and statistical models have been investigated to understand the transmission and spread of novel coronavirus [27, 28], and their vaccination or medication [29–32]. In the meantime, a number of computational and quantitative investigations, have taken into account to study the influence novel coronavirus on the economic progression. As for example, in [33] the authors statistically determined the role of SARS-CoV-2 pandemic on the economy for different countries. Chen et al. [34] studied a network-related epidemic-economic model to estimate the straightforward role of daily labour in each sector appearing from morbidity, mortality as well as lockdown. Altig et al. [35] studied various economic uncertainty indicators for the US and UK before and during the SARS-CoV-2 epidemic. Jena et al. [36] constructed a multilayer artificial neural network-based model to predict the role of novel coronavirus on the GDP of eight different countries including the United States. Xiang et al.[37] amalgamated the theory of economic with an epidemiological model to investigate the long-run role of epidemic on economic progression and the influences of various strategies.

Herein, we investigate a mathematical model to measure the impact of economic development/progression on the transmission dynamics of novel coronavirus that interplay among epidemic outbreak, socio-economic development and the disease management. We have taken into account both the symptomatic and asymptomatic infected individuals in our study, and include the effectiveness of disease control into the respective transmission rates. In the meantime, the factors related with economic development and epidemiology are both incorporated into our proposed model, in which the level of epidemic reduction is highly negatively correlated with the progression of the economic. Moreover, the development of the epidemic and the evolution of the susceptible, infectious and recovered individuals explicitly influences the mitigation and the level of economic development.

The article is organized in the following way. In Section 2, we develop our COVID-19 model with the effect of economic progression under some restrictions. In the next section, we performed basic properties of the mathematical model including boundedness, biologically feasible equilibrium points and their local and global stability analysis. In the same section, we calculate the basic reproduction number by using next generation matrix method. Section 4 explore the extensive numerical simulations of our theoretical findings Finally, in Section 5, we conclude our findings with limitations.

8.2 Mathematical Model

In this section, we formulate a mathematical model for the COVID-19 pandemic by a system of coupled nonlinear ordinary differential equations. We classify the total population into four distinct classes, namely susceptible (S), exposed (A), symptomatic infected (I), and the recovered (R) individuals. A typical characteristics of SARS-CoV-2 is that the asymptomatic and pre-symptomatic infection is common [5], thus the infected population can be contagious even during the latent period. Therefore, we considered that the exposed individuals are capable of transmitting the disease; basically, they are regarded as pre-symptomatic infectious individuals in our investigation. To introduce the effect of mitigation strategies on economic progression, we incorporate two additional components, namely the mitigation level/ effectiveness, denoted by P, and the economic progression level, described by E. We normalize the range of P in such a way that $0 \leq P \leq 1$, where $P = 1$ describing the condition with maximum disease control and $P = 0$ the condition with no disease control at all. In similar way, we normalize E in the range between 0 and 1 where $E = 1$ represents the maximum level of economic progression and $E = 0$ represents the bad situation of economic progression. We consider that the disease transmission rates are modulated by the disease control, that the mitigation level is stimulated by the disease prevalence, and that the economic progression level depends rely the available labour supply. We additionally consider that the disease mitigation level and economic progression level are negatively correlated. Based on the schematic diagram (see Figure 8.1), we have constructed the mathematical model for COVID-19 with special emphasized on economic development. Our epidemic-economic model for COVID-19 transmission model is represented by the following system of ordinary differential equations, with parameters nomenclature are specified in the Table 8.1:

$$
\begin{aligned}
\frac{dS}{dt} &= \Lambda - (\beta_A A + \beta_I I)\frac{S}{1+\theta P} - \delta S,\\
\frac{dA}{dt} &= (\beta_A A + \beta_I I)\frac{S}{1+\theta P} - (\rho + \sigma + \delta)A,\\
\frac{dI}{dt} &= \rho A - (\omega + \mu + \delta)I,\\
\frac{dR}{dt} &= \mu I + \sigma A - \delta R,\\
\frac{dP}{dt} &= \alpha I - d_p P - h_e E,\\
\frac{dE}{dt} &= \theta_s S + \theta_a A + \theta_r R - d_e E - f_p P.
\end{aligned}
\tag{8.1}
$$

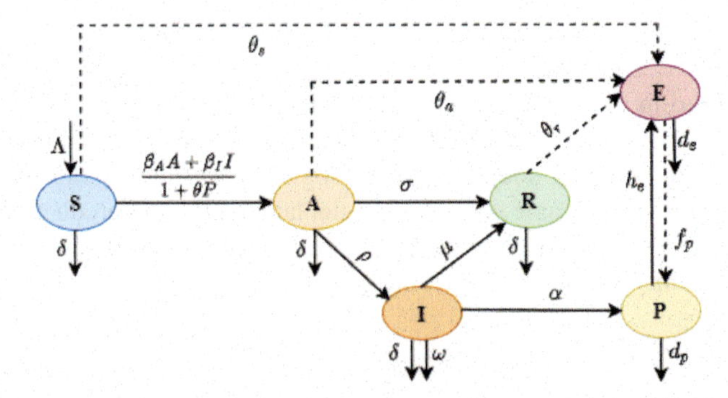

Fig. 8.1: Schematic diagram of the mathematical model for the transmission dynamics of the novel coronavirus.

The last two equations of the model (8.1) represents the negative correlation among the level of mitigation and the level of economic progression, that is if we increase one variable it would tend to decrease the other. This supposition has been influenced by empirical observations of the epidemic management. Particularly, under the influence of novel coronavirus, the gross domestic product (GDP) in the first quarter of 2020 experienced a mitigation of nearly 5% from the preceding quarter, and the second quarter GDP plunged nearly 32%. Such mitigation was greatly due to the closure of businesses, implementation of stay-at-home orders, and other pandemic policies that begun in March 2020 and extended to May/June 2020. To perform the model analysis we have taken the parameters from the existing real-life data and literature.

8.3 Mathematical Analysis

In order to determine a feasible region for the model system (8.1) we now added the first four equations in the $SAIRPE$ model (8.1), and we obtain

$$S + A + I + R \leq \frac{\Lambda}{\delta}. \tag{8.2}$$

Again we added first two equations from the model system (8.1) and we get

$$S + A \geq \frac{\Lambda}{\rho + \sigma + \delta}. \tag{8.3}$$

Next, we take some conditions to verify $0 \leq P \leq 1$ and $0 \leq E \leq 1$. For $P \geq 0$, we need $(dP)/(dt) \geq 0$, when $P = 0$. This yields $\alpha I - h_e E \geq 0$, which satisfies for all $I \geq 0$ and $E \leq 1$ if

$$\alpha \frac{\Lambda}{\delta} - h_e \geq 0. \tag{8.4}$$

Again, $P \leq 0$, we need $(dP)/(dt) \leq 0$, when $P = 1$. This leads to $\alpha I - d_p - h_e E \leq 0$, which satisfies for all $I \leq \Lambda/\delta$ and $E \geq 0$ if

$$\alpha \frac{\Lambda}{\delta} - d_p \leq 0. \tag{8.5}$$

With the same process, we can established certain $E \geq 0$ if

$$\theta_m \frac{\Lambda}{\rho + \sigma + \delta} - f_p \geq 0, \quad \text{where } \theta_m = \min\{\theta_s, \theta_a, \theta_r\}, \tag{8.6}$$

by using condition (8.3), and ensure $E \leq 1$ if

$$\theta_M \frac{\Lambda}{\delta} - d_e \leq 0, \quad \text{where } \theta_M = \max\{\theta_s, \theta_a, \theta_r\}, \tag{8.7}$$

by using condition (8.2).

Thus, the above conditions (8.2)–(8.7), the biologically significant domain

$$\Pi = \{(S, A, I, R, P, E) : S, A, I, R \geq 0, S + A + I + R \leq \frac{\Lambda}{\delta}, 0 \leq P \leq 1, 0 \leq E \leq 1\}. \tag{8.8}$$

Therefore, Π is invariant Set with respect to the vector field of $SAIRPE$ model (8.1).

Noticeably, the model system (8.1) have unique disease free equilibrium as follows

$$\Phi_0 = (S_0, 0, 0, 0, 0, 0, 0) = (\Lambda/\delta, 0, 0, 0, 0, 0, 0)$$

Using disease free equilibrium point, the basic reproduction number of the $SAIRPE$ model (8.1) based on the next generation matrix method calculated in [38].

Let $x_0 = (A, I)^T$, then model system (8.1) we can be written as

$$\frac{dx}{dt} = \mathcal{G}(x) - \mathcal{H}(x),$$

where,

$$\mathcal{G}(x) = \begin{pmatrix} \frac{\beta_A SA}{1+\theta P} + \frac{\beta_I SI}{1+\theta P} \\ 0 \end{pmatrix}, \quad \mathcal{H}(x) = \begin{pmatrix} \rho + \sigma + \delta \\ -\rho A + \omega + \mu + \delta \end{pmatrix}$$

The Jacobian matrices of $\mathcal{G}$ and $\mathcal{H}$ at DFE $\Phi_0(S_0, 0, 0, 0, 0, 0)$ are given respectively,

$$G = \begin{pmatrix} \beta_A S_0 & \beta_I S_0 \\ 0 & 0 \end{pmatrix}, \quad H = \begin{pmatrix} \rho + \sigma + \delta & 0 \\ -\rho & \omega + \mu + \delta \end{pmatrix}.$$

Therefore the next generation matrix is

$$GH^{-1} = \begin{pmatrix} \frac{\beta_A S_0}{\rho+\sigma+\delta} + \frac{\rho\beta_I S_0}{(\rho+\sigma+\delta)(\omega+\mu+\delta)} & \frac{\beta_I S_0}{\omega+\mu+\delta} \\ 0 & 0 \end{pmatrix},$$

Now, the basic reproduction number is given by

$$\mathcal{R}_0 = \frac{\beta_A S_0}{\rho + \sigma + \delta} + \frac{\rho\beta_I S_0}{(\rho + \sigma + \delta)(\omega + \mu + \delta)}. \tag{8.9}$$

8.3.1 Equilibrium and Existence of Endemic Equilibrium

Here we established the existence as well as uniqueness of the endemic equilibrium point $\Phi^*(S^*, A^*, I^*, R^*, P^*, E^*)$ for the $SAIRPE$ model (8.1).

Theorem 8.1 *Assume $\alpha d_e \rho - \theta_a h_e > 0$ and $(\rho + \mu + \delta)(\omega + \mu + \delta)\theta_s > \theta_r(\rho\mu + \sigma(\rho + \mu + \delta))$. If $\mathcal{R}_0 > 1$ the unique endemic equilibrium point $\Phi^*(S^*, A^*, I^*, R^*, P^*, E^*)$ exist define by Eqs.* (8.16)–(8.21).

Proof For an endemic equilibrium $\Phi^*(S^*, A^*, I^*, R^*, P^*, E^*)$ of the SAIRPE model (8.1), we get

$$\Lambda - (\beta_A A^* + \beta_I I^*)\frac{S^*}{1+\theta P^*} - \delta S^* = 0, \tag{8.10}$$

$$(\beta_A A^* + \beta_I I^*)\frac{S^*}{1+\theta P^*} - (\rho + \sigma + \delta)A^* = 0, \tag{8.11}$$

$$\rho A^* - (\omega + \mu + \delta)I^* = 0, \tag{8.12}$$

$$\mu I^* + \sigma A^* - \delta R^* = 0, \tag{8.13}$$

$$\alpha I^* - d_p P^* - h_e E^* = 0, \tag{8.14}$$

$$\theta_s S^* + \theta_a A^* + \theta_r R^* - d_e E^* - f_p P^* = 0. \tag{8.15}$$

Adding (8.10) & (8.11), we can obtain that

$$S^* = S_0 - \frac{\rho + \sigma + \delta}{\delta}A^*. \tag{8.16}$$

From (8.12) & (8.13) we get

$$I^* = \frac{\rho}{\omega + \mu + \delta}A^*, \tag{8.17}$$

and

$$R^* = \left(\frac{\rho\mu}{\delta(\omega + \mu + \delta)} + \frac{\sigma}{\delta}\right)A^*. \tag{8.18}$$

Solving Eqs. (8.14) and (8.15), we obtain

$$P^* = \frac{\alpha d_e I^* - h_e(\theta_s S^* + \theta_a A^* + \theta_r R^*)}{d_p d_e - h_e f_p}, \tag{8.19}$$

and

$$E^* = \frac{d_p(\theta_s S^* + \theta_a A^* + \theta_r R^*) - \alpha f_p I^*}{d_p d_e - h_e f_p}, \tag{8.20}$$

Using Eqs. (8.16)–(8.20) into Eq. (8.11), we can get a unique non-trivial solution for A^*:

$$\begin{aligned}
A^* &= \frac{\beta_A S_0 + \frac{\rho\beta_I S_0}{\omega+\mu+\delta} + \frac{\rho+\mu+\delta\theta h_e S_0}{d_p d_e - f_p h_e} - (\rho+\mu+\delta)}{\beta_A\frac{\rho+\mu+\delta}{\delta} + \beta_I\frac{\rho(\rho+\mu+\delta)}{\rho(\omega+\mu+\delta)} + \frac{\rho+\mu+\delta}{d_p d_e - f_p h_e}\left(\frac{\theta\rho\alpha d_e}{\omega+\mu+\delta} + \frac{\theta h_e\theta_s(\rho+\mu+\delta)}{\delta} - \theta\theta_a h_e - \theta h_e\theta_r\left(\frac{\rho\mu}{\delta(\omega+\mu+\delta)} + \frac{\sigma}{\delta}\right)\right)} \\
&= \frac{(\mathcal{R}_0 - 1) + \frac{(\rho+\mu+\delta)\theta h_e S_0}{d_p d_e - f_p h_e}}{\frac{\beta_A}{\delta} + \frac{\rho\beta_I}{\rho(\omega+\mu+\delta)} + \frac{1}{d_p d_e - f_p h_e}\left(\frac{\theta\rho\alpha d_e}{\omega+\mu+\delta} + \frac{\theta h_e\theta_s(\rho+\mu+\delta)}{\delta} - \theta\theta_a h_e - \theta h_e\theta_r\left(\frac{\rho\mu}{\delta(\omega+\mu+\delta)} + \frac{\sigma}{\delta}\right)\right)} \\
&= \frac{(\mathcal{R}_0 - 1) + \frac{\rho+\mu+\delta\theta h_e S_0}{d_p d_e - f_p h_e}}{\frac{\rho+\mu+\delta}{S_0}\left(\mathcal{R}_0 - 1\right) + \frac{\rho+\mu+\delta}{S_0} + \frac{1}{d_p d_e - f_p h_e}\left(\frac{\theta\rho\alpha d_e}{\omega+\mu+\delta} + \frac{\theta h_e\theta_s(\rho+\mu+\delta)}{\delta} - \theta\theta_a h_e - \theta h_e\theta_r\left(\frac{\rho\mu}{\delta(\omega+\mu+\delta)} + \frac{\sigma}{\delta}\right)\right)},
\end{aligned}$$

For the condition of positive as well as unique endemic equilibrium we get $d_p d_e - f_p h_e > 0, \mathcal{R}_0 > 1$ also $\alpha d_e \rho - \theta_a h_e > 0$ and $(\rho+\mu+\delta)(\omega+\mu+\delta)\theta_s > \theta_r(\rho\mu+\sigma(\rho+\mu+\delta))$ assumption. Using this assumption we can conclude that $\frac{\theta\rho\alpha d_e}{\omega+\mu+\delta} + \frac{\theta h_e \theta_s(\rho+\mu+\delta)}{\delta} - \theta\theta_a h_e - \theta h_e \theta_r\left(\frac{\rho\mu}{\delta(\omega+\mu+\delta)} + \frac{\sigma}{\delta}\right) > 0$ which yields $A^* > 0$ when $\mathcal{R}_0 > 1$. Meanwhile there is only one endemic equilibrium $\Phi^*(S^*, A^*, I^*, R^*, P^*, E^*)$ for the $SAIRPE$ model (8.1) when $\mathcal{R}_0 > 1$. □

Lemma 8.1 *Let ϕ_0 is the DFE of the epidemic system described by $\dot{\varrho} = g(\varrho, \delta)$, for all values of δ. The threshold δ is defined as a bifurcation parameter where for $\delta < 0$, $\mathcal{R}_0 < 1$ and while $\delta > 0$, $\mathcal{R}_0 > 1$. Let the DFE is stable for $\delta < 0$. Consider the zero eigenvalue of $D_\varrho g(\Phi_0, 0)$ (when the parameter δ is equal to zero) would be simple. Also assume that u and v, the left and right null vectors respectively corresponding to that simple eigenvalue be such that*

$$\vartheta_a = \frac{u}{2} D_{\varrho\varrho} g(\Phi_0, 0)v^2 = \frac{1}{2}\sum_{i,j,k=1}^{n} u_i v_j v_k \frac{\partial^2 g_i}{\partial\varrho_j \partial\varrho_k}(\Phi_0, 0), \tag{8.21}$$

$$\vartheta_b = u D_{\varrho\delta} g(\Phi_0, 0)v = \sum_{i,j=1}^{n} u_i v_j \frac{\partial^2 g_i}{\partial_j \partial\delta}(\Phi_0, 0), \tag{8.22}$$

considering $\vartheta_b \neq 0$. Whenever $\delta < 0$, $\vartheta_b > 0$, and there exists $\xi > 0$ such that
(i) endemic equilibria near Φ_0 would be locally asymptotically stable for $0 < \delta < \xi$ and $\vartheta_a < 0$,
(ii) endemic equilibria near Φ_0 would be unstable for $-\xi < \delta < 0$ and $\vartheta_a > 0$.
We employ the Lemma 8.1 to prove the result below.

Theorem 8.2 *Whenever $\mathcal{R}_0 > 1$ and $\mathcal{R}_0 = 1$ is very small, the endemic equilibrium $\Phi^*(S^*, A^*, I^*, R^*, P^*, E^*)$ of the $SAIRPE$ model (8.1) is locally asymptotically stable.*

Proof First we re-write the $SAIRPE$ model Eq. (8.1) as $\dot{\varrho} = g(\varrho, \mathcal{R}_0)$, where $\varrho = [\varrho_1, \varrho_2, \varrho_3, \varrho_4, \varrho_5, \varrho_6]^T = [S, A, I, R, P, E]^T$ and $g = [g_1, g_2, g_3, g_4, g_5, g_6]^T = \left[\frac{dS}{dt}, \frac{dA}{dt}, \frac{dI}{dt}, \frac{dR}{dt}, \frac{dP}{dt}, \frac{dC}{dt}\right]^T$.

To established the characteristic polynomial we consider Jacobian matrix of the $SAIRPE$ model (8.1) at $(\Phi_0, 1)$ is given by

$$D_\varrho g(\Phi_0, 1) = \begin{pmatrix} -\delta & -\beta_A S_0 & -\beta_I S_0 & 0 & 0 & 0 \\ 0 & \beta_A S_0 - (\rho+\sigma+\delta) & \beta_I S_0 & 0 & 0 & 0 \\ 0 & \rho & -(\omega+\mu+\delta) & 0 & 0 & 0 \\ 0 & \sigma & \mu & -\delta & 0 & 0 \\ 0 & 0 & \alpha & 0 & -d_p & -h_e \\ \theta_s & \theta_a & 0 & \theta_r & -f_p & -d_e \end{pmatrix}.$$

Let $\mathcal{R}_0 = 1$. The characteristic polynomial is as:

$$|\lambda I_6 - D_{\varrho} g(\Phi_0, 1)| = -(\delta+\lambda)^2\Big\{\lambda^2 + (d_p + d_e)\lambda + d_p d_e - f_p h_e\Big\}$$
$$\Big\{[\lambda - \beta_A S_0 + (\rho+\sigma+\delta)](\lambda+\omega+\mu+\delta) - \beta_I S_0 \rho\Big\}$$
$$= -(\delta+\lambda)^2\Big\{\lambda^2 + (d_p + d_e)\lambda + d_p d_e - f_p h_e\Big\}$$
$$\Big\{[\lambda^2 - \lambda[\beta_A S_0 - (\rho+\sigma+\delta) - (\omega+\mu+\delta)]$$
$$-(\rho+\sigma+\delta)(\omega+\mu+\delta)(\mathcal{R}_0 - 1)\Big\}$$
$$= -(\delta+\lambda)^2\Big\{\lambda^2 + (d_p + d_e)\lambda + d_p d_e - f_p h_e\Big\}$$
$$\Big\{[\lambda^2 - \lambda[\beta_A S_0 - (\rho+\sigma+\delta) - (\omega+\mu+\delta)].$$

Notable that $\mathcal{R}_0$ is define as

$$\mathcal{R}_{01} = \frac{\beta_A S_0}{\rho+\sigma+\delta}, \quad \mathcal{R}_{02} = \frac{\rho\beta_I S_0}{(\rho+\sigma+\delta)(\omega+\mu+\delta)}.$$

Since $\mathcal{R}_{01} < \mathcal{R}_0 = 1$, we get

$$\beta_A S_0 - (\rho+\sigma+\delta) - (\omega+\mu+\delta) = (\rho+\sigma+\delta)\Big[\mathcal{R}_{01} - 1 - \frac{\omega+\mu+\delta}{\rho+\sigma+\delta}\Big].$$

Therefore, $d_p d_e - f_p h_e > 0$, we can see that the eigen value of $D_{\varrho} g(\Phi_0, 1)$ is simple. All other eigen value of $D_{\varrho} g(\Phi_0, 1)$ have no positive real parts.

Second order partial derivatives of g_i in (8.21) are zero at the DFE except the following:

$$\frac{\partial^2 f_1}{\partial S \partial A}(\Phi_0, 1) = -\beta_E, \quad \frac{\partial^2 f_1}{\partial S \partial I}(\Phi_0, 1) = -\beta_I, \quad \frac{\partial^2 f_1}{\partial A \partial S}(\Phi_0, 1) = -\beta_E, \quad \frac{\partial^2 f_1}{\partial I \partial S}(\Phi_0, 1) = -\beta_I,$$
$$\frac{\partial^2 f_2}{\partial S \partial A}(\Phi_0, 1) = \beta_E, \quad \frac{\partial^2 f_2}{\partial S \partial I}(\Phi_0, 1) = \beta_I, \quad \frac{\partial^2 f_2}{\partial A \partial S}(\Phi_0, 1) = \beta_E, \quad \frac{\partial^2 f_2}{\partial I \partial S}(\Phi_0, 1) = \beta_I,$$

Corresponding first order partial derivatives of g_i in (8.22) are as follows:

$$\frac{\partial f_1}{\partial A}(\Phi_0, 1) = -\beta_A S_0 = -(\rho+\sigma+\delta)\mathcal{R}_{01} = -(\rho+\sigma+\delta)(\mathcal{R}_0 - \mathcal{R}_{02}),$$
$$\frac{\partial f_1}{\partial I}(\Phi_0, 1) = -\beta_I S_0 = -\frac{(\rho+\sigma+\delta)(\omega+\mu+\delta)}{\rho}\mathcal{R}_{02} = -\frac{(\rho+\sigma+\delta)(\omega+\mu+\delta)}{\rho}(\mathcal{R}_0 - \mathcal{R}_{01}),$$
$$\frac{\partial f_2}{\partial A}(\Phi_0, 1) = \beta_A S_0 - (\rho+\sigma+\delta) = (\rho+\sigma+\delta)(\mathcal{R}_{01} - 1) = (\rho+\sigma+\delta)(\mathcal{R}_0 - \mathcal{R}_{02} - 1),$$
$$\frac{\partial f_2}{\partial I}(\Phi_0, 1) = \beta_I S_0 = \frac{(\rho+\sigma+\delta)(\omega+\mu+\delta)}{\rho}\mathcal{R}_{02} = \frac{(\rho+\sigma+\delta)(\omega+\mu+\delta)}{\rho}(\mathcal{R}_0 - \mathcal{R}_{01}),$$

And also non-zero second order partial derivatives of g_i in (8.22) are

$$\frac{\partial^2 f_1}{\partial A \partial \mathcal{R}_0}(\Phi_0, 1) = -(\rho+\sigma+\delta), \frac{\partial^2 f_1}{\partial I \partial \mathcal{R}_0}(\Phi_0, 1) = -\frac{(\rho+\sigma+\delta)(\omega+\mu+\delta)}{\rho},$$
$$\frac{\partial^2 f_2}{\partial A \partial \mathcal{R}_0}(\Phi_0, 1) = (\rho+\sigma+\delta), \frac{\partial^2 f_2}{\partial I \partial \mathcal{R}_0}(\Phi_0, 1) = \frac{(\rho+\sigma+\delta)(\omega+\mu+\delta)}{\rho},$$

We choose u and v such that they are orthogonal to $D_{\varrho}g(\Phi_0, 1)$ (i.e., $u.D_{\varrho}g(\Phi_0, 1) = 0, D_{\varrho}g(\Phi_0, 1).v = 0$), and $v.w = 1$. According to algebraic manipulation, we obtain $u = (0, u_2, u_3, 0, 0, 0)$, where $u_2 = \frac{1}{1+\rho\beta_I S_0} > 0$, $u_3 = \frac{\beta_I S_0}{\omega+\mu+\delta}u_2$ due to $\mathcal{R}_0 = 1$, and $v = (v_1, v_2, v_3, v_4, v_5, v_6)$, where $v_1 = -\frac{\rho+\mu+\delta}{\delta}$, $v_2 = 1$, $v_3 = \frac{\rho}{\omega+\mu+\delta}$, $v_4 = \frac{\sigma(\omega+\mu+\delta)+\mu\rho}{\delta(\omega+\mu+\delta)}$, $v_5 = \frac{\frac{\alpha\rho d_e}{\omega+\mu+\delta}+\frac{\theta_s h_e(\rho+\mu+\delta)}{\delta}-\theta_a h_e-\theta_r h_e\frac{\sigma(\omega+\mu+\delta)+\mu\rho}{\delta(\omega+\mu+\delta)}}{d_e d_p - h_e f_p} > 0$, $v_6 = \frac{-\frac{\theta_s(\rho+\sigma+\delta)}{\delta}+\theta_a d_p+\theta_r d_p\frac{\sigma(\omega+\mu+\delta)+\mu\rho}{\delta(\omega+\mu+\delta)}-\frac{\alpha\rho f_p}{\omega+\mu+\delta}}{d_p d_e - h_e f_p}$. □

From Eq. (8.21), we get

$$\vartheta_a = u_2[v_1 v_2 \beta_E + v_1 v_3 \beta_I] > 0. \tag{8.23}$$

Moreover, from Eq. (8.22), we can get

$$\vartheta_b = u_2(\rho+\mu+\delta)[v_2 + v_3\frac{\omega+\mu+\delta}{\rho}] \; 0. \tag{8.24}$$

Meanwhile, we can established that when $\mathcal{R}_0 - 1$ switch from negative to positive. So a non negative and locally asymptotically stable endemic equilibrium $\Phi^*(S^*, A^*, I^*, R^*, P^*, E^*)$ of the $SAIRPE$ model (8.1) is occurs.

Theorem 8.3 *Let $P = P^*$, When $\mathcal{R}_0 < 1$, the DFE Φ_0 of the turn down system from the $SAIRPE$ model (8.1) is globally asymptotically stable otherwise the DFE Φ_0 unstable.*

Proof If $P = P^*$, the 2nd equation and 3rd equation of (8.1) is implying that

$$\frac{dA}{dt} \leq (\beta_A A + \beta_I I)\frac{S}{1+\theta P^*} - (\rho+\sigma+\delta)A,$$
$$\frac{dI}{dt} \leq \rho A - (\omega+\mu+\delta)I, \tag{8.25}$$

Let $X = (P, C)$. Then the $SAIRPE$ system (8.1) yields

$$\frac{dX}{dt} \leq (F^* - V^*)X, \tag{8.26}$$

Following the Perron-Frobenius theorem, there exists a non negative left eigenvector w of the positive matrix $(V^*)^{-1}F^*$ with respect to the eigenvalue $\mathcal{R}_0 = \rho((V^*)^{-1}F^*) = \rho(F^*(V^*)^{-1})$. Define the Lyapunov function $\mathcal{L} : \Pi \to \mathbb{R}_+^6$ as

$$\mathcal{L} = \kappa^T (V^*)^{-1} X$$

Notable that $\mathcal{L} \geq 0$, and $\mathcal{L} = 0$ with the provision that $X = 0$. Differentiating $\mathcal{L}$ along the solution of the reduced system from (8.1), we can get

$$\mathcal{L}' = \kappa^T (V^*)^{-1} \frac{dX}{dt} \geq \kappa^T (V^*)^{-1} (F^* - V^*) X = (\mathcal{R}_0 - 1) \kappa^T X.$$

Here we find that $\mathcal{L}$ is locally Lipscitz and therefore it can be noticed that $\mathcal{L}' \geq 0$ whenever $\mathcal{R}_0 < 1$. It is notable that $\mathcal{L}' = 0$ indicates $\kappa^T X = 0$, which implies $A = I = 0$. Applying Lyapunov-LaSalle Theorem [39], it is found that every solution starting in Π will go to the invariant set S'(say), where $\mathcal{L}' = 0$ containing only the DFE Φ_0. Therefore, due to LaSalle's Invariance Principle, it is concluded that the DFE Φ_0 of the $SAIRPE$ model (8.1) is globally asymptotically stable. □

Theorem 8.4 *Let $P = P^*$. When $\mathcal{R}_0 > 1$, the one and only endemic equilibrium $\Phi^*(S^*, A^*, I^*, R^*, P^*, E^*)$ of the scale down the $SAIRPE$ model from* (8.1) *is globally asymptotically stable.*

Proof When $P = P^*$, we consider the first three equations of (8.1):

$$\begin{aligned} \frac{dS}{dt} &= \Lambda - \frac{\beta_A AS}{1+\theta P^*} - \frac{\beta_I IS}{1+\theta P^*} - \delta S, \\ \frac{dA}{dt} &= \frac{\beta_A AS}{1+\theta P^*} - \frac{\beta_I IS}{1+\theta P^*} - (\rho + \sigma + \delta)A, \\ \frac{dI}{dt} &= \rho A - (\omega + \mu + \delta)I, \end{aligned} \tag{8.27}$$

We consider the Lyapunov function is as follows:

$$\mathcal{L}_1 = \int_{S^*}^{S} \frac{\kappa - S^*}{\kappa} + \int_{A^*}^{A} \frac{\kappa - A^*}{\kappa} + \frac{\beta_I S^* I^*}{(1+\theta P^*)\rho A^*} \int_{I^*}^{I} \frac{\kappa - I^*}{\kappa}. \tag{8.28}$$

Accordingly, it is easy to verify $\mathcal{L}_1 \geq 0$ and $\mathcal{L}_1 = 1$ as well as $(S, A, I) = (S^*, A^*, I^*)$ and for that the following equations are satisfy:

$$\Lambda - \frac{\beta_A A^* S^*}{1+\theta P^*} - \frac{\beta_I I^* S^*}{1+\theta P^*} - \delta S^* = 0, \tag{8.29}$$

$$\frac{\beta_A A^* S^*}{1+\theta P^*} + \frac{\beta_I I^* S^*}{1+\theta P^*} - (\rho + \sigma + \delta)A^* = 0, \tag{8.30}$$

$$\rho A^* - (\omega + \mu + \delta)I^* = 0, \tag{8.31}$$

Using Eqs. (8.29), (8.30) and (8.31), we can evaluate the derivative of $\mathcal{L}_1$ with the help of subsystem (8.25) is following

$$
\begin{aligned}
\mathcal{L}'|_{(\text{Sys. Eqs.(8.27)})} &= \Big(1-\frac{S^*}{S}\Big)\Big[\Lambda - \frac{\beta_A AS}{1+\theta P^*} - \frac{\beta_I IS}{1+\theta P^*} - \delta S - \Big(\Lambda - \frac{\beta_A A^* S^*}{1+\theta P^*} - \frac{\beta_I I^* S^*}{1+\theta P^*} - \delta S^*\Big)\Big] \\
&+\Big(1-\frac{A^*}{A}\Big)\Big[\frac{\beta_A AS}{1+\theta P^*} + \frac{\beta_I IS}{1+\theta P^*} - (\rho+\sigma+\delta)A \\
&-\Big(\frac{\beta_A A^* S^*}{1+\theta P^*} + \frac{\beta_I I^* S^*}{1+\theta P^*} - (\rho+\sigma+\delta)A^*\Big)\Big] \\
&+\frac{\beta_I S^* I^*}{(1+\theta P^*)\rho A^*}\Big(1-\frac{I^*}{I}\Big)\Big[\rho A - (\omega+\mu+\delta)I - \Big(\rho A^* - (\omega+\mu+\delta)I^*\Big)\Big] \\
&= \frac{\beta_A}{1+\theta P^*}S^*A^*\Big(1-\frac{SA}{S^*A^*} - \frac{S^*}{S} + \frac{A}{A^*}\Big) + \frac{\beta_I}{1+\theta P^*}S^*I^*\Big(1-\frac{SI}{S^*I^*} - \frac{S^*}{S} + \frac{I}{I^*}\Big) \\
&+\delta S^*\Big(2-\frac{S}{S^*}-\frac{S^*}{S}\Big) - \frac{\beta_A}{1+\theta P^*}S^*A^*\Big(1-\frac{SA}{S^*A^*} - \frac{S}{S^*} - \frac{A}{A^*}\Big) \\
&+\frac{\beta_I}{1+\theta P^*}S^*I^*\Big(1-\frac{SI}{S^*I^*} + \frac{SIE^*}{S^*I^*E} - \frac{A}{A^*}\Big) + \frac{\beta_A}{1+\theta P^*}S^*A^*\Big(2-\frac{A^*}{A} - \frac{A}{A^*}\Big) \\
&+\frac{\beta_I}{1+\theta P^*}S^*I^*\Big(2-\frac{A^*}{A} - \frac{A}{A^*}\Big) - \frac{\beta_I}{1+\theta P^*}S^*I^*\Big(1-\frac{A}{A^*} - \frac{I^*}{I} + \frac{AI^*}{A^*I}\Big) \\
&+\frac{\beta_I}{1+\theta P^*}S^*I^*\Big(2-\frac{I^*}{I} - \frac{I^*}{A}\Big) \\
&= \delta S^*\Big(2-\frac{S}{S^*}-\frac{S^*}{S}\Big) + \frac{\beta_A}{1+\theta P^*}S^*A^*\Big(2-\frac{S}{S^*}-\frac{S^*}{S}\Big) \\
&+\frac{\beta_I}{1+\theta P^*}S^*I^*\Big(3-\frac{S}{S^*} - \frac{AI^*}{A^*I} - \frac{SA^*I}{S^*AI^*}\Big) \\
&\le 0.
\end{aligned}
$$

Therefore, $\mathcal{L}'|_{(\text{Sys. Eqs.(8.27)})} = 0$ with the provision that $(S, A, I) = (S^*, A^*, I^*)$. Hence, following the LaSalle's Proncipele, the interior equilibrium (S^*, A^*, I^*) of semi system (8.27) is globally asymptotically stable.

Direct substitution (S^*, A^*, I^*) within the equations for R and E,

$$
\begin{aligned}
\frac{dR}{dt} &= \mu I^* + \sigma A^* - \delta R, \\
\frac{dE}{dt} &= \theta_s S^* + \theta_a A^* + \theta_r R - d_e E - f_p P^*.
\end{aligned}
\tag{8.32}
$$

it is note that (R^*, E^*) of system (8.32) is globally asymptotically stable. Results of subsystems (8.27) and (8.32) is combining then complete the proof. □

8.4 Numerical Illustrations

We undertake numerical illustrations for the proposed model (8.1) to reinforce the theoretical analysis and get further insight into the model behavior. We utilize MATLAB solver ode45 to solve the system of nonlinear ordinary differential equations for the set parameters are specified in the Table 8.1.

Table 8.1: Description of the model (8.1) parameters and their values.

Parameters	Description	Value
Λ	influx rate of susceptible population	100
β_A	disease transmission rate from S to A	6.05×10^{-3}
β_I	disease transmission rate from S to A	1.49×10^{-4}
θ	implementation rate of disease mitigation	0.4
δ	natural decay rate	2.74×10^{-1}
ρ	reciprocal of the incubation period	0.8
σ	disease recovered rate from A to R	0.5
ω	disease-induced death rate	0.01
μ	disease recovered from infected class	1/14
α	mitigation strength stimulated by infected class	0.95
d_p	reduction rate due to mitigation	0.51
h_e	decline rate of mitigation due to economic activities	4.21×10^{-4}
θ_s	labor contribution rate from S compartment	2.05×10^{-4}
θ_a	labor contribution rate from A compartment	2.00×10^{-2}
θ_r	labor contribution rate from R compartment	3.99×10^{-3}
d_e	natural reduction rate of economic progression	0.15292
f_p	decline rate of economic growth due to mitigation	2.59×10^{-2}

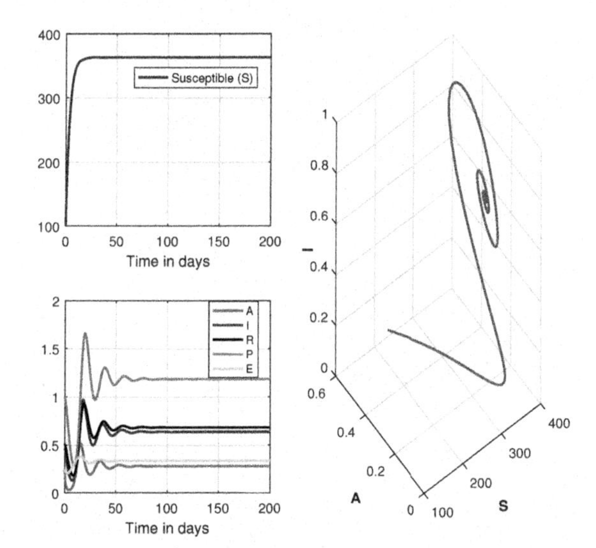

Fig. 8.2: The left panel represents the time series evolution of susceptible (S), exposed (A), symptomatic infected (I), recovered (R) individuals, mitigation level/effectiveness (P) and economic development (E); whereas the right panel represents the 3-dimensional phase-portrait, with initial values: $S_0 = 100$, $A_0 = 0.25$, $I_0 = 0.45$, $R_0 = 0.50$, $P_0 = 1.0$, $E_0 = 0.25$ and the parameters value are given in the Table 8.1.

For the set of parameter values specified in Table 8.1, the components of the endemic equilibrium point ϕ^*E are obtained as,

$$S^* = 363.34, \;\; A^* = 0.282696, \;\; I^* = 0.636293, \;\; R^* = 0.681743,$$
$$P^* = 1.18497, \;\; E^* = 0.341145,$$

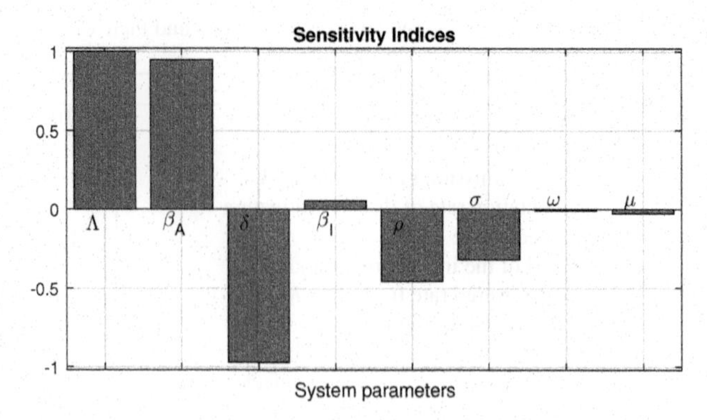

Fig. 8.3: Bar diagram represents the sensitivity indices of the parameters related to the basic reproduction number $\mathcal{R}_0$ and the parameters are given in the Table 8.1.

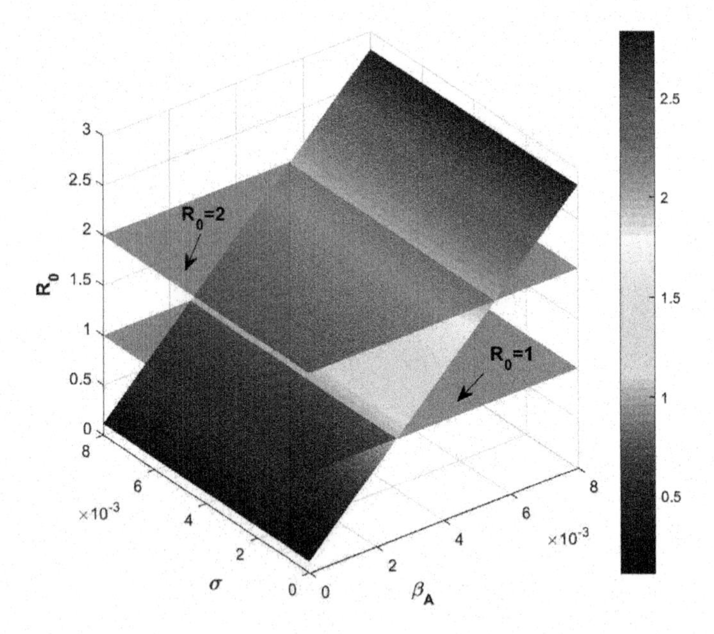

Fig. 8.4: The figure represents the basic reproduction number $\mathcal{R}_0$ when β_A (disease transmission rate) and σ (rate of transition from exposed to recovered class) varies. Other parameters are given in the Table 8.1.

and the corresponding eigenvalues of the Jacobian matrix of the proposed system (8.1) evaluated around the interior equilibrium ϕ^* are given by,

$$-0.811767, \quad -0.0685882 \pm 0.331293i, \quad -0.274376, \quad -0.274, \quad -0.15292.$$

The endemic equilibrium point ϕ^* is locally asymptotically stable as the eigenvalues are either negative and have negative real parts. The time series solution and 3-dimensional phase portrait diagram (see the Figure

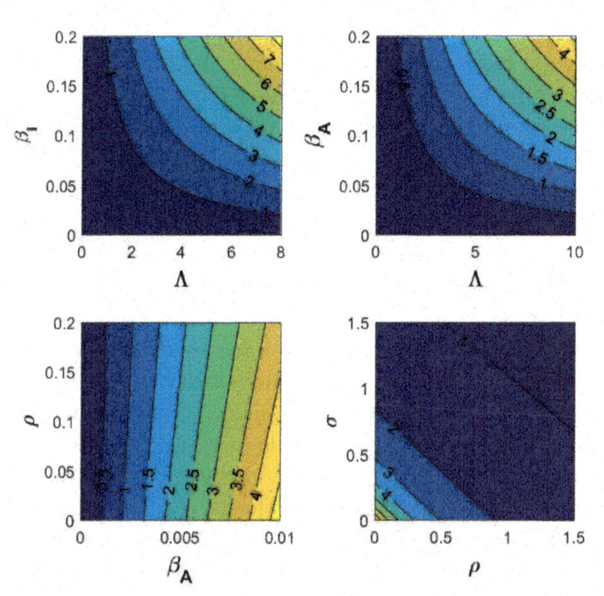

Fig. 8.5: The figure represents the contour plot for $\mathcal{R}_0$ with respect to β_I (disease transmission rate from susceptible to asymptomatic class) versus λ (constant influx rate of susceptible individuals); β_A (disease transmission rate from susceptible to asymptomatic individuals) versus λ; ρ (reciprocal of latent period) versus β_A and ρ versus σ (disease recovered from asymptotic to recovered class). Other parameters are specified in the Table 8.1.

8.2) also verified that the proposed model system is locally asymptotically stable for the specified model parameters in the Table 8.1.

By using expression (8.9) for the basic reproduction number R_0, we get its values for the parametric set up in the Table 8.1 as $R_0 = 1.48058$, which shows the substantial outbreak of the novel coronavirus or disease persist in the system. The disease outbreak can be controlled by bringing the magnitude of the basic reproduction number R_0 below unity.

To control the COVID-19 diseases, we plot the normalized forward sensitivity indices to visualize the most sensitive parameters with respect to the basic reproduction number R_0. From the sensitivity indices (see the Figure 8.3) it is clear that Λ (constant source rate of susceptible individual) and β_A (diseases transmission rate from susceptible to asymptomatic individuals) are highly positively correlated sensitive parameters whereas δ (natural death rate) is highly negatively correlated sensitive parameter. Thus, to control the novel coronavirus we must have to control the parameters Λ and β_A.

By using the parameters in Table 8.1, we compute $R_0 = 1.48058$ that indicates substantial outbreak of novel coronavirus. To better visualize the threshold parameter R_0, we plot the 3-dimensional phase portrait for R_0 with respect to β_A and σ in the Figure 8.4.

Better understand the transmission dynamics of novel coronavirus, we have drawn the contour plot for the basic reproduction number R_0 with respect to Λ (constant influx rate of susceptible individual) - β_I (disease transmission rate from susceptible to asymptomatic individual); Λ - β_A (disease transmission rate from susceptible to asymptomatic individual); β_A - ρ (reciprocal of the latent period) and ρ - σ (disease recovery rate from asymptotic individuals to recovered class) in the Figure 8.5.

8.5 Conclusion

The novel coronavirus is the most significant global pandemic after the second world war, and has affected almost all the countries throughout the world. To maintain the COVID-19 outbreak, it is important to comprehend how the virus is transmitted to a susceptible population and eventually in the community. The primary transmission pathway of novel coronavirus is human-to-human transmission through infectious droplets. While human-to-human transmission dynamics is well recognized, little attention has been given to indirect transmission of the virus through surfaces such as door handles, at least from the mathematical point of view. It is well-established that the novel coronavirus can survive on hard surfaces and in the environment, and as such, environmental factors may have a great impact on the transmission dynamics of the disease. A substantial amount of money have been spent on disinfecting surfaces and work places. In the present study, we investigated a mathematical model for the transmission dynamics of novel coronavirus by considering its spread via direct contact of susceptible with infected individuals. The mathematical computations of the proposed model includes the finding of the basic reproduction number using the next generation matrix method, and it has been noticed that the epidemic threshold depends on both the transmission rate of direct contact and social economy. Disease-free and the endemic steady state of the proposed system are obtained, and global stability of the latter has been performed analytically as well as numerically. Numerically, it is shown that the disease-free and endemic equilibria of the system; the former exists and is stable for $R_0 < 1$ while the latter remain in the system whenever $R_0 > 1$. This shows the necessity of the precautionary measures which can drive the value of R_0 below 1.

For the set of model parameters, we have calculated the basic reproduction number R_0 which is greater than 1 that shows the substantial outbreak of the novel coronavirus. Thus, to control the epidemic outbreak, we must have to control the basic reproduction number R_0 that should be less than 1. So, we have drawn the contour plot (see the Figure 8.5). From the contour plot, we can get an idea about the disease control as the parameters are related to the basic reproduction number R_0. Importantly, we observed that to lessen the direct contacts between susceptible and infected individuals the population must have to use face mask, arranging online classes/seminars, strict lockdown and other measures; disinfecting surfaces also play major role in suppressing the prevalence of COVID-19.

References

[1] Else, H. 2020. How a torrent of COVID science changed research publishing—In seven charts. Nature, 553.

[2] Huang, C., Y. Wang, X. Li, L. Ren, J. Zhao, Y. Hu, L. Zhang, G. Fan, J. Xu, X. Gu, Z. Cheng, T. Yu, J. Xia, Y. Wei, W. Wu, X. Xie, W. Yin, H. Li, M. Liu, Y. Xiao, H. Gao, L. Guo, J. Xie, G. Wang, R. Jiang, Z. Gao, Q. Jin, J. Wang and B. Cao. 2020. Clinical features of patients infected with 2019 novel coronavirus in Wuhan, China. Lancet, 395: 497–506.

[3] Bera, S., S. Khajanchi and T.K. Roy. 2022. Dynamics of an HTLV-I infection model with delayed CTLs immune response. Appl. Math. Comput., 430: 127206.

[4] Dwivedi, A., R. Keval and S. Khajanchi. 2022. Modeling optimal vaccination strategy for dengue epidemic model: A case study of India. Phys. Scr., 97(8): 085214.

[5] Rothe, C., M. Schunk, P. Sothmann, G. Bretzel, G. Froeschl, C. Wallrauch, T. Zimmer, V. Thiel, C. Janke, W. Guggemos, M. Seilmaier, C. Drosten, P. Vollmar, K. Zwirglmaier, S. Zange, R. Wölfel and M. Hoelscher. 2020. Transmission of 2019-nCoV infection from an asymptomatic contact in Germany. N. Engl. J. Med., 382 970–971.

[6] Prather, B.K.A., C.C. Wang and R.T. Schooley. 2020. Reducing transmission of SARS-CoV-2. Science, 368: 1422–1424.
[7] Van Doremalen, N., T. Bushmaker, D. Morris, M. Holbrook and A. Gamble. 2020. Aerosol and Surface Stability of SARS-CoV-2 as compared with SARS-CoV-1. N. Engl. J. Med., 382: 1564–1567.
[8] Samui, P., J. Mondal and S. Khajanchi. 2020. A mathematical model for COVID-19 transmission dynamics with a case study of India. Chaos Soliton Fractal, 140: 110173.
[9] Cotman, Z.J., M.J. Bowden, B.P. Richter, J.H. Phelps and C.J. Dibble. 2021. Factors affecting aerosol SARS-CoV-2 transmission via HVAC systems; a modeling study. PLoS Comput. Biol., 17: e1009474.
[10] Mondal, J. and S. Khajanchi. 2022. Mathematical modeling and optimal intervention strategies of the COVID-19 outbreak. Nonlinear Dyn.
[11] Zhou, B., D. Jiang, Y. Dai and T. Hayat. 2021. Stationary distribution and density function expression for a stochastic SIQRS epidemic model with temporary immunity. Nonlinear Dyn., 105: 931–955.
[12] Zhai, S., G. Luo, T. Huang, X. Wang, J. Tao and P. Zhou. 2021. Vaccination control of an epidemic model with time delay and its application to COVID-19. Nonlinear Dyn., 106: 1279–1292.
[13] Khajanchi, S. and K. Sarkar. 2020. Forecasting the daily and cumulative number of cases for the COVID-19 pandemic in India. Chaos, 30(7): 071101.
[14] Vilar, J.M.G. and L. Saiz. 2021. Reliably quantifying the evolving worldwide dynamic state of the COVID-19 outbreak from death records, clinical parametrization, and demographic data. Sci. Rep., 11: 19952.
[15] Khajanchi, S., K. Sarkar, J. Mondal, K.S. Nisar and S.F. Abdelwahab. 2021. Mathematical modeling of the COVID-19 pandemic with intervention strategies. Results Phys., 25: 104285.
[16] Khyar, O. and K. Allali. 2020. Global dynamics of a multi-strain SEIR epidemic model with general incidence rates: Application to COVID-19 pandemic. Nonlinear Dyn., 102: 489–509.
[17] Rai, R.K., S. Khajanchi, P.K. Tiwari, E. Venturino and A.K. Misra. 2022. Impact of social media advertisements on the transmission dynamics of COVID-19 pandemic in India. J. Appl. Math. Comput., 68: 19–44.
[18] Keeling, M.J. and P. Rohani. 2011. Modeling Infectious Diseases in Humans and Animals. Princeton University Press, Princeton, NJ, USA.
[19] Oraby, T., M.G. Tyshenko, J.C. Maldonado, K. Vatcheva, S. Elsaadany, W.Q. Alali, J.C. Longenecker and M. Al-Zoughool. 2021. Modeling the effect of lockdown timing as a COVID-19 control measure in countries with differing social contacts. Sci. Rep., 11: 3354.
[20] Benjamin, M.F. and D. Brockmann. 2020. Effective containment explains subexponential growth in recent confirmed COVID-19 cases in China. Science, 368: 742–746.
[21] Kermack, W.O. and A.G. McKendrick. 1927. A contribution to the mathematical theory of epidemics. Proceedings of the Royal Society of London Series A, Mathematical and Physical Sciences, 115: 700–721.
[22] Newman, M.E.J. 2002. The spread of epidemic disease on networks. Phys. Rev. E, 66: 016128.
[23] Schutz, G.M., M. Brandaut and S. Trimper. 2008. Exact solution of a stochastic susceptible-infectious-recovered model. Phys. Rev. E, 78: 061132.
[24] Harko, T., F.S.N. Lobo and M.K. Mak. 2014. Exact analytical solutions of the susceptible-infected-recovered (SIR) epidemic model and of the SIR model with equal death and birth rates. Appl. Math. Comput., 236: 184.
[25] Khajanchi, S., K. Sarkar and S. Banerjee. 2022. Modeling the dynamics of COVID-19 pandemic with implementation of intervention strategies. Eur. Phys. J. Plus, 137: 129.

[26] Vespignani, A., H. Tian, C. Dye, J.O. Lloyd-Smith, R.M. Eggo, M. Shrestha, S.V. Scarpino, B. Gutierrez, M.U.G. Kraemer, J. Wu, K. Leung and G.M. Leung. 2020. Modelling COVID-19. Nat. Rev. Phys., 2: 279–281.

[27] Li, R., S. Pei, B. Chen, Y. Song, T. Zhang, W. Yang and J. Shaman. 2020. Substantial undocumented infection facilitates the rapid dissemination of novel coronavirus (SARS-CoV2). Science, 368: 489–493.

[28] Read, J.M., J.R.E. Bridgen, D.A.T. Cummings, A. Ho and C.P. Jewell. 2021. Novel coronavirus 2019-nCoV (COVID-19): Early estimation of epidemiological parameters and epidemic size estimates. Philos. Trans. R. Soc. B, 376: 20200265.

[29] Sarkar, K., J. Mondal and S. Khajanchi. 2022. How do the contaminated environment influence the transmission dynamics of COVID-19 pandemic? Eur. Phys. J.: Spec. Top. https://doi.org/10.1140/epjs/s11734-022-00648-w.

[30] Bubar, K.M., K. Reinholt, S.M. Kissler, M. Lipsitch, S. Cobey, Y.H. Grad and D.B. Larremore. 2021. Model-informed COVID-19 vaccine prioritization strategies by age and serostatus. Science, 371: 916–921.

[31] Saad-Roy, C.M., C.E. Wagner, R.E. Baker, S.E. Morris, J. Farrar, A.L. Graham, S.A. Levin, M.J. Mina, C.J.E. Metcalf and B.T. Grenfell. 2020. Immune life history, vaccination, and the dynamics of SARS-CoV-2 over the next 5 years. Science, 370: 811–818.

[32] Sarkar, K., S. Khajanchi and J.J. Nieto. 2020. Modeling and forecasting the COVID-19 pandemic in India. Chaos Soliton Fractal, 139: 110049.

[33] de la Fuente-Mella, H., R. Rubilar, K. Chahuan-Jimenez and V. Leiva. 2021. Modeling COVID-19 cases statistically and evaluating their effect on the economy of countries. Mathematics, 9: 1558.

[34] Chen, J., A. Vullikanti, J. Santos, S. Venkatramanan, S. Hoops, H. Mortveit, B. Lewis, W. You, S. Eubank, M. Marathe, C. Barrett and A. Marathe. 2021. Epidemiological and economic impact of COVID-19 in the US. Sci. Rep., 11: 20451.

[35] Altig, D., S. Baker, J.M. Barrero, N. Bloom, P. Bunn, S. Chen, S.J. Davis, J. Leather, B. Meyer, E. Mihaylov, P. Mizen, N. Parker, T. Renault, P. Smietanka and G. Thwaites. 2020. Economic uncertainty before and during the COVID-19 pandemic. J. Public Econ., 191: 104274.

[36] Jena, P.R., R. Majhi, R. Kalli, S. Managi and B. Majhi. 2020. Impact of COVID-19 on GDP of major economies: Application of the artificial neural network forecaster. Econ. Anal. Policy, 69: 324–339.

[37] Xiang, L., M. Tang, Z. Yin, M. Zheng and S. Lu. 2021. The COVID-19 pandemic and economic growth: Theory and simulation. Front. Public Health, 9: 741525.

[38] Van den Driessche, P. and J. Watmough. 2002. Reproduction numbers and sub-threshold endemic equilibria for compartmental models of disease transmission. Mathematical Biosciences, 180: 29–48.

[39] La Salle, J.P. 1976. The stability of dynamical systems. Society for Industrial and Applied Mathematics.

Chapter 9

Growth Analysis of Covid-19 Cases Using Fractal Interpolation Functions

M.P. Aparna and *P. Paramanathan**

9.1 Introduction

Over the past few decades, there have been a number of pandemics around the world, including the Russian Flu (1977–1979), the London Flu (1972–1973), and Hong Kong Flu (1968). In 2019, Wuhan city of China, identified the outbreak of another contagious disease identified as a form of coronavirus, later named Covid-19. It began to develop as an epidemic at the beginning of 2020, affecting most parts of China, Vietnam, and Japan. A few instances were documented in a few other regions, including France, Spain, Italy, and Europe. The sickness brought on by SARS-CoV-2 spread through extensive travel networks quickly around the world. According to the latest information, there have been 649,753,806 confirmed cases of Covid-19 globally until December 20, 2022, including 6,648,457 deaths [4].

Considering the case of India, coronavirus infections first appeared as a result of foreign links. On January 30, Kerala experienced the first three cases of Covid-19, which were brought on by a traveller from China's Wuhan city [9]. A 14-day self-quarantine period for all international visitors has been mandated by the Indian government, similar to the restrictions imposed during the Ebola outbreak. As a continuation of the controlling tactics, the Indian government is compelled to apply lockdowns that prevent citizens from leaving their homes. Additionally, several test facilities have been implemented, such as Real-time PCR tests, Point-of-Care molecular diagnostic assays, rapid antibody tests, and rapid antigen detection tests for early detection of COVID-19 [10–15]. As of December 20, 2022, 43319396 confirmed cases had been reported in India with 856843574 tests.

Ever since the emergence of Covid-19, scientists worldwide have conducted several studies to identify the cause of the disease and monitor the spread pattern. Authors have developed a number of models [5] to predict how the condition will grow and spread. One of the remarkable models among them, the SIR (Susceptible, Infectious Recovery) model, categorizes people into three groups: those who are at risk of getting infected, those already infected with the disease, and those who have recovered. According to the world health organization (WHO), these mathematical models help identify the disease's transmission rate, the time the infection reaches its peak, and how long it sustains. Recognizing the fractal characteristics of

Department of Mathematics, Amrita School of Physical Sciences, Coimbatore, Amrita Vishwa Vidyapeetham, India.
Email: mp_aparna@cb.students.amrita.edu
* Corresponding author: p_paramanathan@cb.amrita.edu

Covid-19 data, [16] formulated a new model similar to SIR. As a result, these models indirectly assist in taking the necessary safety measures to fend off the outbreak. Reconstruction of the death rate for the USA, Brazil, India, and Russia is done in [17] using fractal interpolation, followed by estimating the correlation fractal dimension. The graph of seven-day moving averages for the countries India, Denmark, Netherlands, UK, South Africa, and Germany is investigated in [18] using fractal interpolation functions. Assuming that the infection rate exhibits a power law behaviour, [19] uses a multifractal formalism for Covid-19 data. To investigate the dynamics of novel coronavirus disease, [21] suggests a new SITR model with fractal parameters. In [22], a generalized mathematical model that uses a fractal fractional operator is presented to analyze the current outbreak of this disease in India. For the nations of Romania, Italy, Spain, and Germany, a reconstruction of the epidemic curve is offered in [2] from the perspective of fractal interpolation. In [20], the SIR and fractal interpolation models are used to estimate the epidemic curve and anticipate the number of positive cases in India.

Besides these mathematical models, statisticians have formulated several metrics to assess the growth rate and complexity of the spread pattern of Covid- 19. An indicator of the transmission rate is the ratio of the number of positive cases confirmed in a day to the total number of tests conducted. This ratio is known as the positivity rate. The relation between the positivity rate and the number of deaths is explored in [6].

The fundamental aim of the present work is to analyze the growth rate and spread pattern of the coronavirus in India from Jun 1, 2020, to May 31, 2022. The growth rate will be evaluated every six months throughout the monitoring period. In contrast to the usual methods, this chapter measures the growth rate by considering the population of the country and the number of cumulative Covid-19 cases every six months. The cumulative number of cases is calculated as the area under the curve representing the number of Covid-19 cases per day using fractal numerical integration. The ordinate of the curve denotes the number of Covid-19 cases per day, and the abscissa represents the respective dates. The curve is obtained as the attractor of an iterated function system formulated from the Covid-19 data set with zero vertical scaling factor. Using a similar method, the curves representing the daily number of Covid-19 tests are reconstructed with fractal interpolation functions for each half-year. Approximating these curves through a fractal point of view helps to evaluate the data's randomness and predict the future disease trend. The advantages of employing fractal interpolation techniques in reconstructing are as follows:

- The daily number of Covid 19 cases is irregular and unpredictable. Since fractal analysis deals with signals of uneven characteristics, it will be more appropriate to choose fractal interpolation techniques to process these data sets.
- Fractal interpolation techniques helps to retrieve the missing information from inadequate testing.
- The self similarity property of fractals provides a fresh perspective on how to forecast the course of an epidemic. The fractal architecture of the epidemic curves enables the assessment of the current state of the disease and the prediction of upcoming changes.

The chapter is organized as follows: following the introduction, the second section of the chapter briefly revises the fundamentals of the fractal theory, which are essential in understanding the rest of the sequel. The third section explains the methodology adopted in calculating the growth rate and plotting the graphs. The fourth section displays all the computation results, along with the discussion on the observed points. Finally, the chapter concludes in section five by summarizing the obtained results.

9.2 Preliminaries

This section provides a brief recap of the basics of the fractal interpolation theory.

9.2.1 Fractal Interpolation Functions [1]

Let $\{(t_n, x_n)\}$ be the given set of data points where $t_0 < t_1 < ... < t_N$ representing the input values. $x_n, n = 0, 1, ..., N$ denotes the function values at these points. Set $I = [t_0, t_N]$ and define N number of contractive homeomorphisms $L_n : I \to I_n$ where $I_n = [t_{n-1}, t_n]$, for $n = 1, 2, ..., N$. The map L_n should satisfy

$$L_n(t_0) = t_{n-1}, \quad L_n(t_N) = t_n \tag{9.1}$$

and the contractivity condition

$$| L_n(c_1) - L_n(c_2) | \leq l \mid c_1 - c_2 \mid, \tag{9.2}$$

for some l such that $0 \leq l < 1$ and $c_1, c_2 \in I$ The map L_n considered here is given by

$$L_n(t, x) = a_n t + b_n, \tag{9.3}$$

where a_n and b_n are obtained by solving the conditions (9.1). Choose a number α_n from $(-1, 1)$. This number is the vertical scaling factor for the construction and numerical integration of fractal interpolation functions corresponding to the data set $\{(t_n, x_n) : n = 0, 1, ..., N\}$. Set $F = I \times R$ and define N mappings $F_n : F \to R$ such that

$$F_n(t_0, x_0) = x_{n-1}, \quad F_n(t_N, x_N) = x_n \tag{9.4}$$

and

$$| F_n(t, x) - F_n(t, y) | \leq | \alpha_n || x - y | \tag{9.5}$$

for $n = 1, 2, ..., N$. The function F_n used here is

$$F_n(t, x) = q_{n1} t + q_{n0} + \alpha_n x, \tag{9.6}$$

the coefficients q_{n1} and q_{n2} are obtained by solving (9.4). Now, the iterated function system for this data set is given by

$$w_n(t, x) = (L_n(t), F_n(t, x)), \text{ for } n = 1, 2, ..., N. \tag{9.7}$$

Define an operator $W = \cup_n w_n(t, x)$ on the space of all nonempty, compact subsets of $I \times R$. Then, the unique, fixed point of this operator is known as the attractor of the IFS. Note that the attractor of the IFS (9.7) is the graph of a continuous function interpolating the given data set $\{(t_n, x_n) : n = 0, 1, 2, ..., N\}$. This continuous function is defined to be the fractal interpolation function for the data set $\{(t_n, x_n) : n = 0, 1, 2, ..., N\}$.

Example 9.1 Let $\{(2.7, 0.8395), (3.5, -1.1339), (4.3, 0.0647), (5.1, -1.8872), (5.9, 0.3553), (6.7, 0.0693), (7.5, 0.8056)\}$ be the given data set. The fractal interpolation function corresponding to the given data can be constructed using the iterated function system given as follows:

$$w_n(t, x) = (L_n(t), F_n(t, x)), \quad n = 1, 2, ..., N.$$

Using the conditions (9.1), (9.4) and considering the given data set, this IFS becomes:

$$\{(0.1667t + 2.25, 0.2210x - 0.4096t + 1.7595),$$
$$(0.1667t + 3.05, -0.0985x + 0.2490t - 1.7235),$$
$$(0.1667t + 3.85, 0.0175x - 0.4065t + 1.1476)$$
$$(0.1667t + 4.65, 0.1599x + 0.4683t - 3.2859)$$
$$(0.1667t + 5.45, -0.2366x - 0.0613t + 0.7193),$$
$$(0.1667t + 6.25, 0.2594x + 0.1552t - 0.5676)\}$$

Figure 9.1 shows the attractor obtained for this iterated function system.

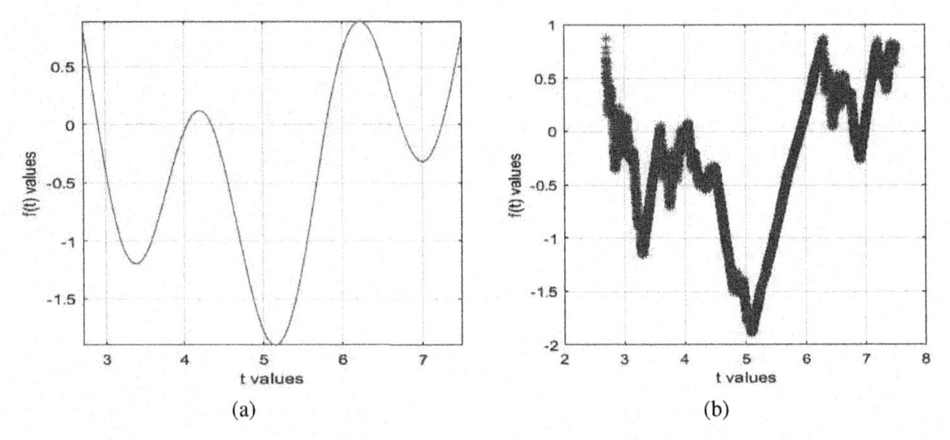

Fig. 9.1: Original graph and attractor of the iterated function systems for Example 9.1 (a) Original graph of the function, (b) Attractor the IFS.

Example 9.2 Consider the data set $\{(2.7, 2.5648), (3.5, 0.1788), (4.3, 0.9113), (5.1, -1.5420), (5.9, 0.1742), (6.7, -0.6566), (7.5, -0.4794)\}$. Then, the iterated function system for this data set is :

$$w_n(t, x) = (L_n(t), F_n(t, x)), \;\; n = 1, 2, ..., N.$$

Using the conditions (9.1), (9.4) and considering the given data set, this IFS becomes:

$$\{(0.1667t + 2.25, 0.2288x - 0.3519t + 2.9281),$$
$$(0.1667t + 3.05, -0.1054x + 0.0858t + 0.2175),$$
$$(0.1667t + 3.85, 0.0169x - 0.5004t + 2.2189)$$
$$(0.1667t + 4.65, 0.1666x + 0.4632t - 3.2198)$$
$$(0.1667t + 5.45, -0.2489x - 0.3309t + 1.7060),$$
$$(0.1667t + 6.25, 0.2714x + 0.2090t - 1.9170)\}$$

The attractor obtained is plotted in Figure 9.2.

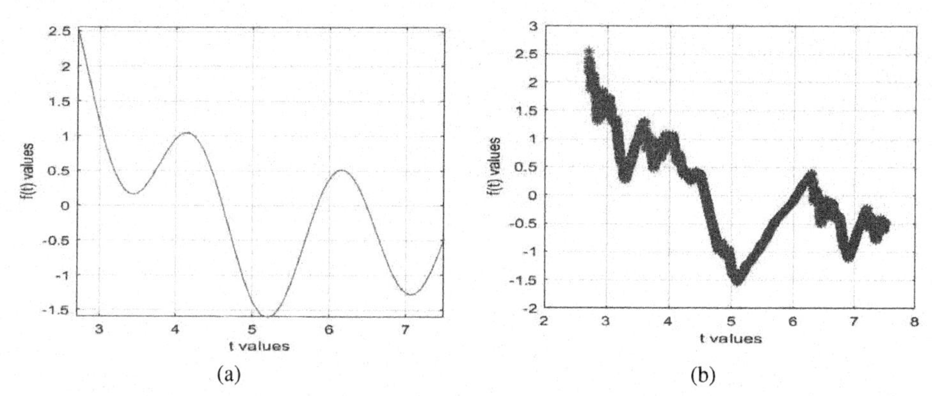

Fig. 9.2: Original graph and attractor of the iterated function systems for Example 9.2 (a) Original graph of the function, (b) Attractor the IFS.

9.2.2 Fractal Numerical Integration [3]

The fractal numerical integration formula is defined by :

$$M_0 = \frac{\int_I Q(t)}{1 - \sum_{n=1}^{N} \alpha_n a_n}, \tag{9.8}$$

where $Q(t) = q_{n1}o(L_n^{-1}(t)) + q_{n0}, t \in I_n, n = 1, 2, \ldots, N$.

Fractal numerical integration for Example 9.1

Consider the data set provided in Example 9.1

The numerical integration value for this data set using fractal numerical integration formula (M_0) is given in Table 9.1.

Fractal numerical integration for Example 9.2

Consider the data set given in Example 9.2. The numerical integration value for this data set using fractal numerical integration formula (M_0) is given in Table 9.2.

9.3 Methodology

The first aim of this chapter is to display the curve representing the spread pattern of coronavirus in India from June 1, 2020, to May 31, 2022. The entire period of study is divided into four half-years:

- June 1, 2020 - December 31, 2020.
- January 1, 2021 - May 31, 2021.
- June 1, 2021 - December 31, 2021.
- January 1, 2022 - May 31, 2022.

Table 9.1: Exact integral value and fractal numerical integral for Example 9.1: N = No of subdivisions, W = Exact integral value, M_0=Fractal numerical integral.

N	W	M_0
6	-1.82140	-1.6699
12	-1.82140	-1.7867
18	-1.82140	-1.8062
24	-1.82140	-1.8129
48	-1.82140	-1.8193
96	-1.82140	-1.8209
144	-1.82140	-1.8212
198	-1.82140	-1.8213
246	-1.82140	-1.8213
300	-1.82140	-1.8214

Table 9.2: Exact integral value and fractal numerical integral for Example 9.2: N = No of subdivisions, W = Exact integral value, M_0=Fractal numerical integral.

N	W	M_0
6	-0.354615	-0.1990
12	-0.354615	-0.3192
18	-0.354615	-0.3391
24	-0.354615	-0.3459
48	-0.354615	-0.3525
96	-0.354615	-0.3541
144	-0.354615	-0.3544
198	-0.354615	-0.3545
246	-0.354615	-0.3545
300	-0.354615	-0.3546

The number of confirmed cases is collected from [7] on a daily basis during each of the half-years. Due of the data set's inherent randomness, fractal interpolation functions are used to examine the spread pattern. Fractal interpolation functions are constructed using iterated function systems. The iterated function system considered here is given by:

$$w_n(t,x) = (a_n t + b_n, q_{n1} t + q_{n0} + \alpha_n x) \tag{9.9}$$

for $n = 1, 2, ..., N$ where the coefficients are calculated using the conditions:

$$L_n(t_0) = t_{n-1}, \quad L_n(t_N) = t_n \tag{9.10}$$

and

$$F_n(t_0, x_0) = x_{n-1}, \quad F_n(t_N, x_N) = x_n \tag{9.11}$$

The number α_n corresponds to the vertical scaling factor.

For the curve denoting the number of Covid-19 cases, the t values are $1, 2, 3, ...$ (denoting each day of the half-year) and the x values are the number of Covid-19 cases reported in each of these days. The t values are the same for the curve displaying the number of Covid-19 tests and the x values are the number of tests conducted on each of these days.

The attractor of this iterated function system is the fractal interpolation curve representing the number of confirmed cases in each half-year. The $X-$ axis of the graph represents the day and the $Y-$ axis indicates the daily number of confirmed cases. The fractal interpolation curves obtained during each half-year considered are given in Figure 9.3, Figure 9.4, Figure 9.5 and Figure 9.6.

Proceeding further, the reconstruction of the curves that display the amount of tests conducted over the course of each half-year is studied. The number of tests conducted on each day is obtained from [7]. An IFS similar to the former one has been formulated, and the respective attractors are plotted. Figure 9.7, Figure 9.8, Figure 9.9 and Figure 9.10 represent the fractal interpolation curves for the number of tests during the half-years June 1, 2020 - December 31,2020, January 1, 2021 - May 31,2020, June 1, 2021 - December 31,2021 and January 1, 2022 - May 31,2022 respectively. All the figures displayed in the chapter are drawn using Matlab R2018a.

Growth rate of the virus provides information about how quickly it is spreading throughout the nation. Different formulas have been presented by researchers to assess the growth rate. According to [23], growth rate has been calculated as the difference in number of cases between two consecutive days, divided by the count of infected cases on the previous day of the two days under consideration, multiplied by 100. In [24], the authors proposes a methodology to measure growth rate using regression analysis.

This chapter measures the growth rate by finding the ratio of the cumulative number of cases reported at the end of each half-year to the population of the country. The cumulative number of cases is normally calculated by adding the number of new cases appeared each day. This becomes a tedious process whenever we want to calculate the number of cumulative cases for a long period of time. The present chapter provides an easier and straightforward method to find this value. Firstly, the curve representing the number of Covid-19 cases is reconstructed using fractal interpolation technique. The abscissa of the curve is the particular dates and the ordinate denotes the number of new cases reported on each of these dates. Then, the area under the curve corresponds to the cumulative number. Since the explicit function of the curve is unknown, the area is obtained by numerically evaluating the integral value. The fundamental motivations for employing the fractal numerical integration approach when determining the integral values are as follows:

- The standard numerical integration techniques might not be able to produce an appropriate answer since the data set is unpredictable and complex.
- Fractal numerical integration reduces computation work by achieving the desired results with fewer iterations.
- Since fractal interpolation functions substantially reduce information leakage, the results of fractal numerical integration will be more accurate.

Therefore, fractal numerical integration (9.8) is applied to assess the area under the curve. The formula is based on the coefficients of the iterated function system as explained in Section 9.2.2. The cumulative number of cases obtained is provided in Table 9.3 and Table 9.4 shows the growth rate of the virus in the country during each half-year.

9.4 Results

This section provides the reconstructed curves and numerical integral values.

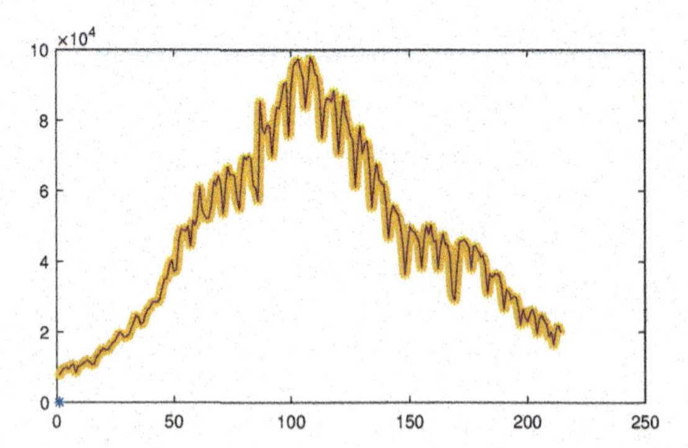

Fig. 9.3: Curves representing the number of confirmed cases from June 1, 2020 to December 31, 2020. Black color denotes the original curve and yellow color denotes the fractal interpolation curve.

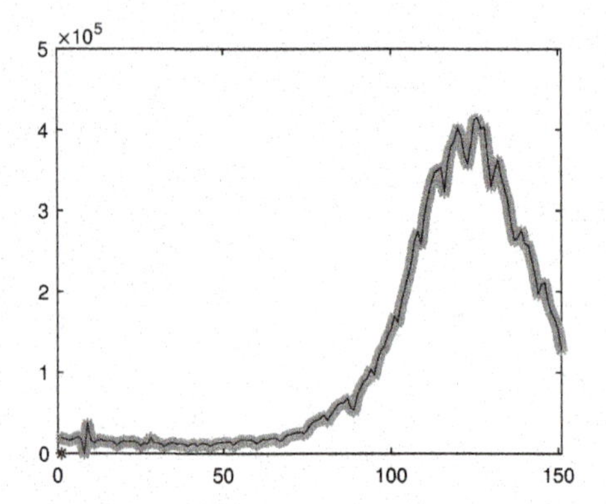

Fig. 9.4: Curves representing the number of confirmed cases from January 1, 2021 to May 31, 2021. Black color denotes the original curve and yellow color denotes the fractal interpolation curve.

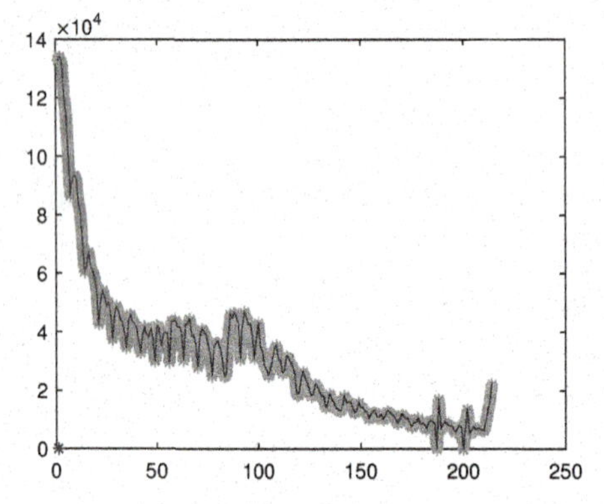

Fig. 9.5: Curves representing the number of confirmed cases from June 1, 2021 to December 31, 2021. Black color denotes the original curve and yellow color denotes the fractal interpolation curve.

9.4.1 Regarding the Curves

On observing the curves, it has been obtained that:

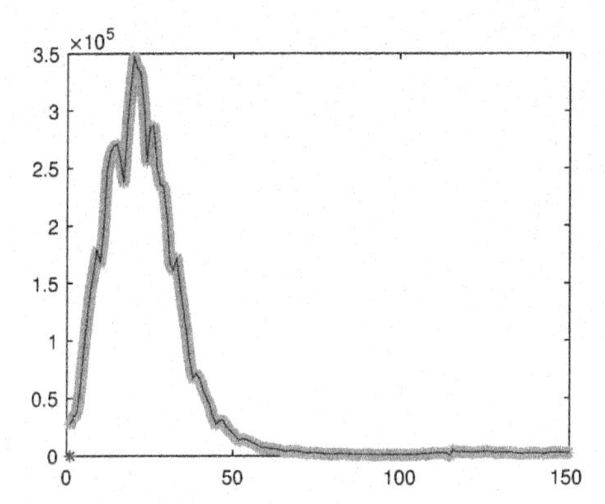

Fig. 9.6: Curves representing the number of confirmed cases from January 1, 2022 to May 31, 2022. Black color denotes the original curve and yellow color denotes the fractal interpolation curve.

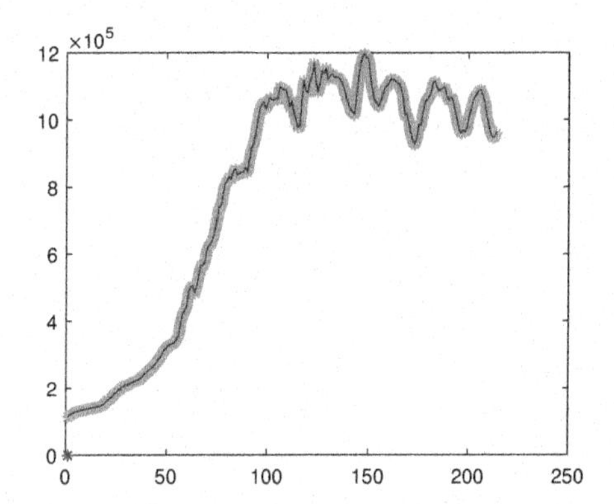

Fig. 9.7: Curves representing the number of daily tests from June 1, 2020 to December 31, 2020. Black color denotes the original curve and yellow color denotes the fractal interpolation curve.

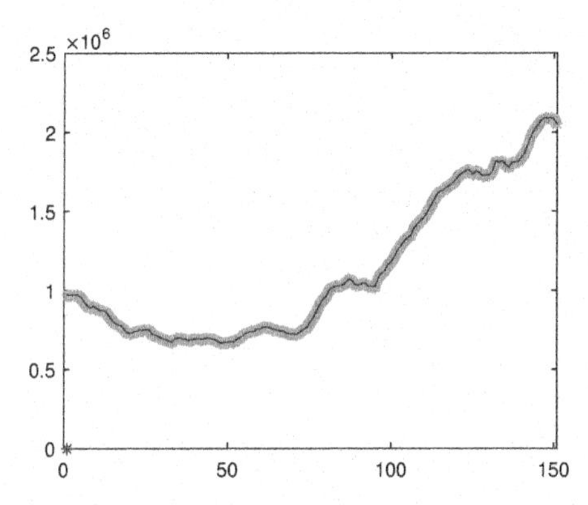

Fig. 9.8: Curves representing the number of daily tests from January 1, 2021 to May 31, 2021. Black color denotes the original curve and yellow color denotes the fractal interpolation curve.

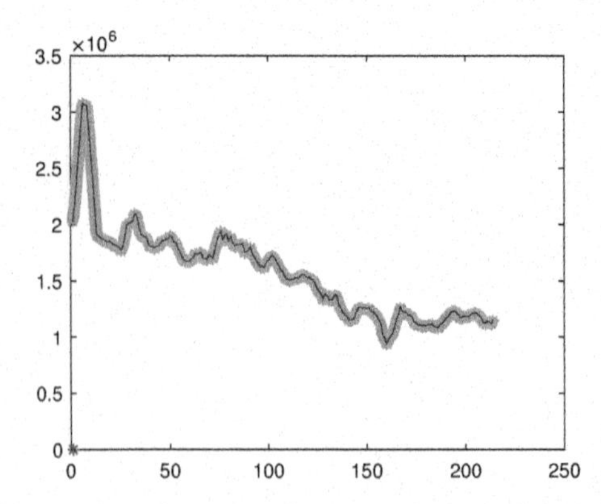

Fig. 9.9: Curves representing the number of daily tests from June 1, 2021 to December 31, 2021. Black color denotes the original curve and yellow color denotes the fractal interpolation curve.

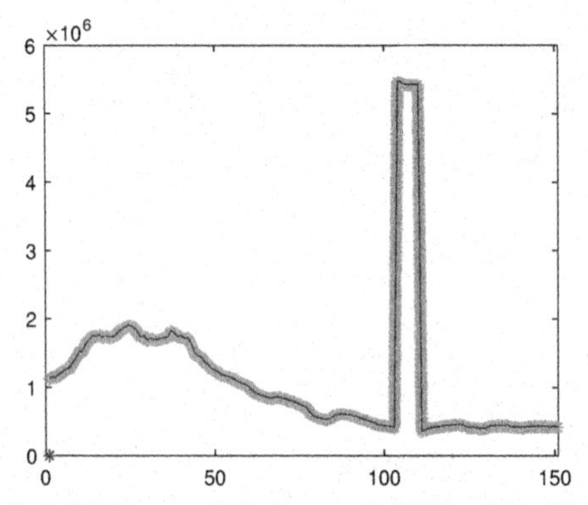

Fig. 9.10: Curves representing the number of daily tests from January 1, 2022 to May 31, 2022. Black color denotes the original curve and yellow color denotes the fractal interpolation curve.

- The curves representing the number of daily confirmed cases exhibit an oscillating behaviour.
- Initially, there was a limited number of Covid-19 tests. The number of tests is increased during the months of September 2020. A sudden increase in the number of Covid-19 tests is visible during February-March 2022.
- The curves showing the number of daily confirmed cases are rather erratic, and fractal interpolation does a better job of capturing this erratic behaviour.

Table 9.3: Table calculating the number of cumulative cases during each half-year (The number is calculated by evaluating the area under the curve using fractal numerical integration).

Area under the curve in Figure 9.3	10082202
Area under the curve in Figure 9.4	17815000
Area under the curve in Figure 9.5	6608800
Area under the curve in Figure 9.6	8284104

Table 9.4: Table showing the ratio of the cumulative number of cases to the population (population is according to [8]).

Period	Population	Cumulative number of cases	$\frac{\text{Cumulative number of cases}}{\text{Population}}$
01/06/2020 - 31/12/2020	1,380,004,385	10082202	0.0073
01/01/2021 - 31/05/2021	1,393,409,038	17815000	0.0128
01/06/2021 - 31/12/2021	1,380,004,385	6608800	0.0047
01/01/2022 - 31/05/2022	1,406,631,776	8284104	0.0059

On observing the table, it is obtained that:

- Almost 0.7% of the population is affected by Covid-19 in India during June 2020 to December 2020.
- The growth rate is slightly increased during January 2021 to May 2021 and around 1.2% of the population is affected during this period.
- The rate began to decline slowly and almost 0.4% is affected during June 2021 to December 2021.
- The portion of the population affected by Covid-19 is around 0.5% during the period January 2022 to May 2022.

9.5 Conclusion

The unexpected increase in Covid instances poses a threat to humanity and negatively impacts the nation's financial, economic, and health conditions. The forecast of the coronavirus's growth rate in the upcoming years will aid humanity in making the necessary preparations and actions to lessen the harm the virus causes. This chapter analyses the spread pattern and growth rate of the Covid-19 pandemic in India from June, 2020 to May 2022 using fractal approach. Using iterated function system, the curves for the number of daily confirmed cases and the number of daily Covid-19 tests have been reconstructed. Drawing these curves through fractal approach helps in retrieving the missing pieces of information and capturing the irregularities within the curves. Reconstructing curves through a fractal approach helps to forecast the upcoming tendencies of the disease. Growth rate is ascertained by ratio of the cumulative number of cases with the population of the country. An alternative method that makes use of fractal numerical integration is proposed to calculate the cumulative number of Covid-19 instances over a period of time.

References

[1] Barnsley, M.F. 1986. Fractal functions and interpolation. Constr. Approx., 2: 303–329.

[2] Cristina-Maria, P. and N. Bogdan-Radu. 2020. An analysis of COVID-19 spread based on fractal interpolation and fractal dimension. Chaos, Solitons Fractals, 139: 110073.

[3] Navascués, M.A. and M.V. Sebastián. 2013. Numerical integration of affine fractal functions. J. Comput. Appl. Math., 252: 169–176.

[4] https://covid19.who.int/.

[5] Awadh Alanazi, S., M.M. Kamruzzaman, M. Alruwaili, N. Alshammari, S.A. Alqahtani and A. Karime. 2020. Measuring and preventing COVID-19 using the SIR model and machine learning in smart health care. Journal of Healthcare Engineering.

[6] Al Dallal, A., U. AlDallal and J. Al Dallal. 2021. Positivity rate: An indicator for the spread of COVID-19. Curr. Med. Res. Opin., 37(12): 2067–2076.

[7] https://ourworldindata.org/covid-cases.

[8] statisticstimes.com/demographics/country/india-population.php.

[9] Patrikar, S., D. Poojary, D.R. Basannar, D.S. Faujdar and R. Kunte. 2020. Projections for novel coronavirus (COVID-19) and evaluation of epidemic response strategies for India. Med. J. Armed Forces India, 76(3): 268–275.

[10] Sharma, S., S. Basu, N.P. Shetti and T.M. Aminabhavic. 2020. Current treatment protocol for COVID-19 in India. Sensors Int., 1: 100013.

[11] Shetti, N.P., R.K. Srivastava, S. Sharma, S. Basu and T.M. Aminabhavi. 2020. Invasion of novel corona virus (COVID-19) in Indian territory. Sensors Int., 1: 100012.

[12] Konwar, A.N. and V. Borse. 2020. Current status of point-of-care diagnostic devices in the Indian healthcare system with an update on COVID-19 pandemic. Sensors Int., 1: 100015.

[13] Mahapatra, S. and P. Chandra. 2020. Clinically practiced and commercially viable nanobio engineered analytical methods for COVID-19 diagnosis. Biosens. Bioelectron., 165: 112361.

[14] Chandra, P., Y. Nee Tan and S.P. Singh. 2017. Next Generation Point-of-care Biomedical Sensors Technologies for Cancer Diagnosis, Springer. 10.1007/978-981-10-4726-8, 2017.

[15] Sudan, P. and B. Bhargava. 2020. Empowering citizens for testing of SARS-CoV-2 virus to save precious lives and contain the virus.

[16] Abbasi, M., A.L. Bollini, J.L.B. Castillo, A. Deppman, J.P. Guidio, P.T. Matuoka, A.D. Meirelles, J.M.P. Policarpo, A.A.G.F. Ramos, S. Simionatto, A.R. Varona, E. Andrade-II, H. Panjeh and L.A. Trevisan. 2020. Fractal signatures of the COVID-19 spread. Chaos, Solitons and Fractals, 140: 110119.

[17] Easwaramoorthy, D., A. Gowrisankar, A. Manimaran, S. Nandhini, L. Rondoni and S. Banerjee. 2021. An exploration of fractal-based prognostic model and comparative analysis for second wave of COVID-19 diffusion. Nonlinear Dyn., 106(2): 1375–1395.

[18] Gowrisankar, A., T.M.C. Priyanka and S. Banerjee. 2022. Omicron: A mysterious variant of concern. Eur. Phys. J. Plus, 137(1): 1–8.

[19] Gowrisankar, A., L. Rondoni and S. Banerjee. 2020. Can India develop herd immunity against COVID-19? Eur. Phys. J. Plus, 135(6): 526.

[20] Kavitha, C., A. Gowrisankar and S. Banerjee. 2021. The second and third waves in India: When will the pandemic be culminated? Eur. Phys. J. Plus, 136(5): 596.

[21] Sanchez, Y.G., Z. Sabir and J.L. Guirao. 2020. Design of a nonlinear SITR fractal model based on the dynamics of a novel coronavirus (COVID-19). Fractals, 28(08): 2040026.

[22] Abdulwasaa, M.A., M.S. Abdo, K. Shah, T.A. Nofal, S.K. Panchal, S.V. Kawale and A.H. Abdel-Aty. 2021. Fractal-fractional mathematical modeling and forecasting of new cases and deaths of COVID-19 epidemic outbreaks in India. Results Phys., 20: 103702.

[23] Gupta, R., S.K. Pal and G. Pandey. 2020. A Comprehensive Analysis of COVID-19 Outbreak situation in India. MedRxiv. 10.1101/2020.04.08.20058347.

[24] Sharma, D.K. and H. Sharma. 2021. A study of trend growth rate of confirmed cases, death cases and recovery cases in view of Covid-19 of top five States of India. Solid State Technology, 64(2): 4526–4541.

Chapter 10

Classification of COVID-19 Time Series Through Hurst Exponent and Fractal Dimension

C. Kavitha, M. Meenakshi and *A. Gowrisankar**

10.1 Introduction

The World Health Organization (WHO) received information on numerous cases of lungs related diseases with unknown causes from China Health Authority(CHA) in Wuhan city, on December 31, 2019. Most people had been affected severely by fever, cold, cough, and body pain, while diagnosing these people with the above-mentioned symptoms it was found that they were commonly affected with new respiratory diseases in Wuhan [1]. A new type of Corona Virus disease(COVID-19), apart from Severe Acute Respiratory Syndrome (SARS) and Middle East Respiratory Syndrome (MERS), was discovered in December 2019. In the initial months of COVID-19, worldwide medical experts, public sectors, and the general public were uncertain about the disease's spread and effect on daily life. The United Nations released fifteen million in amount to assist with the worldwide COVID-19 response on March 2020. From Wuhan city, this disease spread rapidly to two hundred three countries by the end of March 2020 and WHO authoritatively proclaimed this disease as a worldwide pandemic. COVID-19 proceeded from being a significant issue that appeared to be restricted to China to a worldwide health emergency in a short amount of time. In [2] the authors have analyzed the fractal interpolation and SIR models for assessing the epidemic frequency for the second and third waves of COVID-19 in India, including high-impact states such as Tamil Nadu, Delhi, Kerala, Maharashtra, and Karnataka. The results of the SIR and fractal models have shown that the pandemic reached its peak in India around May 2021. They have examined the COVID-19 data day-wise for positive cases, suspected cases, and recovery cases. These techniques of SIR and fractal interpolation have been employed to forecast COVID-19 impact outcomes for the future. Many methods, such as Fuzzy Time Series Modeling, stage-dependent stochastic model, and neutralizing antibodies have been analyzed to forecast the future epidemic of the time series by analyzing the dynamical development of the viral transmission during the second and third waves(In addition information [16]–[23]).

In several countries, the number of cases, hospitalizations, and deaths due to COVID-19 went down because people had to follow rules to stop the virus from spreading. But the $\lambda(C.37)$ variant was found for the first time in Peru, and the United States on May 2020. The WHO says that this variant has now spread

Department of Mathematics, School of Advanced Sciences, Vellore Institute of Technology, Vellore 632 014, Tamil Nadu, India.
Emails: cmallikakavi@gmail.com, meenakshiyayathirajan@gmail.com
* Corresponding author: gowrisankargri@gmail.com

to at least twenty-nine countries. There were more new Covid -19 variants discovered such as $\beta(B.1.351)$ in South Africa on May 2020, $\gamma(B.1.351)$ in Brazil on November 2020, and $\Delta(B.1.617.2)$ in India on October 2020. While the $\alpha(B.1.1.7)$ variant was discovered for the first time in the UK on September 2020. Obtaining these different kinds of the virus has been crucial because it demonstrated that the virus was evolving. As a consequence of this, the indications and diagnosis of the results have changed. For instance, indications have shown that the α variant may increase the risk of terrible COVID-19 effects. As a result of the new variants, COVID-19 cases surged again in several nations, and by September 2020, one million fatalities had been attributed to these viruses (For further information [3]–[5]).

In [6] Gowrisankar et al. have studied a comparison of the seven-day moving average of daily positive Omicron cases for the majority of infected countries such as Germany, Denmark, Netherlands, India, UK, and South Africa. The fractal interpolation was employed to analyze the epidemic curve of the Omicron mutant in these countries. Numerous authors have established the prediction of positive COVID-19 cases based on these models—the fractal models and the fractional models, amongst others, for the first wave, the second wave, and also the new variants such as $\lambda, \beta, \gamma, \Delta$, and Omicron. They have discussed these results for positive cases, fatality cases, and suspected cases from 2020 to 2022. As a characterized the organization of Covid-19 genome sequence based on the fractal scaling analysis. The Authors have compared the Covid-19 with SARS sequence and has portrayed as covid-19 more randomness than SARS.(for more details, [7]–[15]). Numerous methods, such as Fuzzy Time Series Modelling, stage-dependent stochastic model, and neutralizing antibodies have been analyzed to forecast the future epidemic of the time series of COVID-19 by analyzing the dynamical development of the viral transmission during the second and third waves(for further information [16]–[23]).

Harold Edwin Hurst, the British hydrologist was born in 1880 near Leicester and quit school at 15 to become a teacher. Hurst's career began in terrestrial magnetism and astronomy—he was in charge of Egypt's magnetic survey—and become a head of the Egyptian physical department and assigned a work to construct the dam across the river Nile. For this project, he started to collect Nile data, in 1913. He spend his life time for this project. Dr. H. E. Hurst is most known for his long-term studies of the Nile, and he is pioneered the study of persistence in hydro-logical phenomena [24]. Hurst introduced new procedure called rescaled range analysis to find the persistence. Hurst formulated the following estimation

$$\mathcal{K}(t,s) = \frac{\log[\mathcal{R}(t,s)/\mathcal{S}(t,s)]}{\log(s) - \log 2},$$

where s is series of samples with respect the time t and $\mathcal{K}(t,s)$ is later called as Hurst exponent $\mathcal{H}$. It is nothing but a slope of log-log plot trend line [25]. Hurst value must lies between 0 to 1. If the hurst values lies between $0 < \mathcal{H} < 0.5$ then its is persistence especially anti persistence, if $\mathcal{H} = 0$ is random walk, we cannot predict it, if $0.5 < \mathcal{H} < 1$ is persistence and it is called as Brownian motion. Mandelbrot have been provided the relation between Hurst exponent $\mathcal{H}$ and Fractal dimension $\mathcal{D}$ as $\mathcal{H} = E + 1 - \mathcal{D}$, where E is the Euclidean dimension. For a one-dimensional $(1-\mathcal{D})$ function that varies with time, $\mathcal{H} = 2-\mathcal{D}$ or $\mathbb{D} = 2-\mathcal{H}$ (for more details in [26]–[29]). If the time series of fractal dimension D is 1.5, there is no relation between the changes in amplitude that happen at two different time intervals. So, the time series makes it impossible to tell if there is a trend in the amplitude, so the process is unpredictable. But as the fractal dimension goes down to 1, the process gets easier to predict because it stays the same. The fractal dimension goes from 1 to 1.5, the process goes from persistent. As the fractal dimension goes from 1.5 to 2, the process goes from being persistent to not being persistent. As the fractal dimension climbs from 1.5 to 2, anti-persistence is seen. In other words, a drop in the amplitude of the process is more likely to result in a future rise.

Several researchers have estimated the fractal dimension of the predictions through Hurst exponents for COVID-19 cases based on seven days of rolling average data for the positive case, such as the most affected countries and states of countries for the first wave, the second wave, and also the new variants $\lambda, \beta, \gamma, \Delta$, and Omicron. They have taken these data for the month-wise period from 2020 to 2022 and have analyzed affected people for that method of $\mathcal{R}/\mathcal{S}$ for predicting their epidemic curve and Hurt line or trend line for the slope(In addition details [30]–[39]). Wang et al. have analyzed the method of multifractal detrended fluctuation analysis (MF-DFA) for the vaccinated COVID-19 cases and new fatality cases that occurred in nine various countries for the time series from 23 July 2020 to 24 March 2022 [40]. Consequently, illustrating the positive outcomes discovered in various analyses, the problem in the prediction of epidemic time series by the hypothesis of presence of fractal dimension is still open, either for modeling epidemic time series or for trend analysis for epidemic indicators. In order to bridge this knowledge gap, the time series of COVID-19 over the period 2020-2023 is analyzed with the seven days moving average for positive cases, fatality cases, and vaccinated cases of fractal dimension through the Hurst exponent.

This chapter is organised as follow: Section 10.2 provided the methodology of rescaled range analysis, Hurst exponent, fractal dimension for time series. The positive COVID-19 data for total cumulative cases, seven day moving average of positive new daily cases, new fatality case, and vaccinated cases are described and analyzed in Section 10.3. Finally, prescribed COVID-19 times series data corresponding to the evaluate fractal dimension through Hurst exponent.

10.2 Methodology

The statistical method known as rescaled range analysis is employed in the process of identifying the characteristics of a time series as well as analyzing its variability. The Hurst exponent for time series of the COVID-19 positive case can be calculated by rescaled range analysis $\mathcal{R}/\mathcal{S}$ analysis. The following steps are describing the $\mathcal{R}/\mathcal{S}$ analysis as

Step 1: The time series data of COVID-19 positive cases has to be rescaled in powers of 2.

Step 2: Calculate the average for time series data

$$\text{average of Sample} = m_s = \frac{1}{n}\sum_{t=1}^{n} \mathcal{X}_t,$$

where s is series of sample, n is the size of the range of sample, $\mathcal{X}$ is the value of an element in the range.

Step 3: To determine the deviation for each data and define the new time series as

$$\mathcal{Y}_t = \mathcal{X}_t - \bar{\mathcal{X}} \text{ for } t = 1, 2, \ldots, n.$$

Step 4: To find the cumulative series which is the running total of the deviations from the average

$$y = \sum_{i=1}^{t} \mathcal{Y}_t.$$

Step 5: To evaluate the widest difference in the series of deviation by

$$\mathcal{R}_t = \max(\mathcal{Y}_1, \mathcal{Y}_2, \ldots, \mathcal{Y}_t) - \min(\mathcal{Y}_1, \mathcal{Y}_2, \ldots, \mathcal{Y}_t)$$

for $t = 1, 2, \ldots, n$, where $\mathcal{R}_t$ is the range of the time series.
Step 6: To find standard deviation for each range

$$\sigma = \sqrt{\left(\frac{1}{t}\sum_{i=1}^{t}(X_i - m_s)^2\right)}.$$

Step 7: Calculate the rescaled range for each range in the time series

$$(\mathcal{R}/\mathcal{S})_t = \frac{\mathcal{R}_t}{\sigma_t} \text{ for } t = 1, 2, \ldots, n$$

where $(\mathcal{R}/\mathcal{S})_t$ is the rescaled range for each range in time series, $\mathcal{R}_t$ is the range created with respected to the described time series, σ is the standard deviation for the range under consideration. Next, average the rescaled range values for each region to summarize each range. Now have rescaled range in the time series. Then calculate the Hurst exponent $\mathcal{H}$,

$$(\mathcal{R}/\mathcal{S})_t = ct^{\mathcal{H}}$$

where $(\mathcal{R}/\mathcal{S})$ denotes rescaled range, n denotes the duration of individual short time series, c is a constant and $\mathcal{H}$ denotes the Hurst exponent. take logarithims on both sides of the above equation, it become as:

$$\log(\mathcal{R}/\mathcal{S})_t = \log c + \mathcal{H}\log t.$$

if replace the log values as $y = \log(\mathcal{R}/\mathcal{S})_t, x = \log(t), C = \log c$, then it gives equation of straight line with slope and y-intercept as

$$y = \mathcal{H}x + C.$$

From this equation, is clearly understood that $\mathcal{H}$ hurst exponent is just the slope of the ordinary line equation that is obtained by plotting the $\log(\mathcal{R}/\mathcal{S})_t$ *versus* $\log(t)$.

In [29]. Let D be any non empty bounded subset of $\mathbf{R}^n$ and let $N_\gamma(D)$ be the minimum number of square boxes of sides at most γ parallel to the axes which can cover D. The lower and upper box – counting dimensions of D respectively are defined as

$$\underline{\dim}_B(D) = \underline{\lim}_{\gamma\to 0}\frac{\log N_\gamma(D)}{-\log\gamma},$$

$$\overline{\dim}_B(D) = \overline{\lim}_{\gamma\to 0}\frac{\log N_\gamma(D)}{-\log\gamma}.$$

If $\underline{\dim}_B(D) = \overline{\dim}_B(D)$, the common value is termed as the box dimension for D,

$$\dim_B(D) = \lim_{\gamma\to 0}\frac{\log N_\gamma(D)}{-\log\gamma}.$$

Mandelbrot et al. have introduced the concept of fractal dimension via Hurst exponent. They have analyzed the interaction between fractal dimension and Hurst exponent [26]. A fractal dimension $\mathbb{D}$ is defined by the Hurst coefficient $\mathcal{H}$ as $\mathcal{H} = E + 1 - \mathbb{D}$, where E is the Euclidean dimension and $E = 0$ for a point, 1 for a line, and 2 for a surface. When $\mathcal{H}$ is less than 1, the item invades the next dimension, much as a curved or rough surface must be embedded in three-dimensional space to be perceived. The fractal theory has confirmed the direction of COVID-19's spread, providing more evidence of the virus's transmission method. If the plot of the logarithm of the size (x – axis) of each series versus the logarithm of the rescaled range (y – axis). The slope of the trend line from the log – log plot is Hurst exponent $\mathcal{H}$. Mandelbrot(1983) indicated that the exponent $\mathcal{H}$ in the interval $0 < \mathcal{H} < 1$ is related to the fractal dimension $\mathbb{D}$ by

$$\mathbb{D} = 2 - \mathcal{H}, \tag{10.1}$$

which leads to the values of $\mathbb{D}$ in the interval $1 < \mathbb{D} < 2$.

As part of the analysis of this chapter, the rescaled range analysis focuses on the relationship between the proportions of seven days moving average($\mathcal{R}$) and standard deviation ($\mathcal{S}$, where t is a time series,) to the concentration of the statistics length((n)). Then the constructed model for Covid-19 as the time series through Hurst exponent ($\mathcal{H}$) and fractal dimension

$$\log(\mathcal{R}/\mathcal{S})_t = \log c + \mathcal{H}\log(t). \tag{10.2}$$

The Moving average is a statistical technique employed to analyze the prescribed data through computing the time series of average of the various subsets of the whole set of data. This is generally computed to decrease unpredictability and short-term inconsistency of the data and to determine the curve tendency of provided data. It is considered as a tendency following indicators since it is based on the past data.

In this chapter, the 7-day rolling average of the daily positive cases and death cases is determined by taking the average of the past seven-day data by using the following formula,

$$\text{Seven days moving average} = \frac{\text{Sum of data over 7-days}}{7}.$$

The following Section 10.3 is discussing for COVID-19 data interpretation with the graph of epidemic curve and table.

10.3 Data Description

The COVID-19 data set has been received from the COVID-19 data repository by the Center for Systems Science and Engineering (CSSE) at Johns Hopkins University (https://ourworldindata.org). It is a set of data have presented daily updated details on COVID-19 for the world and most countries. This data portal has been developed and hosted by the Center for Systems Science and Engineering (CSSE) at Johns Hopkins University [3]. In this analysis, the seven-day moving average of daily positive cases, death cases, newly vaccinated cases, and boosted cases for the world, and five countries(the USA, India, the UK, France, and China) is discussed through the Hurst exponent and fractal dimension. Further, the fractal curves are derived from data points such as time (in days) and the 7-day moving average (in days).

Based on the total number of cases infected with corona (COVID-19) disease in the world, we know from the data graph that this disease is more prevalent in other countries than China. Especially, when this study examine available data's of the 5 Countries, the United States of America, India, France, the United Kingdom, and China from the date 25/1/2020 ton 25/1/2023. According to the basic data available, the United States of America is at the first place and India is at the second place followed by France and the United Kingdom. China, which is considered to be the origin of this disease is in the last place in the comparison chart. Looking at this graph, there are a lot of fluctuations in the curves. Short rise and declines or sudden peak rise and very small decline are detected in the early period. According to the graph of 2020, America is considered to be the country that has suffered the most from this disease with India following in second.

Table 10.1 described the data values of total cumulative cases and the 7-day rolling average of Covid-19 for the years 2020-2023 and the corresponding figures prescribed in Figure 10.1. The total cumulative cases data and the 7 days moving average data are picturized for the affected countries such as United States of America, India, the United Kingdom, France, and China. Figure 10.2 portrays the epidemic curve of an interpretation of the COVID-19 positive new smoothed daily cases for the years 2020–2023 for the highly affected countries such as the United States of America, France, China, India, and the United Kingdom. For instance, the fluctuation of the epidemic curve shows fractals and is inducing to find the fractal dimension for these countries. The USA country attained a tiny peak at the end of March, between July and August, and has progressively increased from October through December 2020. The USA is one of the most affected countries and reached its highest peak in late 2020. Similarly, other countries also have described the fluctuation of positive cases of the graphical approaches that have shown year-wise.

Table 10.1: Year wise Total cumulative positive cases and seven-day moving average.

	Years	Total cumulative cases	Seven days moving average
	2020	22151716	238554
World	2021	183913763	554652
	2022	546858621	981919
	2020	5011672	57615
USA	2021	36351456	92843
	2022	88219631	124476
	2020	3217448	30803
India	2021	25246782	67367
	2022	43363015	25427
	2020	514867	7078
UK	2021	6125060	27725
	2022	21977808	28150
	2020	606222	8146
France	2021	5841655	19744
	2022	30762528	77241
	2020	83004	238554
China	2021	103074	554652
	2022	884324	981919

The next graph to attract notice is India's, which reaches its high in September 2020. In the beginning, the number of cases in India is quite low. However, by the first week of April, it has increased considerably and continues to grow until it reaches its peak in September. In addition, it has begun to decline again gradually. Examining this epidemic curve more closely indicates that while the country's incidence was modest during the early March-April phase, it has subsequently been maintained under control and has begun to prevail from August to December. This is true despite the fact that it was only marginally apparent at the beginning of the period in March-April. The location that is recognized in China as the point of origin is subject to stringent regulation; this is evident from the epidemic curve, which shows that China's graph always lies on the x-axis.

The positive instances of COVID-19 from 2019 to 2023 are shown in Figure 10.3, and it can be seen that the United States is always the first country to be impacted by COVID-19. It attains the highest Himalayan peak from February to March 2022. The count of affected people is 8×10^5. By that time, all countries had

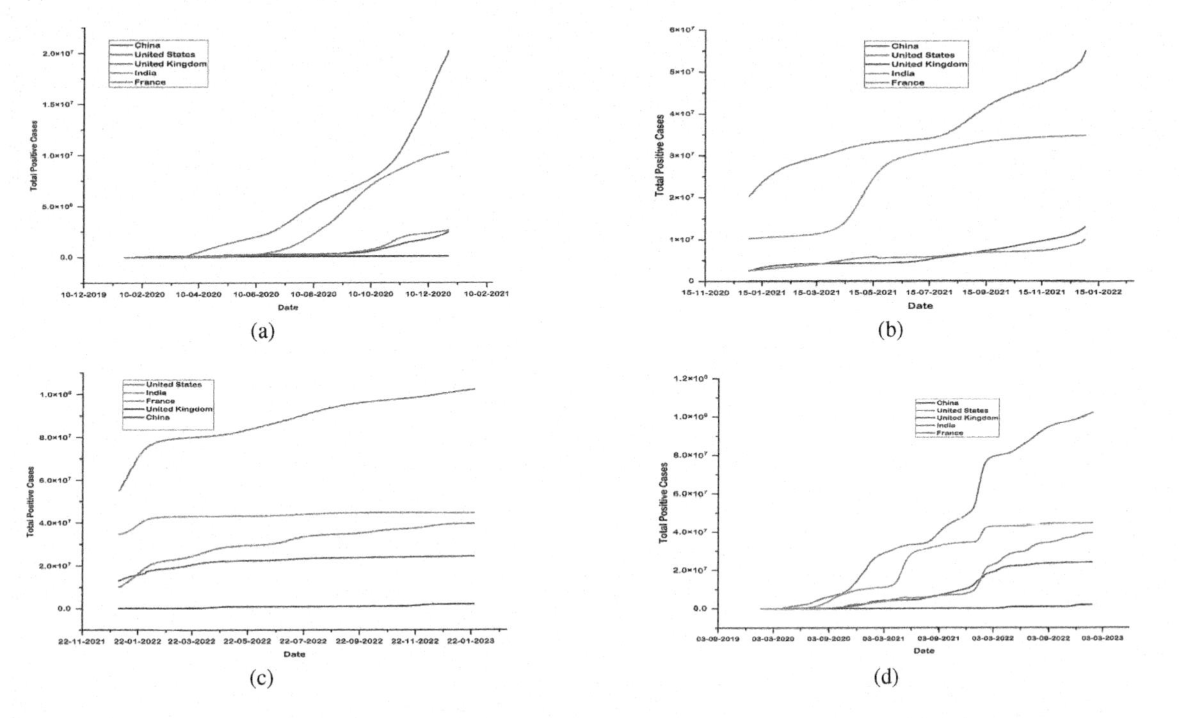

Fig. 10.1: Total cumulative positive cases of Covid-19 for USA, India, UK, France, and China during 2020–2023: (a) 2020–2021, (b)2021–2022, (c)2022–2023, (d)2020–2023.

reached their respective apex. For France and the UK, it attains the first highest peak by this period. The epidemic curve of India attains its first peak on end of May 2020 with 4×10^5 cases and the second maximum level obtained on the period on May to June 2020. Thereafter, the epidemic curve drops progressively until the end, indicating that the influence of COVID-19 diminishes.

10.4 Result and Discussion

The obtained data of positive confirmed COVID-19 cases for the years 2020 to 2023 and, year-wise separately, with the Hurst exponent $\mathcal{H}$ is calculated using rescaled range analysis. The fractal dimension is computed by using the formula $\mathbb{D} = 2 - \mathcal{H}$. The gained values of the Hurst exponent and fractal dimension for worldwide data (USA, UK, India, France, and China) are tabulated below. The graphs below depict the Hurst exponent value and a rescaled range curve with a normal line fit.

Table 10.2 presents the data gathered between 2020 and 2022 with varying sample sizes of Hurst value and Fractal dimension. It illustrates graphical methods in Figure 10.2 of the Hurst value using Origin and Matlab software. In the $\mathcal{R}/\mathcal{S}$ study of its computed Hurst of total confirmed cases in the World, the $\mathcal{H}$ estimates in the early stage have been estimated to be 0.9109, which is more than 0.5, indicating that the future time series has a positive association with fractal properties. The $\mathcal{H}$ value for second stage is 0.9663, which is approximately one, indicating that the future pandemic situation is completely unavoidable. The Hurst exponent and $\mathcal{R}/\mathcal{S}$ are the graphs representing the world Covid-19 data for 2020-2023 illustrated

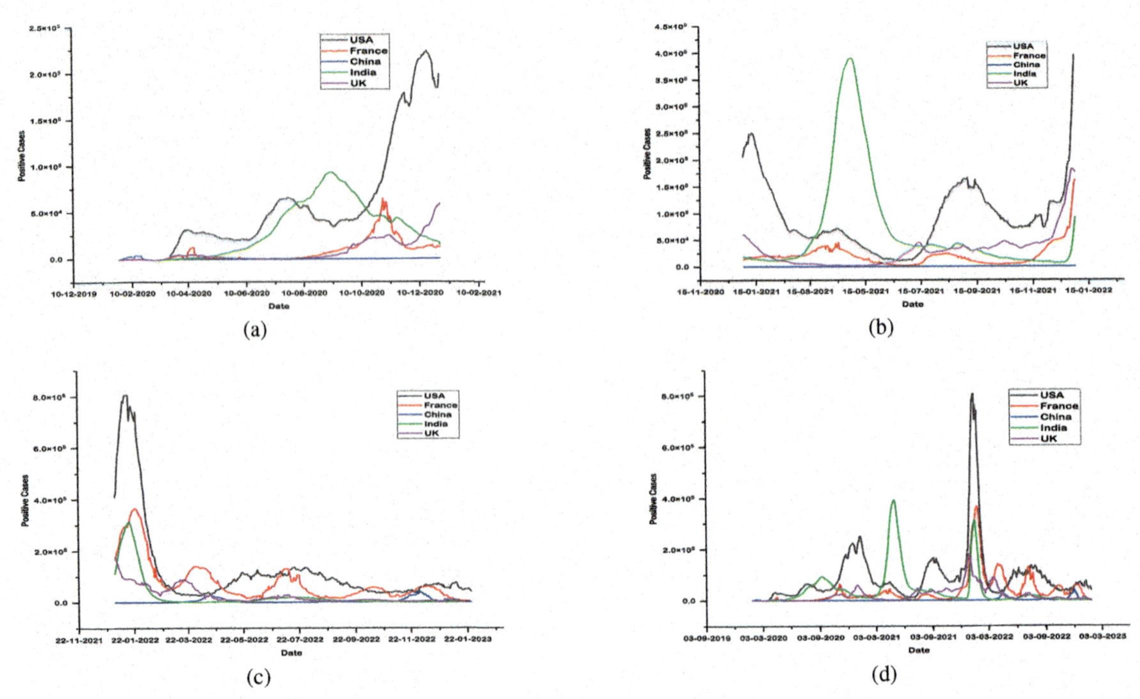

Fig. 10.2: Total cumulative positive cases of Covid-19 for USA, India, UK, France, and China during 2020–2023: (a) 2020–2021, (b)2021–2022, (c)2022–2023, (d)2020–2023.

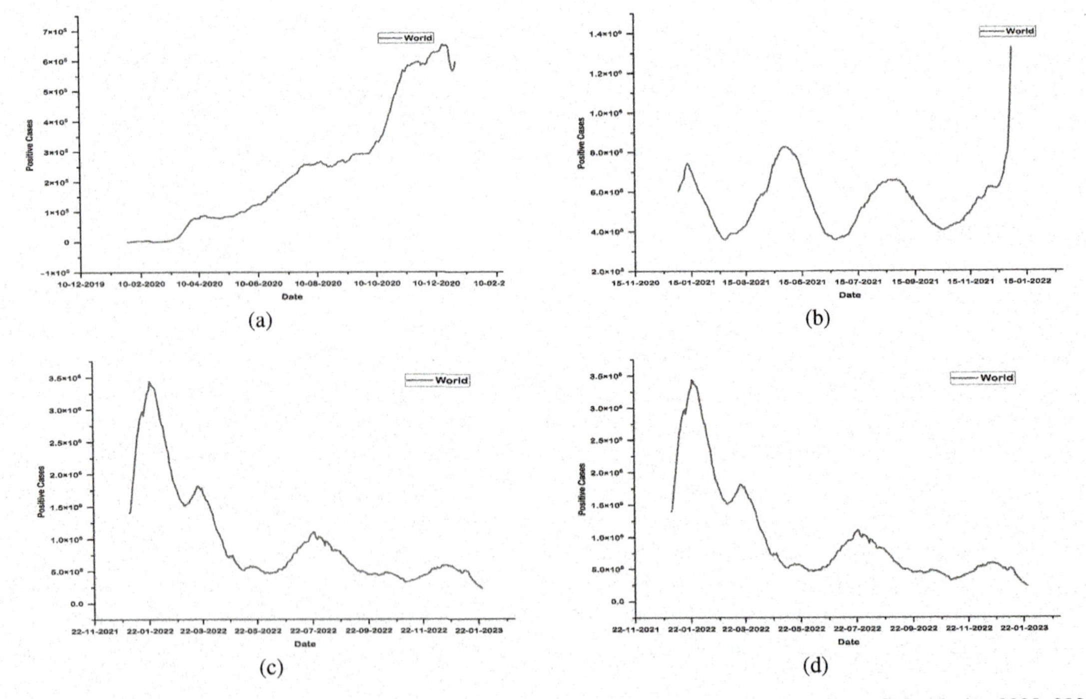

Fig. 10.3: Seven day moving average for positive cases of Covid-19 for USA, India, UK, France, and China during 2020–2023: (a) 2020–2021, (b) 2021–2022, (c) 2022–2023, (d)2020–2023.

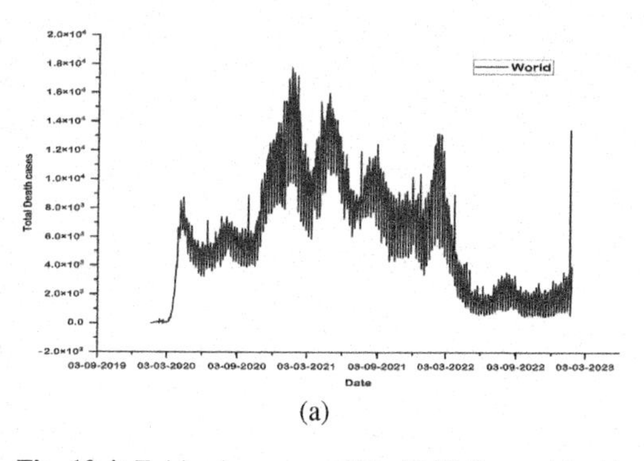

(a)

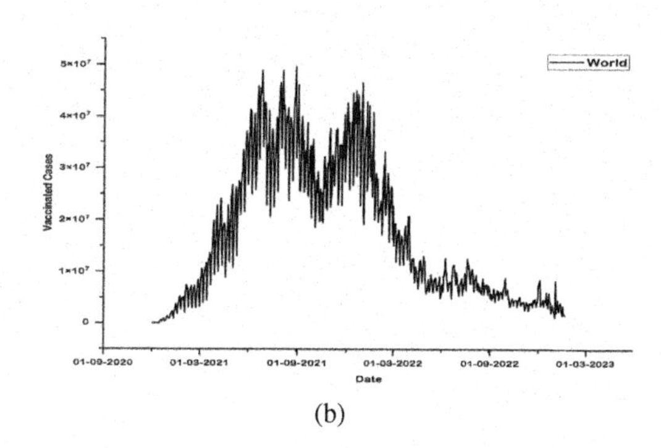

(b)

Fig. 10.4: Epidemic curves of Covid-19 for world wide data: (a) total death cases over the period 2020–2023, (b) vaccinated cases data from 2021 to 2023.

Table 10.2: Hurst exponent and fractal dimension of World wide Covid-19 positive cases and vaccinated cases.

World	Years	Hurst exponent	Fractal Dimension
Seven days moving average positive cases	2020	0.9109	1.0891
	2021	0.7823	1.2177
	2022	0.9663	1.0337
	2020-2023	0.8814	1.1186
Total Vaccinated cases	2021	0.9952	1.0048
	2022	0.9757	1.0243
Total boosted cases	2021	0.9953	1.0047
	2022	0.9606	1.0394

in Figure 10.5. The Hurst exponent and fractal dimension corresponding to the both total vaccinated and boosted people for the world sample data provided between 2021-2022. The graph portrays the simulation of the Hurst model in Figure 10.3. World wide death cases and vaccinated cases of Covid-19 are represented in Figure 10.4. The $\mathcal{H}$ estimate of the $\mathcal{R}/\mathcal{S}$ study of total confirmed cases for the world, is determined to be 0.9953, which is more than 0.5, implying that the future trend analysis has a positive association fractal properties. The $\mathcal{H}$ value in the following stage is 0.9952, which is less than 1, indicating that the future pandemic situation is completely preventable.

Table 10.3 depicts the data generated from 2020 and 2022 with vastly different sample sizes of Hurst value and Fractal dimension. It presents simulation models of Hurst value in Figure 10.6. Hurst exponent associated with the total confirmed cases of Covid-19 for UK, India, France and China are respectively provided in Figures 10.7, 10.8, 10.9 and 10.10 for three different time intervals. The $\mathcal{H}$ estimate of the $\mathcal{R}/\mathcal{S}$ study of total confirmed cases for the highly affected countries such as the USA, India, UK, France, and China, determined to be 0.9921, which is more than 0.5, implying that the future trend analysis has a positive association fractal properties. The $\mathcal{H}$ value in the following stage is 0.9929, which is approximately one, so their fluctuation of epidemic curve indicating that future pandemic situations are completely unpreventable.

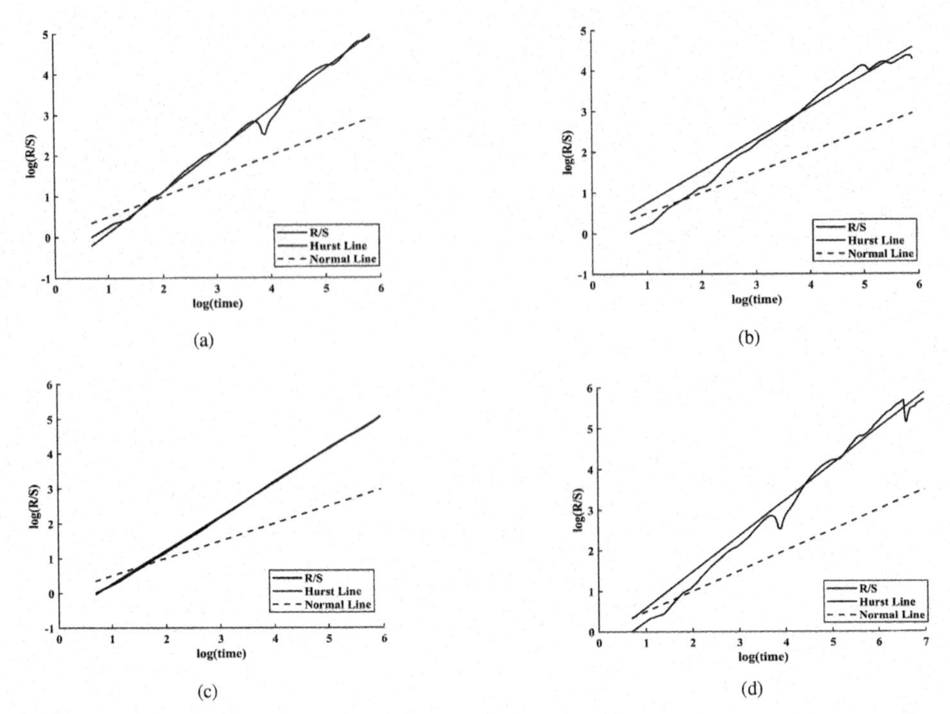

Fig. 10.5: Hurst exponent corresponding to the seven Total cumulative positive cases of Covid-19 for USA, India, UK, France, and China during 2020–2023: (a) 2020–2021, (b) 2021–2022, (c) 2022–2023, (d) 2020–2023.

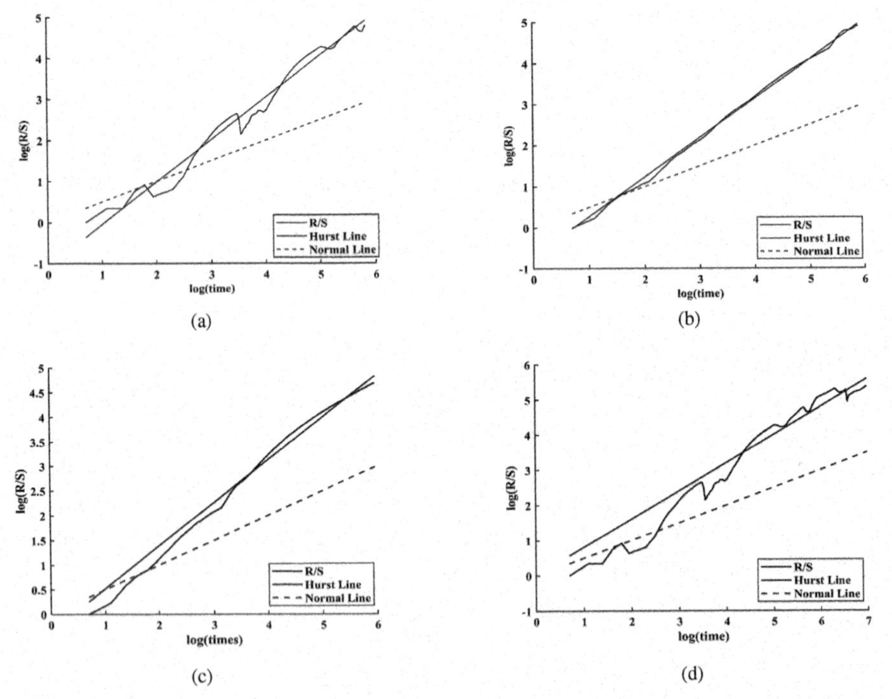

Fig. 10.6: Hurst exponent associated with the total confirmed cases of Covid-19 for USA over the period of three years: (a) 2020–2021, (b) 2021–2022, (c) 2022–2023, (d) 2020–2023.

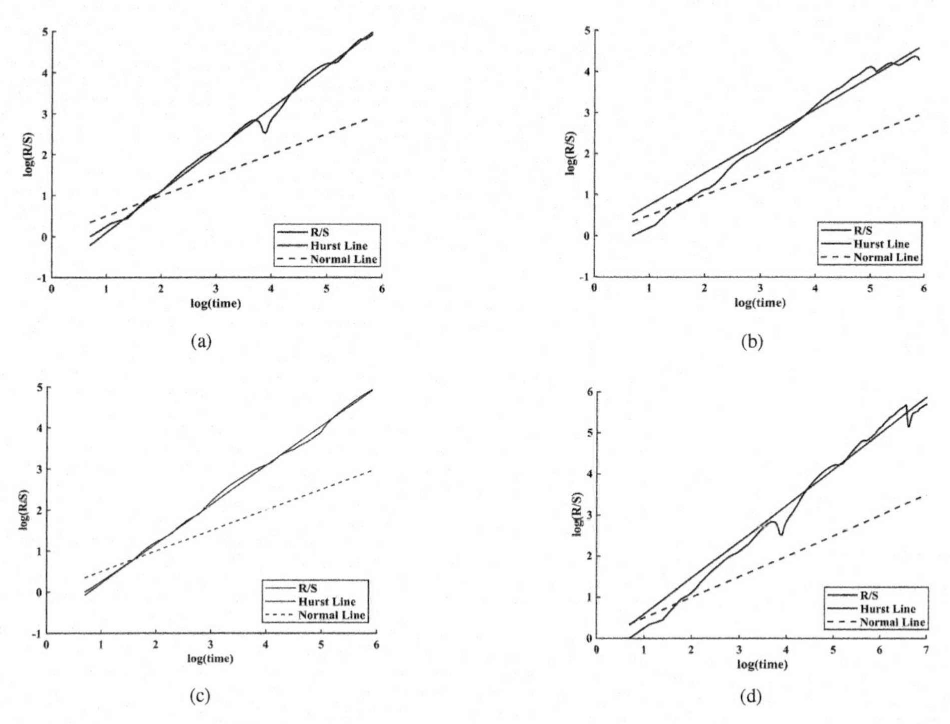

Fig. 10.7: Hurst exponent associated with the total confirmed cases of Covid-19 for UK over the period of three years: (a) 2020–2021, (b) 2021–2022, (c) 2022–2023, (d) 2020–2023.

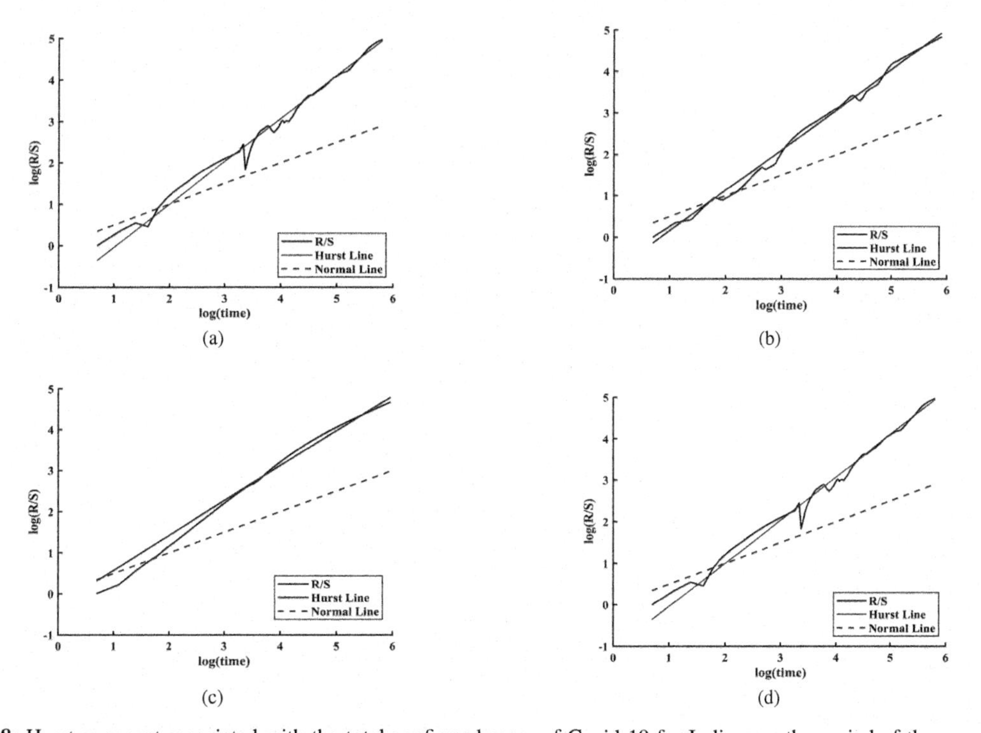

Fig. 10.8: Hurst exponent associated with the total confirmed cases of Covid-19 for India over the period of three years: (a) 2020–2021, (b) 2021–2022, (c) 2022–2023, (d) 2020–2023.

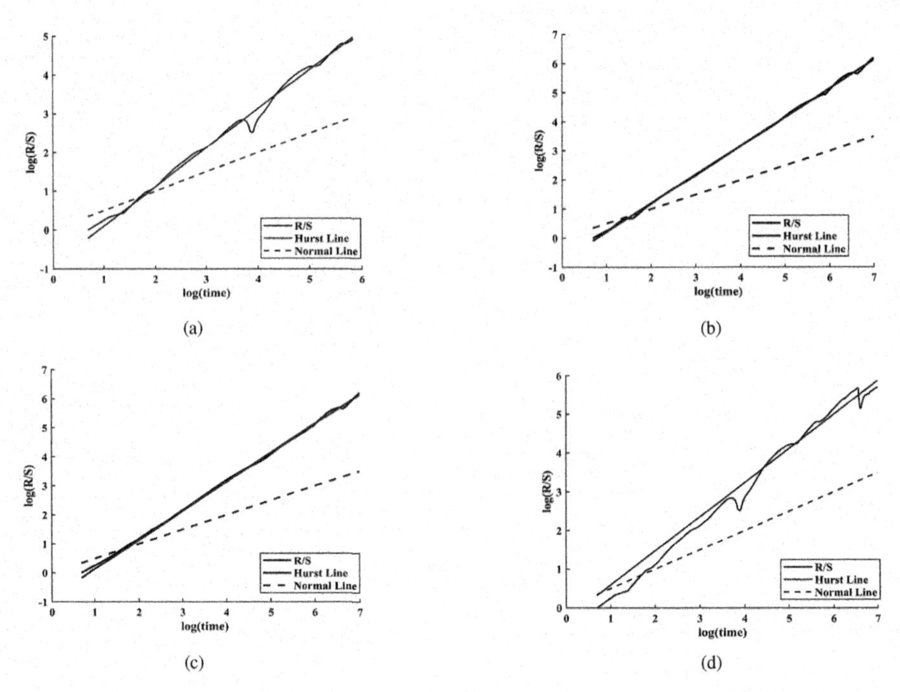

Fig. 10.9: Hurst exponent associated with the total confirmed cases of Covid-19 for France over the period of three years: (a) 2020–2021, (b) 2021–2022, (c) 2022–2023, (d) 2020–2023.

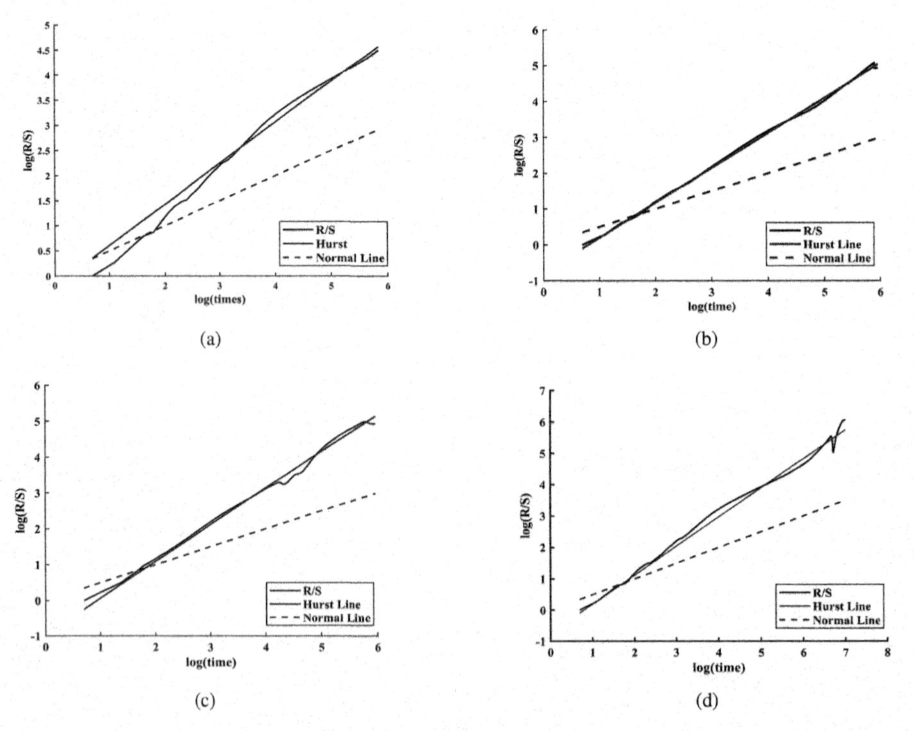

Fig. 10.10: Hurst exponent associated with the total confirmed cases of Covid-19 for China over the period of three years: (a) 2020–2021, (b) 2021–2022, (c)2022–2023, (d) 2020–2023.

Table 10.3: Hurst exponent and fractal dimension of Total confirmed case for prescribed Covid-19 data.

Countries	Years	Hurst Exponents	Fractal Dimension
	2020	0.9897	1.0103
USA	2021	0.9555	1.0455
	2022	0.8682	1.1318
	2020-2023	0.8814	1.1186
	2020	0.9723	1.0277
India	2021	0.8486	1.1514
	2022	0.9374	1.0626
	2020-2023	0.8637	1.1363
	2020	0.9897	1.0103
UK	2021	0.9929	1.0071
	2022	0.9562	1.0438
	2020-2023	0.9179	1.0027
	2020	0.9921	1.0009
France	2021	0.9947	1.0053
	2022	0.8940	1.0026
	2020-2023	0.9046	1.0027
	2020	0.8196	1.1804
China	2021	0.9747	1.0253
	2022	0.9179	1.0821
	2020-2023	0.9268	1.0732

10.5 Conclusion

This chapter categorizes the COVID-19 cases from 2020 to 2023 that used the fractal dimension via the Hurst exponent. The time series data of positive newly confirmed COVID-19 cases, fatality COVID-19 cases from January 2020 to January 2023, and vaccinated and boosted cases from 2021 to 2023 for the world and most affected countries, including United States, India, United Kingdom, France, and China have been analyzed via Hurst exponent. The obtained analysis results range between 0.5 and 1, indicating persistence, and the value of the fractal dimension ranges between 1 and 1.5, indicating that more fluctuations were attained for prescribed COVID-19 cases.

References

[1] WHO, Coronavirus Disease (COVID-2019) Situation Reports. https://www.who.int/emergencies/diseases/ novel-coronavirus-2019/situation-reports/.

[2] Kavitha, C., A. Gowrisankar and S. Banerjee. 2021. The second and third waves in India: when will the pandemic be culminated? The European Physical Journal Plus, 136(5): 596.

[3] COVID-19 Data Repository by the Center for Systems Science and Engineering (CSSE) at Johns Hopkins University. https://github.com/CSSEGISandData/COVID-19.

[4] Roser, M., H. Ritchie, E. Ortiz-Ospina and J. Hasell. 2020. Coronavirus Pandemic (COVID-19). OurWorldInData.org. https://ourworldindata.org/coronavirus.

[5] Ranjan, R., A. Sharma and M.K. Verma. 2021. Characterization of the Second Wave of COVID-19 in India. MedRxiv, 2021-04.
[6] Gowrisankar, A., T.M.C. Priyanka and S. Banerjee. 2022. Omicron: A mysterious variant of concern. The European Physical Journal Plus, 137(1): 1–8.
[7] Păcurar, C.M. and B.R. Necula. 2020. An analysis of COVID-19 spread based on fractal interpolation and fractal dimension. Chaos, Solitons and Fractals, 139: 110073.
[8] Bazargan, M., R. Elahi and A. Esmaeilzadeh. 2022. OMICRON: Virology, immunopathogenesis, and laboratory diagnosis. The Journal of Gene Medicine, 24(7): e3435.
[9] Burabari Konne, J., R.N. Nwalozie, A. Paago and C. Ugochukwu Nyenke. 2022. Current issue on Omicron COVID-19 variants. Asian Journal of Medical Principles and Clinical Practice, 5(4): 250–259.
[10] Easwaramoorthy, D., A. Gowrisankar, A. Manimaran, S. Nandhini, B. Santo and R. Lamberto. 2021. An exploration of fractal based prognostic model and comparative analysis for second wave of COVID-19 diffusion. https://doi.org/10.21203/rs.3.rs-178464/v1.
[11] National Informatics Centre, Ministry of Electronics and Information Technology, Government of India. https://www.mygov.in/covid-19.
[12] Gowrisankar, A., L. Rondoni and S. Banerjee. 2020. Can India develop herd immunity against COVID-19? The European Physical Journal Plus, 135(6): 526.
[13] Rafiq, D., S.A. Suhail and M.A. Bazaz. 2020. Evaluation and prediction of COVID-19 in India: A case study of worst hit states. Chaos, Solitons and Fractals, 139: 110014.
[14] Pai, C., A. Bhaskar and V. Rawoot. 2020. Investigating the dynamics of COVID-19 pandemic in India under lockdown. Chaos, Solitons and Fractals, 138: 109988.
[15] Arora, P., H. Kumar and B.K. Panigrahi. 2020. Prediction and analysis of COVID-19 positive cases using deep learning models: A descriptive case study of India. Chaos, Solitons and Fractals, 139: 110017.
[16] Krishnamurthy, S., S.S. Kar, R. Dhodapkar and N. Parameswaran. 2022. Comparison of COVID-19 infection in children during the first and second wave. Indian Journal of Pediatrics, 89(10): 1016–1018.
[17] Kumar, N., H. Kumar and K. Kumar. 2022. A study for plausible third wave of COVID-19 in India through fuzzy time series modelling based on particle swarm optimization and fuzzy c-averages. Mathematical Problems in Engineering.
[18] Loginov, K.K. and N.V. Pertsev. 2021. Direct statistical modeling of the spread of the epidemic based on a stage-dependent stochastic model. Mathematical Biology and Bioinformatics, 16(2): 169–200.
[19] Gowrisankar, A., T.M.C. Priyanka, A. Saha, L. Rondoni, M. Kamrul Hassan and S. Banerjee. 2022. Greenhouse gas emissions: A rapid submerge of the world. Chaos: An Interdisciplinary Journal of Nonlinear Science, 32(6): 061104.
[20] Rehman, A.U. and R. Singh. 2022. Dynamics of coronavirus and malaria diseases: Modeling and analysis. In Nonlinear Dynamics and Applications: Proceedings of the ICNDA 2022 (pp. 1449–1464). Cham: Springer International Publishing.
[21] Jelley, L., J. Douglas, X. Ren, D. Winter, A. McNeill, S. Huang and J.L. Geoghegan. 2022. Genomic epidemiology of Delta SARS-CoV-2 during transition from elimination to suppression in Aotearoa New Zealand. Nature Communications, 13(1): 4035.
[22] Ray, D., R.N. Quijano and I. Andricioaei. 2022. Point mutations in SARS-CoV-2 variants induce long-range dynamical perturbations in neutralizing antibodies. Chemical Science, 13(24): 7224–7239.
[23] Liu Zhirui, Xiao Dian and Zhou Xinbo. 2022. The latest research progress of Remdesivir in the treatment of novel coronavirus pneumonia. Journal of Clinical Drug Therapy, 20(5): 6–11.

[24] Sutcliffe, J., S. Hurst, A.G. Awadallah, E. Brown and K. Hamed. 2016. Harold Edwin Hurst: The Nile and Egypt, past and future. Hydrological Sciences Journal, 61(9): 1557–1570.

[25] Mandelbrot, Benoit B. and James R. Wallis. and quot;Some long-run properties of geophysical records.and quot; Water resources research 5.2 (1969): 321-340.

[26] Mandelbrot, B.B. and J.R. Wallis. 1969. quot;Some long-run properties of geophysical records.and quot; Water resources research 5.2, 321–340.

[27] Kavitha, C., T.M.C. Priyanka, C. Serpa and A. Gowrisankar. 2022. Fractional calculus for multivariate vector-valued function and fractal function. In Applied Fractional Calculus in Identification and Control (pp. 1–23). Singapore: Springer Nature Singapore.

[28] Banerjee, S., M.K. Hassan, S. Mukherjee and A. Gowrisankar. 2020. Fractal Patterns in Nonlinear Dynamics and Applications. CRC Press.

[29] Falconer, J. 1990. Fractal Geometry: Mathematical Foundations and Applications. John Wiley Sons Inc., Newyork.

[30] Radiom, M. and J.F. Berret. 2020. Common trends in the epidemic of Covid-19 disease. The European Physical Journal Plus, 135: 1–11.

[31] Kale, M.D. and F.B. Butar. 2005. Fractal analysis of time series and distribution properties of Hurst exponent (Doctoral dissertation, Sam Houston State University).

[32] Raj, V., A. Renjini, M.S. Swapna, S. Sreejyothi and S. Sankararaman. 2020. Nonlinear time series and principal component analyses: Potential diagnostic tools for COVID-19 auscultation. Chaos, Solitons and Fractals, 140: 110246.

[33] Balcı, M.A., L.M. Batrancea, Ö. Akgüller, L. Gaban, M.I. Rus and H. Tulai. 2022. Fractality of Borsa Istanbul during the COVID-19 Pandemic. Mathematics, 10(14): 2503.

[34] Ghatak, S., S. Chakraborti, M. Gupta, S. Dutta, S.K. Pati and A. Bhattacharya. 2022. Fractal dimension-based infection detection in chest X-ray images. Applied Biochemistry and Biotechnology, 1–20.

[35] Kumar, G.J. and G. Jayalalitha. 2021. Fractal approach and evaluation of mathematical model of Covid-19 in Tamil Nadu. Elementary Education Online, 20(4): 1413–1413.

[36] Meraz, M., R. Carbó, E. Rodriguez and J. Alvarez-Ramirez. 2023. Fractal correlations in the Covid-19 genome sequence via multivariate rescaled range analysis. Chaos, Solitons and Fractals, 113132.

[37] Wang, J., W. Shao, Y. Yan and J. Kim. 2021. The effect of "Wuhan Closure" on the COVID-19 pandemic in China. Fluctuation and Noise Letters, 20(06): 2150052.

[38] Thangaraj, C. and D. Easwaramoorthy. 2022. Generalized fractal dimensions based comparison analysis of edge detection methods in CT images for estimating the infection of COVID-19 disease. The European Physical Journal Special Topics, 231(18): 3717–3739.

[39] Rong, Q., C. Thangaraj, D. Easwaramoorthy and S. He. 2021. Multifractal based image processing for estimating the complexity of COVID-19 dynamics. The European Physical Journal Special Topics, 230(21): 3947–3954.

[40] Wang, J., W. Jiang, X. Wu, M. Yang and W. Shao. 2023. Role of vaccine in fighting the variants of COVID-19. Chaos, Solitons and Fractals, 113159.

Chapter 11

A Study on the Variants and Subvariants of a Solitary Virus

A.A. Navish[*] and *R. Uthayakumar*

11.1 Introduction

SARS Cov-2 is changing day-by-day and becoming more dangerous by its increasing transmissibility and severity of the disease. These variants are made by the virus mutation process and vaccines may be less effective against them [1].

In brief, when a person is affected by Covid-19, the virus hijacks the cells to create a copy of itself by transmitting copies of the virus's genetic material. Suppose the genetic material is copied improperly, which is known as a mutation (Figure 11.1). In most cases, the mutated viruses died, while others spread to other cells in the body and eventually to other people. On rare occasions, one of these genetic mistakes can result in a virus modification that may result in the fast spread of the disease by effectively dominating the human immune system.

The SARS Cov-2 variants are the versions of the coronavirus which have a genetic change, i.e., it has a different genome sequence distinct from its original sequence which was discovered when the first time the coronavirus variant was identified [3].

The variants that are currently causing the most concern around the world are essentially the same virus that causes the same sickness. But SARS Cov-2 variants are significantly varied from their original and cause severe disease with unique symptoms compared with the original SARS Cov-2 [2].

A SARS Cov-2 lineage is a genetically linked collection of viral variations formed from a common ancestor that creates a new branch of its epidemiological family tree, whereas subvariants and recombinants are produced by combining two variants. So far numerous variants of SARS Cov-2 have been discovered and named using Greek alphabets. Among which alpha, beta, delta and omicron are prominent variants. Currently, the omicron and omicron variants are dominating worldwide [4].

A visually insignificant modification in the examined object can significantly impact its fractal measure. Consequently, fractals are aiding in numerous protein and genome research to reveal the characteristics and distinguish defective genome and proteins. In this line, some researchers have computed the fractal dimension of proteins using invariant parameters such as fluorescence energy transfer [12], dihedral angles [10] and

Department of Mathematics, The Gandhigram Rural Institute - Deemed to be University, Dindigul, Tamil Nadu-624 302, India.
Email: uthayagri@gmail.com
* Corresponding author: aa.navish2@gmail.com

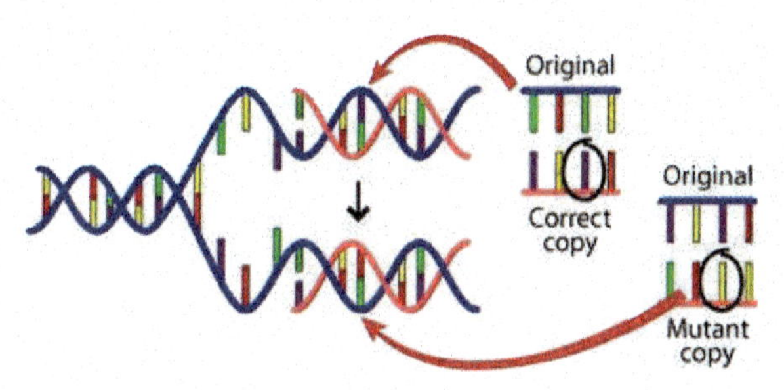

Fig. 11.1: Mutation in the genetic sequences.

provided globally acceptable results. However, few researchers have simply discovered any fractal dimension for the backbone images or the 3D view of the proteins and protein surfaces [8]. Though these are unique, their shapes are variants under rotation. In that case, the gathered results would be authentic only locally rather than globally. Also, research on the protein-protein interaction networks attained a significant reach in a short period as they are helpful in drug developments [6]. At the same time, there is a lot of research done on the mathematical descriptions of genetic sequences [9]. Through this research, the complexity and similarity of protein and genetic sequences are explored [7, 11].
This work is based on two main concepts:

(i) Identify the variation between spike proteins of the SARS Cov-2 variants, namely alpha, beta, delta and omicron.
(ii) Examine the variation between the variants (BA.2 and BA.5) and subvariants of omicron (including BQ.1, BQ.1.1, BF.7, XBB.1.5).

In this instance, the distinct translation and rotational invariance graphs of protein and genetic sequences are modelled and their fractal dimensions are measured. Finally, to refine the precise character of the fractal dimensions, the SSIM between the obtained CGR graph interpretation is measured. For time consumption and accuracy, some software has been used. The software detail and the corresponding findings are provided in the following table.

Table 11.1: Software and findings.

Software	**Findings**
Matlab R2021a	Zig-zag curve and its dimension, Structural Similarity Index Measure (SSIM)
NAPS	Protein Contact Map (PCM)
C-GREx	Chaos Game Representation (CGR)
ImageJ	Mass dimension, Box dimension

11.2 Preliminaries

11.2.1 Relationship between Genetic Codes and Proteins

Every living thing has a distinct genetic code, or genome made up of nucleotide bases namely A, T, G and C. In which a base pair(bp) is made up of joining the two nucleotides together by hydrogen bonds. Based on the conventional Watson–Crick base pairing, A forms a base pair with T using two hydrogen bonds,

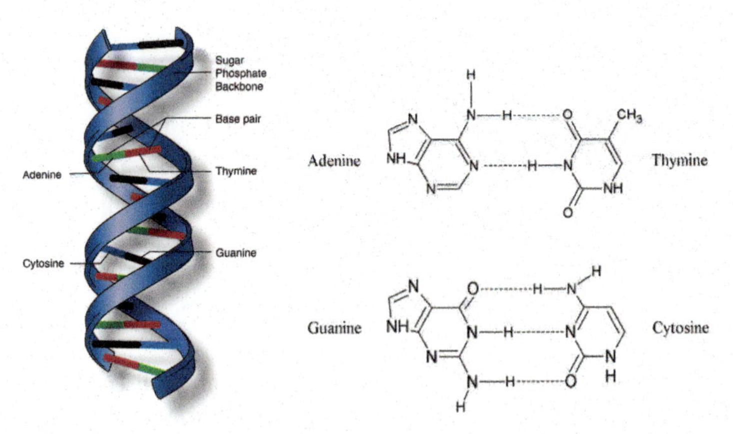

Fig. 11.2: DNA structure and basic pairing.

whereas G forms a base pair with C using three hydrogen bonds. Consequently, A and T are complementary to one another, just as C and G. To know the sequence of the bases in an organism, one should identify its unique DNA fingerprint or pattern. This process is called sequencing and this is done with the aid of a laboratory procedure. Protein plays numerous roles in the biological world, such as transporting nutrients and constructing the structures of living things. It will perform its functions by interacting with other molecules such as DNA or RNA proteins and small molecules. Descriptively, genes instruct cells to produce particular proteins, which in turn determine traits.

In view of this concept, this work has been developed and examined the variation between the variants and subvariants of the SARS Cov-2. Also, the raw data related to this work is described as follows.

11.2.2 Raw Data Description

The 3D proteins of the SARS Cov-2 variants used in this investigation were downloaded from the RCSB PDB website. Moreover, the genetic sequences employed in this work were gathered from the NCBI website under the Genome Project. All of the genetic sequences are the complete sequences decoded from the subvariants of Omicron. For more detail, the PDB Id for spike proteins and accession number for genetic sequences are provided in the table of results and discussion section.

11.3 Analyzing Chaotic Characteristics of SARS Cov-2 Variants and Subvariants

11.3.1 Examine the Spike Protein of SARS Cov-2 and its Variants

There are different types of viral proteins exist. Particularly this study focuses on one of the structural proteins of the coronavirus. Structural proteins act a fundamental role in forming cells, tissues and organisms. All the viruses that belong to the Coronaviridae family have four structural proteins Spike (S), Envelope (E), Membrane (M), and Nucleocapsid (N). Among that the S protein is a crucial multifunctional and clover-shaped protein that interacts with particular cellular receptors to indicate the host-specificity of coronaviruses. Thus, a single amino acid change in the spike protein affects the host's immune response in addition to the virus's ability to replicate and infect new cells [5].

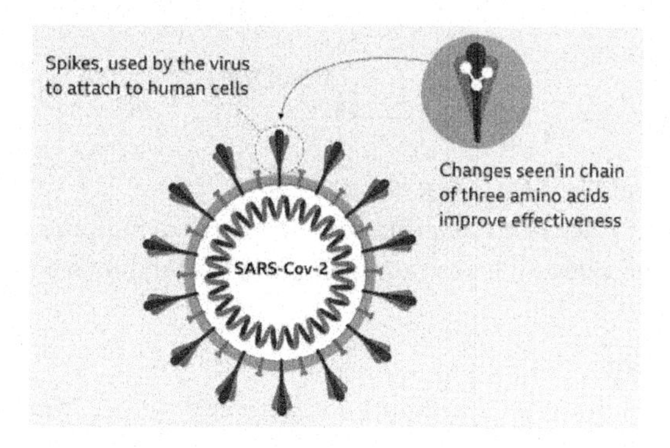

Fig. 11.3: Mutation in the spike protein.

In a nutshell, a change/mutation in the genome impacts the physicochemical properties and structure of the protein which subsequently impacts the behavior of the virus.

In this sub section, the various invariant graph interpretations of the spike proteins of distinct variants are carried out. As some of these graphs are chaotic in nature or self-similar, the fractal dimensions are used as a parameter to examine the variation between the spike proteins of distinct variants. Basically, these variations result from mutations in the spike proteins.

11.3.2 Zig-zag Curve Representation

It is a simplistic indication of 3D spike proteins, enabling the polymer chain structure to be formed by connecting the alpha carbons of the proteins [13]. Proteins are made up of amino acids, while alpha carbons are part of the structure of amino acids. When missense mutations in DNA make different amino acids, they subsequently impact the alpha carbons. The MATLAB molviewer acquired the zig-zag curve by taking the homology modelled .pdb file as input [14].

11.3.3 Method 1: Fractal Dimension

In this method, the protein molecule is considered a function of the fineness or coarseness of the scale r [15]. This is similar to the walker dimension method. Herewith, the zig-zag curve is acquired by connecting the alpha atoms of the proteins with the interval of r residues starting from the alpha atoms of the N-terminal residue. Continue the process until spot the less residues to make the next move. Repeat the process with different residues r.

The length of the protein molecule on a scale of r, $L(r)$ is obtained by the sum of the length of the zig-zag line L_z and the correction term C_t, which are calculated using the following equations:

$$L(r) = L_z + C_t$$

with

$$C_t = \frac{N(u)}{r+1} \times L_m$$

Here $N(u)$ indicates the number of remaining disconnected residues and L_m represents the average length of the fractional lines that make up the zig-zag lines. Then the fractal dimension is acquired by using the relation

$$N = \left(\frac{L(r)}{r}\right)^{\mathrm{FracDim}_Z}$$

where N represents the total number of residues.

Here, the fractal dimension is measured in terms of alpha carbons. Suppose the considered spike proteins are the same, then they have the same alpha carbons and same fractal dimension.

11.3.4 Protein Contact Map

It was possible to predict whether the considered spike protein is different from the original SARS Cov-2 spike protein by noticing the number of residues and the number of interactions of amino acids. However, there are different proteins with the same number of amino acid interactions. In that case, the amino acids may have been misplaced compared with the original. Consequently, mutations cannot be identified using the number of interactions between protein sequences alone. We need some further classification to confirm the protein sequence variation of SARS Cov-2 variants. So we need to verify whether the amino acids correctly interact with the appropriate amino acids.

To resolve this mess, over the last three decades, the research on PRN have evolved. Initially, this is a kind of mathematical formulation of 3D proteins derived from graph theory. In this sequence, PCM is used to explore the contact/connectivity between all possible amino acid residue pairs in a three-dimensional protein structure using a two-dimensional binary matrix. In other words, this is a kind of adjacency matrix representation of PRN. This can be expressed as follows.

Let r_m, r_n be any two residues. The edge between any two residues are denoted by $e_{r_m r_n}$. Then, the PCM of a 3D protein is defined as

$$\mathrm{PCM} = \begin{cases} 1 & \text{if } e_{r_m r_n} \text{ exists} \\ 0 & \text{Otherwise} \end{cases}$$

With the help of contact maps, the similarity between proteins are quickly evaluated. Moreover, the contact maps are translation and rotation invariant. As a consequence, the coordinates of proteins are reconstructed without interruption. Both PRN and PCM are acquired from NAPS [16], a web-based tool that provides the desired output by giving input or uploading the PDB file on the web page.

11.3.5 Method 2: Mass Dimension

The mass dimension is like a traditional box dimension. Instead of counting the boxes (with size $\breve{\varepsilon}$) that covers the taken object, we count the average number of pixels $\mu_{\breve{\varepsilon}}$ in the boxes. It quantifies the connectivity of PRN and can be calculated for each pixel in a given image and used to identify the irregularities of heterogeneous geometrical objects. The following equation can be used to calculate $\mathrm{FracDim}_M$.

$$\mathrm{FracDim}_M = \lim_{\breve{\varepsilon} \to 0} \frac{ln\ \mu_{\breve{\varepsilon}}}{ln\ \breve{\varepsilon}}$$

Fractal dimension is not only a measure to quantify the similarity but also a measure of the space-filling property. If the mutation affects the connectivity between the amino acid residues, the resultant PCM of the spikes may look the same with a minute difference. In that case, the mass dimension is utilized to explore its variation.

11.3.6 Chaos Game Representation

The CGR could be used to translate the amino acid sequence into bi-dimensional real values. It helps to preserve the statistical properties of the sequences and offers information on the global and local patterns of the sequences. Each sequence member has a corresponding point representation in CGR. As a result, each amino sequence has a unique CGR [17] through that a change in the amino sequences is discovered.

Initially, protein sequences consist of 20 different amino acids, including phenylalanine (F), histidine (H), isoleucine (I), lysine (K), leucine (L), methionine (M), threonine (T), valine (V), tryptophan (W), alanine (A), aspartic acid (D), glutamic acid (E), asparagine (N), serine (S), cysteine (C), glycine (G), proline (P), glutamine (Q), arginine (R) and tyrosine (Y). Among these, the first nine amino acids are essential, the succeeding five are non-essential amino acids and the remaining six are conditional amino acids.

These sequences can be represented as a CGR graph using the HP model. It is a lattice-based model introduced in the year of 1985 in which the amino acids are categorized into four groups: the eight amino acids A, I, L, M, F, P, W, and V are categorized as a non-polar class; the seven amino acids N, C, Q, G, S, T, and Y are labelled as an uncharged polar class; the three amino acids R, H, and K are considered a positive polar class; and the remaining two amino acids D and E are designated as a negative polar class. The only premise is that two non-polar amino acids interact iff they are spatially close to each other, whereas the other techniques are based on statistically predicting interactions from the primary sequence. Thus, the HP model is more precise and that is why the HP model is widely chosen [19].

To convert a given protein's amino acid sequence into CGR coordinates, consider the given protein sequence as follows:

$$\text{Seq} = \{S_1 S_2 ... S_N\} \tag{11.1}$$

where S_i, $i = 1, 2, ...N$ indicates the elements in the amino acid sequence and N represents the length of the sequence.

Let

$$s_i = \begin{cases} 0 \text{ if } S_i \text{ is non polar} \\ 1 \text{ if } S_i \text{ is negative polar} \\ 2 \text{ if } S_i \text{ is uncharged polar} \\ 3 \text{ if } S_i \text{ is positive polar} \end{cases}$$

Then the Eq. (11.1) is reconstructed as

$$\mathcal{X}(S) = s_1 s_2 ... s_N, \quad s_i \in \{0, 1, 2, 3\} \tag{11.2}$$

To plot the CGR consider the $[0, 1] \times [0, 1]$ square, with 4 corners that reflects the values $0, 1, 2$ and 3. Then, plot the first element in the sequence $\mathcal{X}(S)$ by positioned the point halfway between the centre of the square. Similarly, plot the ith point in the halfway between the $(i-1)^{th}$ point. Continuing in this way, the desired CGR of the protein sequence is constructed.

The sample protein sequence and the corresponding reconstructed sequences are presented in the following Figures 11.4 and 11.5. This interpretation is made via the software C-GREx.

MKSSHHHHHHENLYFQSNATKKSAAEASKKPRQKRTATKAYNVTQAFGRRGPEQTQGNFGDQELIRQGTDYKHW
PQIAQFAPSASAFFGMSRIGMEVTPSGTWLTYTGAIKLDDKDPNFKDQVILLNKHIDAY

Fig. 11.4: Amino acid representation of sample protein.

03223333331202022202332001023303233202302202200233201212222021210032221233002
002000202000202302010202220022220030113102031200002330102

Fig. 11.5: A reconstructed sequence representation of Fig 11.4.

11.3.7 Examine the Genetic Sequences of the Omicron Variants and its Subvariants

As far as SARS CoV-2 variants go, Omicron and its subvariants top the list. After the initial Omicron B.1.1.529 was discovered in South Africa in November 2021, cases immediately spread and multiplied in other nations. By December of that year, Omicron was driving up the number of cases reported every day and was also spawning variants and subvariants. In this sequence, BA.5 became the most common viral variant, whereas BF.7 is its shortened version. Following that, in November, the BA.5 is replaced by two subvariants known as BQ.1 and BQ.1.1. Moreover, at the beginning of 2023, a new subvariant known as XBB.1.5, which is a sublineage of XBB and a subvariant of two BA.2 sublineages, began to emerge.

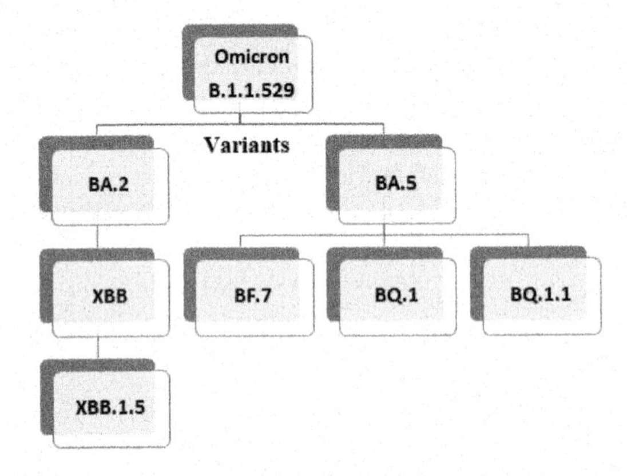

Fig. 11.6: Omicron variants and its subvariants focused in this work.

In this sub section, the CGR of the genome sequence is formulated to explore how the Omicron variants are distinct from the subvariants. As subvariants are a recombination of the variants, they are also affected by the mutation of genome sequences.

11.3.8 Chaos Game Representation

Chaos game theory is a very popular procedure to produce many complex patterns. However, one of the specific applications of this theory in the medical field is that it can be used to convert the DNA sequence into bi-dimensional real values for easy handling. By doing so, one may retrieve the exact statistical properties and global and local patterns of the sequences. In this procedure, every element in the DNA sequence has its matching point representation, which leads to the existence of a unique CGR of each sequence [18]. Assume the following sequence is undertaken for the evaluation:

$$\text{Seq} = \{q_1 q_2 ... q_n ... q_N\}$$

Then mathematically, q_n is the nth element of the sequence and is mapped with $(q_x(n), q_y(n))$.

Herein,

$$q_x(n) = \begin{cases} 1 \ if \ q_n = A \\ -1 \ if \ q_n = T \\ -1 \ if \ q_n = C \\ 1 \ if \ q_n = G \end{cases}$$

and

$$q_y(n) = \begin{cases} 1 \ if \ q_n = A \\ 1 \ if \ q_n = T \\ -1 \ if \ q_n = C \\ -1 \ if \ q_n = G \end{cases}$$

Each component of the DNA sequence $(q_x(n), q_y(n))$ can be converted as a chaos game representation $(G_x(n), G_y(n))$ with the initial condition $(G_x(0), G_y(0)) = (0, 0)$.

$$G_x(n) = \frac{1}{2}[q_x(n) + G_x(n-1)] \quad n = 1, 2, 3, ..., N$$

$$G_y(n) = \frac{1}{2}[q_y(n) + G_y(n-1)] \quad n = 1, 2, 3, ..., N$$

The graphical description gives the frequencies of occurrence of a genetic signature by partitioning the CGR space. This action is done with the appropriate grid size and calculating the number of occurrences in each quadrant. Moreover, every sub-square contributes to this computation in a significant way. The actual procedure of doing the division of the quadrants and the evaluation of the number of occurrences is explained below.

At the first, the CGR is split into four quadrants. Here, the top right quadrant indicates the points for which the sub-sequences end with G as a midway between any other point in the square. Thus, the G-corner square lies in this quadrant. Then, the counting of occurrences in this quadrant will be based on the number of bases G in the sequence. Split this quadrant into four sectors once again in the clockwise direction and it will give the sub sequences end with GG, TG, AG and CG. Summing up the points in the quadrant will impact the 2-mer count. Repetition of this procedure will show the count of n-mer. The pictorial representation of this procedure is given below.

One of the special features of CGR is that the images collected from various genome sections have the same structure as the entire genome. Hence, we gain a genetic signature from the assessing portion of a genome. In the case of accessibility of portions of a genome, it helps in comparing the non-homologous genetic sequences.

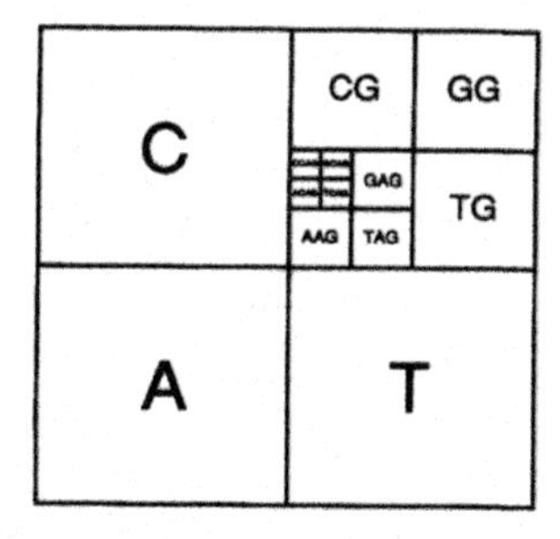

Fig. 11.7: Relevance between n-mer and the sub squares of CGR.

11.3.9 Method 3: Box Counting Dimension

The fractal dimension of CGR is determined using the standard box count approach, where the provided CGR is covered by tiny boxes of size $(\breve{\varepsilon})$. The number of boxes $(\mathcal{N}(\breve{\varepsilon}))$ that cover the item varies depending on the box size. The following expression can be used to compute the box dimension:

$$FracDim_B = \lim_{\breve{\varepsilon}\to 0} -\frac{log\ \mathcal{N}(\breve{\varepsilon})}{log\breve{\varepsilon}}$$

Here, the variation in the fractal dimension of the proteins reflects that the spike proteins of the variants are not same.

11.3.10 Comparing the Similarity Between Obtained Graphs using Structural Similarity Index Measure

The structural similarity index is one of the most accepted image classification methods, introduced in the 2004 IEEE paper [20]. It is a perception-based model that quantifies the similarity between two considered images. It classifies the images based on essential features such as luminance, contrast and structure which makes the method more accurate.

The luminance represents the average of all pixel values. Let x and y be the images with size $N \times N$. Then the luminance (μ) of any image is expressed as follows:

$$\mu_j = \frac{1}{N}\sum_{i=1}^{N} j_i$$

where $j = x, y$.
The luminance comparison function $L(x, y)$ is given by

$$L(x, y) = \frac{2\mu_x\mu_y + c_1}{\mu_x^2 + \mu_y^2 + c_1} \tag{11.3}$$

The contrast is nothing but the standard deviation of total pixel values. The contrast of any image can be defined as

$$\sigma_j = \left(\frac{1}{N-1}\sum_{i=1}^{N}(j_i - \mu_j)^2\right)^{\frac{1}{2}}$$

Besides, the contrast comparison is given by

$$C(x, y) = \frac{2\sigma_x\sigma_y + c_2}{\sigma_x^2 + \sigma_y^2 + c_2} \tag{11.4}$$

Similarly, the structural comparison is measured based on the standard deviation of the considered images and expressed as

$$S(x, y) = \frac{\sigma_{xy} + c_3}{\sigma_x\sigma_y + c_3}$$

hither

$$\sigma_{xy} = \frac{1}{N-1}\sum_{i=1}^{N}(x_i - \mu_x)(y_i - \mu_y) \tag{11.5}$$

On the basis of the above (11.3)(11.4) and (11.5), the required SSIM can be obtained using the following expression:

$$\mathrm{SSIM}(x, y) = [L(x, y)]^{\alpha}[C(x, y)]^{\beta}[S(x, y)]^{\gamma} \tag{11.6}$$

where $\alpha, \beta, \gamma > 0$. To generate the simplified form of (11.6), assume that $\alpha = \beta = \gamma = 1$ and $c_3 = c_2/2$. Then the Eq. (11.6) is written as

$$\mathrm{SSIM}(x, y) = \frac{(2\mu_x\mu_y + c_1)(2\sigma_{xy} + c_2)}{(\mu_x^2 + \mu_y^2 + c_1)(\sigma_x^2 + \sigma_y^2 + c_2)}$$

The range of $\mathrm{SSIM}(x, y)$ is $[-1, 1]$. It represents the similarity level between the images x and y. If the $\mathrm{SSIM}(x, y)$ is 1, then the images x and y are the same, whereas the value –1 indicates that the images are totally different. In precisely, we can consider its range in $[0, 1]$, since the $\mathrm{SSIM}(x, y)$ reflects that there is no similarity between images.

11.4 Results and Discussion

Different objects may have the same fractal dimensions. If similar objects have the same dimension, then they must be identical. Most of our acquired graphs are visually the same, but they have distinct fractal dimensions. As a result, they have minute variations. These minor variations are caused by changes or mutations in the corresponding protein or genetic sequences.

The possible way of graph interpretations of spike protein are presented in Figure 11.8. The differences between the graphs in Figure 11.9 can be visually identified. But there are many visually similar structures with unidentified variations. So in that situation, using fractal dimensions and SSIM to discover the differences between the obtained graphs can enrich the findings.

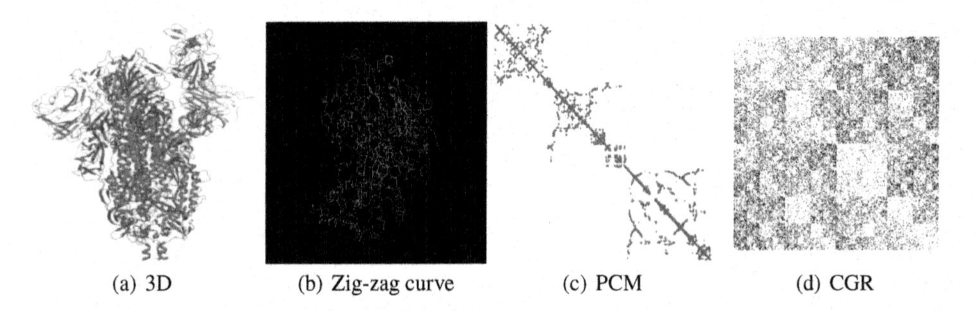

(a) 3D (b) Zig-zag curve (c) PCM (d) CGR

Fig. 11.8: Distinct graph representation of SARS Cov-2 spike protein.

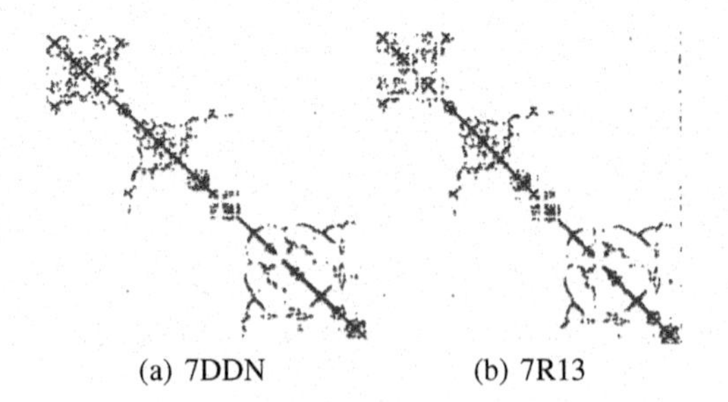

(a) 7DDN (b) 7R13

Fig. 11.9: Sample visually similar PCM graphs.

Table 11.2: Spike proteins of various coronavirus and the fractal dimension of its various graph interpretations.

Corona Virus	PDB ID	$FracDim_Z$	$FracDim_M$	$FracDim_B$	r	nz
SARS Cov-2	7DDN	1.4508	1.3650	1.5716	25049	25664
Alpha	7R13	1.4231	1.3381	1.5593	24303	24939
Beta	7VX1	1.4635	1.3796	1.6023	25362	25992
Delta	7W92	1.4592	1.3645	1.5932	25071	25689
Omicron	7WVN	1.4438	1.3460	1.5687	24805	25423

r-Number of residues
nz-Number of interaction between amino acids

Table 11.3: SSIM between SARS Cov-2 and its variants.

SARS Cov-2 variants	SSIM (CGR)
Alpha	0.9699
Beta	0.9802
Delta	0.9868
Omicron	0.9524

Tables 11.1 and 11.2 show how the number of residues and the number of interactions of amino acids are related to the fractal dimensions. Consequently, we can assure they are positively correlated, i.e., As, the zig-zag curve, PCM and CGR modelled based on the number of residues and interactions, they impact its fractal dimension.

Moreover, Table 11.2 shows that the SSIM between CGR of SARS Cov-2 and Omicron is more, compared with others, which means that the spike protein of the Omicron is a little more distinct/mutated from the SARS Cov-2.

Similarly, Table 11.3 shows that the bp of subvariants and box dimensions are positively correlated.

The SSIM between the CGR of Omicron variants, Omicron subvariants and omicron is provided in Table 11.4. while the SSIM between BA.2 and BA.5 and its subvariants are described in Tables 11.5 and 11.6. These reflect the fact that the Omicron variants and its subvariants have only minute variations in their structure compare with the variation between Omicron and its variants.

Table 11.4: FracDim$_B$ of Omicron variants and its subvariants.

Omicron variants and subvariants	Accession Number	bp	FracDim$_B$
B.1.1529	OQ318440	29684	1.8602
BA.2	OQ333099	29794	1.8598
BA.5	OQ322609	29853	1.8599
BF.7	OQ325599	29718	1.8597
BQ.1	OQ327091	29856	1.8599
BQ.1.1	OQ318809	29639	1.8596
XBB	OQ329134	29721	1.8344
XBB.1.5	OQ318730	29794	1.8598

Table 11.5: SSIM between SARS Cov-2 and Omicron variants and subvariants.

Omicron variants and subvariants	SSIM (CGR)
BA.2	0.9768
BA.5	0.9710
BF.7	0.9751
BQ.1	0.9708
BQ.1.1	0.9724
XBB	0.9721
XBB.1.5	0.9710

Table 11.6: SSIM between Omicron variant BA.5 and its subvariants.

Omicron subvariants	SSIM (CGR)
BF.7	0.9900
BQ.1	0.9870
BQ.1.1	0.9846

Table 11.7: SSIM between Omicron variant BA.2 and its subvariants.

Omicron subvariants	SSIM (CGR)
XBB	0.9872
XBB.1.5	0.9902

11.5 Conclusion

Through this work, we have identified that the visually similar graphs or the graphs with negligible changes are not identical. Minute changes are reflected in its fractal dimensions. The number of alpha carbons and interactions, bp are proportional to the fractal dimension of obtained graphs. Thus, instead of counting them, quantifying the fractal dimension reflect whether the considered protein or genetic sequences are large or small. Also, we discovered that the Omicron's spike protein is a bit more distinct from SARS Cov-2 spike protein. Also, Omicron subvariants are only very little bit different/mutated from their variants. As a result, these types of studies are fruitful in making comparative research since the above-described graphs are exactly the same for identical proteins or genetic sequences.

References

[1] https://ec.europa.eu/research-and-innovation/en/horizon-magazine/covid-19-variants-five-things-know-about-how-coronavirus-evolving.
[2] https://www.cdc.gov/coronavirus/2019-ncov/variants/variant-classifications.html#:~:text=Lineage\%3A\%20A\%20lineage\%20is\%20a,contain\%20one\%20or\%20more\%20mutations.
[3] https://en.wikipedia.org/wiki/Variants_of_SARS-CoV-2.
[4] https://www.yalemedicine.org/news/covid-19-variants-of-concern-omicron.
[5] Ding, C., J. He, X. Zhang, C. Jiang, Y. Sun, Y. Zhang, Q. Chen, H. He, W. Li, J. Xie and Z. Liu. 2021. Crucial mutations of spike protein on SARS-CoV-2 evolved to variant strains escaping neutralization of convalescent plasmas and RBD-specific monoclonal antibodies. Frontiers in Immunology, 12: 693775.
[6] Navish, A.A. and R. Uthayakumar. 2022. An exploration on the topologies of SARS-CoV-2/human protein-protein interaction network. Journal of Biomolecular Structure and Dynamics, 1–13.
[7] Navish, A.A. and R. Uthayakumar. 2022. A chaotic approach to recognize the characteristics of genetic codes of covid patients. Computer Methods in Biomechanics and Biomedical Engineering: Imaging & Visualization, 1–14.
[8] Craciun, D., A. Isvoran and N. Avram. 2008. Fractal characteristics of proteins surfaces. Annals of the West University of Timisoara. Physics Series, 52: 116.
[9] Arniker, S.B. and H.K. Kwan. 2009, June. Graphical representation of DNA sequences. In 2009 IEEE International Conference on Electro/Information Technology (pp. 311–314). IEEE.
[10] Peng, X., W. Qi, M. Wang, R. Su and Z. He. 2013. Backbone fractal dimension and fractal hybrid orbital of protein structure. Communications in Nonlinear Science and Numerical Simulation, 18(12): 3373–3381.
[11] Cattani, C. 2010. Fractals and hidden symmetries in DNA. Mathematical Problems in Engineering.
[12] Dewey, T.G. and M.M. Datta. 1989. Determination of the fractal dimension of membrane protein aggregates using fluorescence energy transfer. Biophysical Journal, 56(2): 415–420.
[13] Rout, R.K., P. Pal Choudhury, S.P. Maity, B.S. Daya Sagar and S.S. Hassan. 2018. Fractal and mathematical morphology in intricate comparison between tertiary protein structures. Computer Methods in Biomechanics and Biomedical Engineering: Imaging & Visualization, 6(2): 192–203.
[14] Niknam, N., H. Khakzad, S.S. Arab and H. Naderi-Manesh. 2016. PDB2Graph: A toolbox for identifying critical amino acids map in proteins based on graph theory. Computers in Biology and Medicine, 72: 151–159.

[15] Torrens, F. 2002. Fractal hybrid orbitals analysis of the tertiary structure of protein molecules. Molecules, 7(1): 26–37.

[16] Chakrabarty, B., V. Naganathan, K. Garg, Y. Agarwal and N. Parekh. 2019. NAPS update: Network analysis of molecular dynamics data and protein–nucleic acid complexes. Nucleic Acids Research, 47(W1): W462–W470.

[17] Yu, Z.G., V. Anh and K.S. Lau. 2004. Chaos game representation of protein sequences based on the detailed HP model and their multifractal and correlation analyses. Journal of Theoretical Biology, 226(3): 341–348.

[18] Nair, A.S., V.V. Nair, K.S. Arun, K. Kant and A. Dey. 2009. Bio-sequence signatures using chaos game representation. In Bioinformatics: Applications in Life and Environmental Sciences (pp. 62–76). Springer, Dordrecht.

[19] Dill, K.A. 1985. Theory for the folding and stability of globular proteins. Biochemistry, 24(6): 1501–1509.

[20] Wang, Z., A.C. Bovik, H.R. Sheikh and E.P. Simoncelli. 2004. Image quality assessment: From error visibility to structural similarity. IEEE Transactions on Image Processing, 13(4): 600–612.

Chapter 12

Mathematical Modelling of Multicellular Tumor Spheroid Growth Using Lambert Function

C. Aishwarya and *P. Paramanathan**

12.1 Introduction

With the advancement of technology and resources over the last decade, mathematical modelling of tumor growth has become a popular and developing field. The rate of tumor growth is critical information for doctors in determining how aggressive the tumor growth may be and devising the best treatment plan for the patient. Tumor is a term that describes swelling or a lumpy bloated state that is usually connected with inflammation. Excessive cell division or growth in the body, hereditary factors, Ultraviolet light exposure, toxins, smoking and viruses are all prominent causes of tumor development [8].

Tumor cells divide and expand uncontrollably, infecting normal tissues and organs before spreading throughout the body. It occurs when tumor cells multiply at an uncontrollable rate. As a result of cumulative irregularities in multiple cell regulatory systems, the cells show a generalized loss of growth control, which is reflected in several aspects of cell behavior that distinguish tumor cells from their aberrant counterparts [7, 21]. As a tumor grows, it begins to spread throughout the body, consuming all of the nutrients and space available to it.

To understand the precise growth of each tumor, growth rate equations are employed to calculate the volume of tumor cells over time. Exponential, logistic, linear, surface and Gompertz are examples of growth models. These growth models are essential for building an engineering background for tumor treatment. The physiological processes as well as the observations are described in a well-defined tumor growth model [1]. The tumor information can be extracted using a variety of techniques. Researchers employ image fusion for diagnosis, tumor treatment, analysis and radiotherapy but it is not widely recognized due to time, computer complexity and scarcity of medical images [5, 6]. The majority of research in the early 1970s used 2D monolayer tumor data. These models as Brohem pointed out, fail to represent the complex and dynamic conditions found in vivo tissues [23]. According to recent research, multicellular tumor spheroids (MTS) is the best option to be used in the biomedical field since they exhibit better tissue structure complexity and maintain a variety of cell connections [17].

Department of Mathematics, Amrita School of Physical Sciences, Coimbatore, Amrita Vishwa Vidyapeetham, India.
Email: chulliyilaishwarya1@gmail.com
* Corresponding author: p_paramanathan@cb.amrita.edu

The Gompertz function can well represent tumor growth in rats, mice and rabbits that is marked by a constant slowing from the early times of observation [1]. Stimulation of natural growth suppressing factors could be useful in lowering the incidence of clinical tumors. However, there is no consensus on how to interpret the growth parameters utilized in the Gompertz equation and how they effect tumor growth. In recent research, the Gompertz model is the best alternative for describing Multicellular tumor spheroids (MTS) growth data and it has considerable flexibility to adapt its predictions to the volume of growth data variability observed in the simulated spheroids [2]. However, the study does not explain how the characteristics interact and how this may be utilized to forecast the next stage of tumor growth.

In this chapter, we estimate the parameters of the Gompertz equation and explain how it is used to forecast tumor growth using multicellular spheroid tumor data. Rest of the chapter is organized as follows: The Gompertz equation, Lambert function, the structure and use of 3D multicellular tumor spheroids (MTS) are discussed in Section 2. In Section 3, the mathematical formulation for obtaining the parameters of the Gompertz equation using the Lambert W function is illustrated. The results and discussion are presented in Section 4. Section 5 describes the conclusion.

12.2 Materials and Methods

12.2.1 Gompertz Function

The Gompertz function is a sigmoid function that is utilized to explain animal and plant growth, as well as the number and volume of bacteria. Growth is described as being slowest at the beginning and end of a time period. Benjamin Gompertz proposed the law of mortality to explain the increasing death rate as a function of age in 1825. This was utilized by the insurance business to forecast death risk at the time. In 1964, Laird A.K. demonstrated how the Gompertz equation can be utilized to match tumor progression [1], i.e.,

$$W(t) = W_0\, e^{\frac{L}{k}\left(1-e^{(-kt)}\right)} \tag{12.1}$$

where W_0 is the initial tumor size, L is the initial specific growth rate and k is the coefficient of specific growth rate [2].

12.2.2 Lambert W Function

The Lambert W function is defined to be the multivalued inverse function of the mapping:

$$x \mapsto xe^x \tag{12.2}$$

The following Eq. 12.3 is solved to produce solution in the form of the Lambert W function, i.e., Eq. 12.4

$$ye^y = x \tag{12.3}$$

$$y = W(x) \tag{12.4}$$

Based on Eq. 12.3 we can write the following relation,

$$W(x)e^{W(x)} = x. \tag{12.5}$$

There is no unique inverse of the xe^x function since the mapping in Eq. 12.2 is not injective (except at the minimum). It is used when variable is both a base and an exponent and the equations cannot be solved using elementary functions.

The Lambert W function is mostly used and discussed with great detail in computational sciences and mathematical physics. But the function not demonstrated well in biochemistry and biotechnology. For tumor growth, we have decomposed Gompertz function at the inflection point and the parameters are equated using Lambert W function [3, 4].

12.2.3 Dataset Description

We consider multicellular tumor spheroid(MTS) data for our model [14]. The three-dimensional tumor cell cultures are cultivated using several vitro methods such as liquid overlay, spinning flask, and gyratory rotation systems on monolayer tumor cells. These cells reproduce and mimic the features of real cells, resulting in enhanced cell-to-cell interactions, which is critical for studying tumor growth and response to various medication testing. It also has superior accuracy than typical 2D cell culture findings since it ignores aspects of cell growth such as heterogeneity and the *in vivo* environment, resulting in low model accuracy.

A tumor spheroid in Figure 12.1 is an abnormal clump of rapidly dividing cells that looks to be tumor [20]. An exterior shell of proliferating cells, an inner layer of quiescent cells that are dormant but viable, and a central core of necrotic material make up a typical multi-cell spheroid. With limited food supply, the cells mutate into quiescent as the spheroid size grows. Long-term food restriction causes the core of the tumor to die, resulting in a collection of dead cells known as the necrotic core [5]. The cells in the proliferative zone are constantly growing because they have access to the nutrients essential for proliferation.

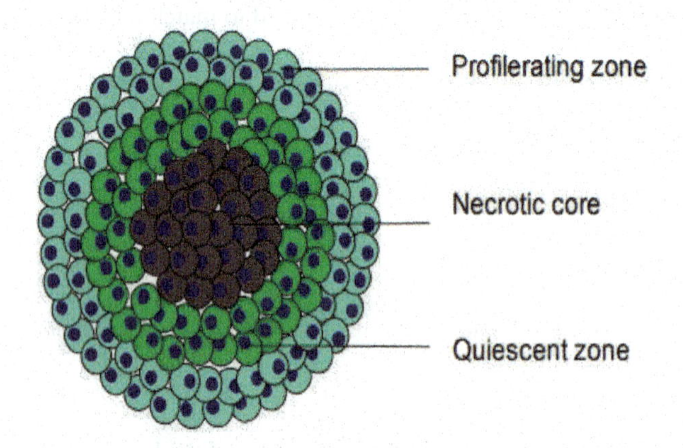

Fig. 12.1: Structure of tumor spheroid.

As the tumor spheroid develops, the cells closer to the center and core have a harder time acquiring nutrition [9].

12.3 Model Formulation

We have found how well the multicellular tumor spheroid data fits into gompertz equation, and also how using lambert function, the growth rate is measured. It is found that the parameters k and L, i.e., initial specific growth rate and coefficient of growth rate are dependent variables.The gompertz function when decomposed till inflection point discover parameter L in terms of k, i.e., we can see how negatively they are correlated in 12.13. Gomepertz Laird equation in general:

$$f(t) = W_0 \, e^{\frac{L}{k}\left(1-e^{(-kt)}\right)} \tag{12.6}$$

First-derivative of Eq. 12.6 can be obtained as:

$$\begin{aligned} f'(t) &= W_0 e^{\frac{L}{k}\left(1-e^{(-kt)}\right)} \frac{d}{dt}\left[\frac{L}{k}\left(1-e^{(-kt)}\right)\right] \\ f'(t) &= W_0 \frac{L}{k}\left[\left(-e^{(-kt)}\right)\right] e^{\frac{L}{k}\left(1-e^{(-kt)}\right)} \frac{d}{dt}[-kt] \end{aligned} \tag{12.7}$$

The above equation can be re-written as:

$$f'(t) = W_0 L e^{\frac{L}{k}\left(1-e^{(-kt)}\right)-kt} \tag{12.8}$$

Also the second derivative of Eq. 12.6 is obtained as:

$$f''(t) = W_0 L \frac{d}{dt}\left[e^{\frac{L}{k}\left(1-e^{(-kt)}\right)-kt}\right] \tag{12.9}$$

$$f''(t) = W_0 L e^{\frac{L}{k}\left(1-e^{(-kt)}\right)-kt} \frac{d}{dt}\left[\frac{L}{k}\left(1-e^{(-kt)}\right)-kt\right] \tag{12.10}$$

Then we obtain the following equation:

$$f''(t) = W_0 L e^{\frac{L}{k}\left(1-e^{(-kt)}\right)-kt}\left[Le^{(-kt)}-k\right] \tag{12.11}$$

The gompertz function decomposed at inflection point is expressed as:

$$\begin{aligned} W_0 L &= 0 \\ or\ Le^{(-kt)} - k &= 0 \\ or\ e^{\frac{L}{k}\left(1-e^{(-kt)}\right)} &= 0 \\ Le^{(-kt)} - k &= 0 \end{aligned}$$

Let $u = kt$, then equation is transformed into the form of Lambert W function.

$$L = Ke^{(kt)} \tag{12.12}$$

$$\begin{aligned} L &= \frac{u}{t} e^{u} \\ Lt &= ue^{u} \\ u &= W(Lt) \end{aligned}$$

$$k = \frac{W(Lt)}{t} \tag{12.13}$$

Lambert function approximated for the parameters 12.13 is used for further study of tumor growth rate in MTS datasets.

12.4 Results and Discussion

The three MTS data with growth in the range of 24–79 days are fitted into Gompertz function using R studio. For each tumor data, the growth rate is found using MS Excel from the Gompertz equations 12.1 decomposed till second derivatives producing lambert function 12.2 at inflection point 12.13. This moment represents the point in time when the growth rate is at its highest. Used the statistical indicators as Root-mean-square error (RMSE), Coefficient of determination (r^2) and Correlation coefficient (r) to evaluate performance of the models.

12.4.1 U87 Multicellular Tumor Spheroid (MTS)

The MTS data is fitted on Gompertz equation using R studio. According to Aggrey [13], L is the instantaneous growth rate (per day) and k is the rate of exponential decay of the initial specific growth rate for the Gompertz - Laird model and that explains the decreasing values of k with time found in Table 12.1. The values of L

Table 12.1: Volume vs time with k and L values calculated for U87.

Time(days)	Volume	L	k
3	149.2063	1.4490	0.5220
5	203.1746	3.3298	0.3778
7	274.6031	7.6517	0.3019
9	339.682	17.58295	0.2540
11	369.841	40.4040	0.2206
13	379.3650	92.8448	0.195
15	404.761	213.3491	0.1766
17	411.1111	490.2571	0.161
19	422.2222	1126.5667	0.1485
21	439.6825	2588.7488	0.1379
24	450.7936	9017.5682	0.1248

and k are calculated using 12.13 with the help of MS Excel where $k = 0.416$ and $L = 2.5$ are fixed at a time. U87 MTS has highest specific growth rate around 9015.1 on 24 day, while the exponential decay of growth rate or the coefficient of growth rate seems to be lowest on the same day in Table 12.1.

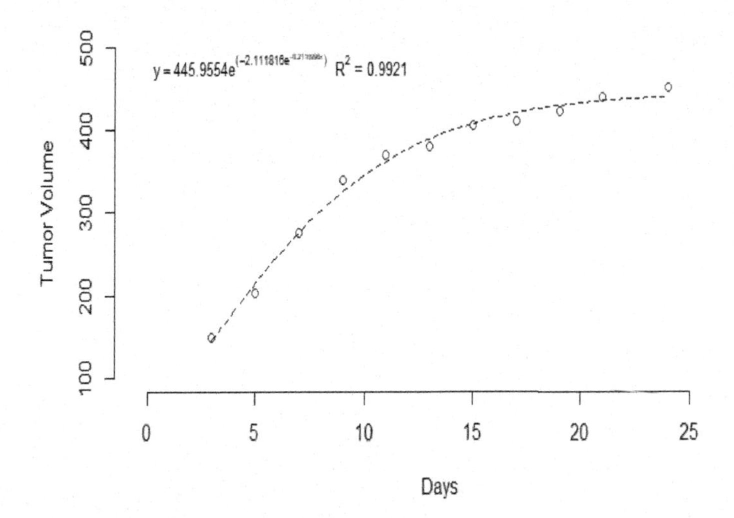

Fig. 12.2: U87 MTS volume against time plot.

Using R studio, gompertz equation 12.1 is curve fitted on U87 MTS to capture the trend in the tumor to allow us to make predictions of how the tumor growth will behave in the future. The fitting of gompertz equation for U87 MTS data in Figure 12.2 shows R squared value 0.99, i.e., almost perfect fit.

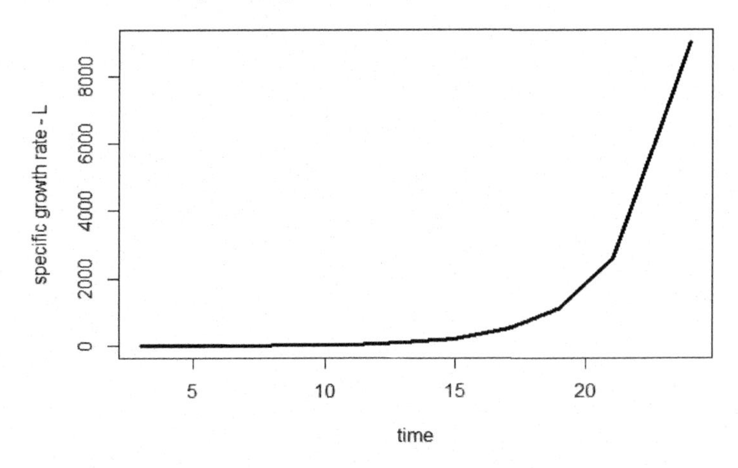

Fig. 12.3: Specific growth rate of U87 MTS.

The experimental points are taken from Mascheroni et al. (2016) [19] and Figure 12.3 represents the exponential growth rate of U87 spheroids when $k = 0.416$.

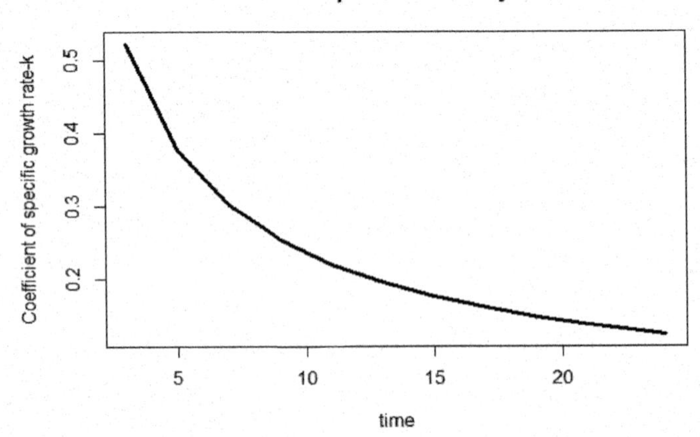

Fig. 12.4: Gompertz-Laird parameter k against time for U87 MTS.

Figure 12.4 plots the coefficient of specific growth rate k found using 12.13 when $L = 2.5$ which results in exponential decrease.

12.4.2 9L Multicellular Tumor Spheroid (MTS)

The regression line doesn't quite fit the gompertz equation correctly on 9L MTS compared to the other two datasets as there is perturbation due to periodic change of growth medium [15].

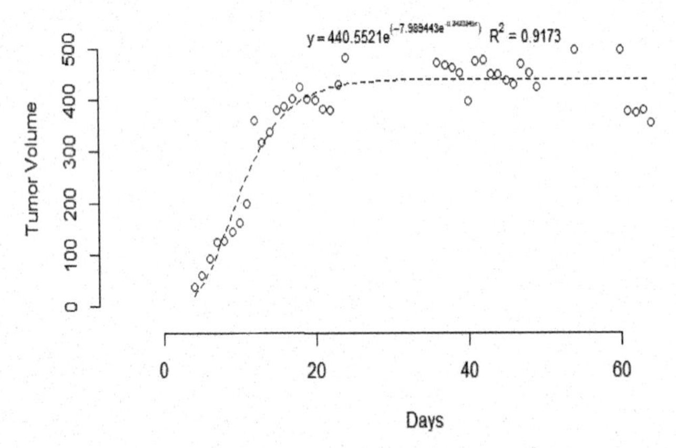

Fig. 12.5: 9L MTS volume against time plot.

The experimental points are taken from Chignola et al. (1998) [15] and represent the growth trend and curve fitting of 9L spheroids in Figure 12.5.

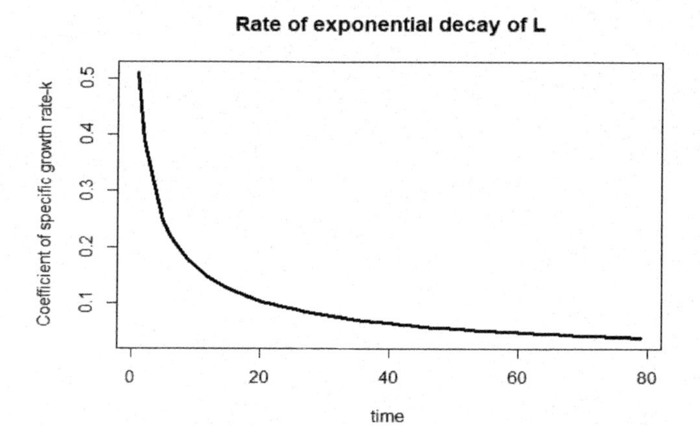

Fig. 12.6: Gompertz-Laird parameter k against time for 9L MTS.

Figure 12.6 presents the coefficient of specific growth rate found using 12.13 when $L = 0.85$.

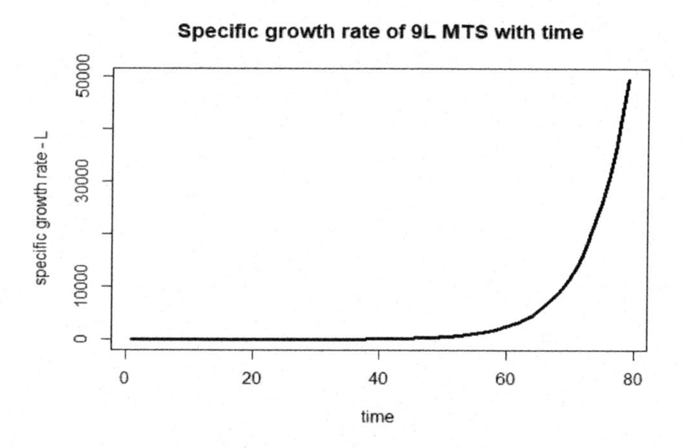

Fig. 12.7: Specific growth rate of 9L MTS.

Specific growth rate seen in Figure 12.7 is constant till 45 days and increases rapidly after the 60 days of growth with sharp exponential curve in the end. The initial specific growth rate L and coefficient of specific growth rate k of 9L MTS is found using Microsoft Excel. The values of L and k are calculated using 12.13 with $k = 0.16$ and $L = 0.85$ fixed at a time in Table 12.2.

12.4.3 Rat1-T1 Multicellular Tumor Spheroid (MTS)

The experimental points are taken from Leoni A. Kunz-Schughart et al. (1997) [18] and represent the growth of Rat1-T1 spheroids. The initial specific growth rate L and coefficient of specific growth rate k of Rat1-T1

Table 12.2: Volume vs time with k and L values calculated for 9L.

Time(days)	Volume	L	k
1	4.64	0.187762	0.510279
2	13.2	0.22034	0.389801
5	21.5	0.356087	0.247094
6	37.1	0.417871	0.223006
7	47.2	0.490377	0.203926
8	59	0.575462	0.18836
9	72.5	0.675311	0.175371
12	88	1.091353	0.146511
13	96.5	1.280715	0.139186
14	96.5	1.502933	0.13267
15	106	1.763708	0.126827
16	115	2.069731	0.121555
19	147	3.344839	0.108393
20	159	3.925205	0.104705
21	159	4.606271	0.101295
22	172	5.405509	0.098133
23	185	6.343423	0.09519
26	214	10.25144	0.087463
27	214	12.03018	0.085196
28	214	14.11755	0.08306
29	214	16.5671	0.081043
30	214	19.44167	0.079136
33	245	31.41918	0.073982
34	199	36.87075	0.07243
35	199	43.26823	0.07095
36	214	50.77573	0.069538
40	214	96.29521	0.064474
41	199	113.0035	0.063336
42	214	132.6108	0.062243
43	214	155.6202	0.061191
44	245	182.622	0.06018
47	245	295.1308	0.05736
48	245	346.3392	0.056485
49	229	406.4328	0.05564
50	214	476.9533	0.054823
51	199	559.7099	0.054032
54	199	904.5328	0.051809
55	185	1061.479	0.051113
56	214	1245.657	0.050438
57	159	1461.792	0.049782
58	199	1715.429	0.049146
62	185	3253.279	0.046773
63	199	3817.758	0.04622
64	172	4480.18	0.045681
65	185	5257.54	0.045156
68	214	8496.576	0.043659
69	199	9970.824	0.043185
70	199	11700.87	0.042722
71	172	13731.1	0.04227
72	159	16113.59	0.041829
75	147	26040.77	0.040565
76	185	30559.12	0.040162
77	185	35861.46	0.039768
78	185	42083.82	0.039383
79	214	49385.82	0.039006

MTS is found using MS Excel. The values of L and k are calculated using 12.13 with k = 0.416 and L = 2.5 fixed at a time in Table 12.3. Figure 12.8 shows the gompertz equations curve fitting on Rat1-T1 MTS growth. The regression line has good fit on the tumor growth with best RMSE value compared to other two datasets.

Table 12.3: Volume vs time with k and L values calculated for Rat1-T1.

Time(days)	Volume	L	k
1	250.7632	0.125273	0.123269
2	323.9875	0.14012	0.111556
3	373.8318	0.156726	0.102521
4	404.9844	0.1753	0.095259
5	427.4455	0.196075	0.089246
6	467.2897	0.219313	0.084157
7	505.134	0.245304	0.079775
8	520.134	0.274376	0.075948
9	570.0935	0.306893	0.072568
10	598.8224	0.343264	0.069554
11	616.8224	0.383945	0.066844
12	630.2835	0.429447	0.06439
13	651.7445	0.480342	0.062155
14	685.3209	0.537269	0.060107
15	700.6667	0.600942	0.058223
16	722.7414	0.672162	0.056482
17	728.972	0.751821	0.054867
18	741.433	0.840922	0.053363
19	772.5857	0.940582	0.051958
20	778.8162	1.052053	0.050642
21	800.6231	1.176735	0.049407
22	794.3925	1.316193	0.048244
23	809.9688	1.472179	0.047147
24	797.5078	1.646651	0.046109

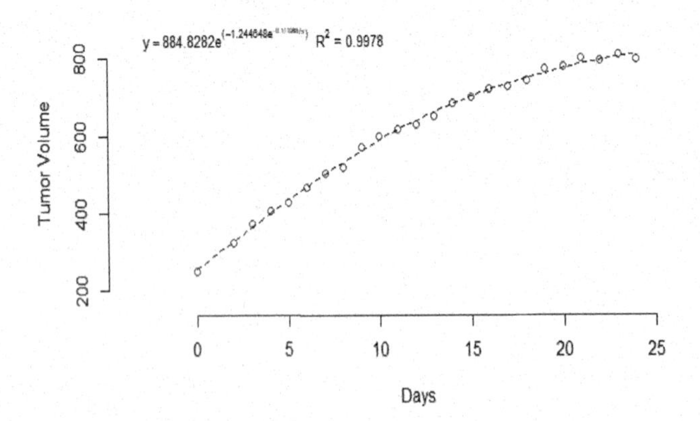

Fig. 12.8: Rat1-T1 MTS volume against time plot.

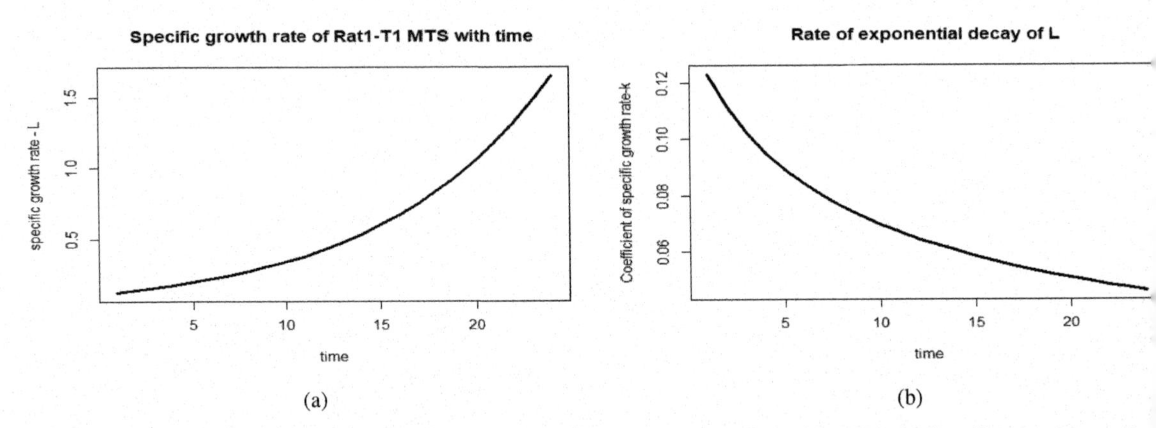

Fig. 12.9: Specific growth rate and exponential decay of specific growth rate for Rat1-T1 MTS, (a) Specific growth rate of Rat1-T1 MTS, (b) Gompertz- Laird parameter k against time for Rat1-T1 MTS.

In Figure 12.9(a), the specific growth rate when $k = 0.416$ shows sharper increase over time. Also,the coefficient of specific growth rate in Figure 12.9(b) found using 12.13 when $L = 2.5$ has exponential decay, as with time, the measure of k value decreases rapidly.

12.4.4 Growth Rate Stages

For U87 MTS follows exponential growth, yet has a small deviation in between the smooth growth. The instantaneous increase in growth is shown only after 21 days of time. The data in Figure 12.10 is segmented into three parts, with stage 1 having first 3–9 days data, stage 2 with 11–17 days data and stage 3 with 19–24 days data. The growth rate for the three stages are found using 12.13. In all the three stages, growth rate

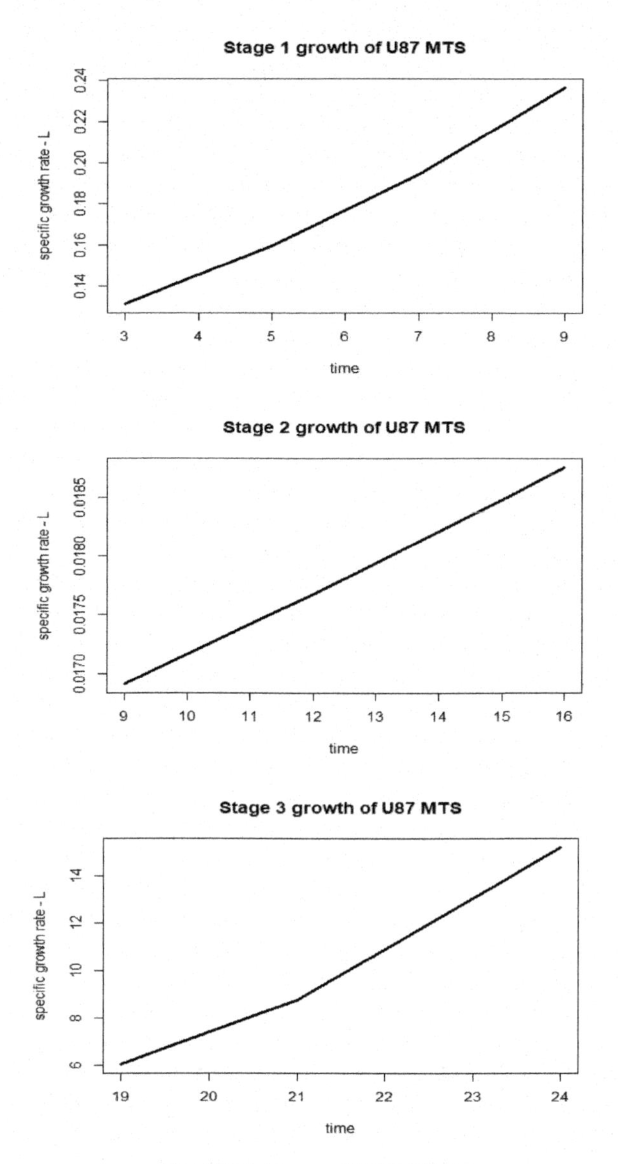

Fig. 12.10: Stages of U87 MTS data.

appears to be linear, except the third stage, that has a small deviation at 21st day and after that the growth rate is increasing exponentially. The growth rate seems to be maximum in the third stage ranging from 23–24/day.

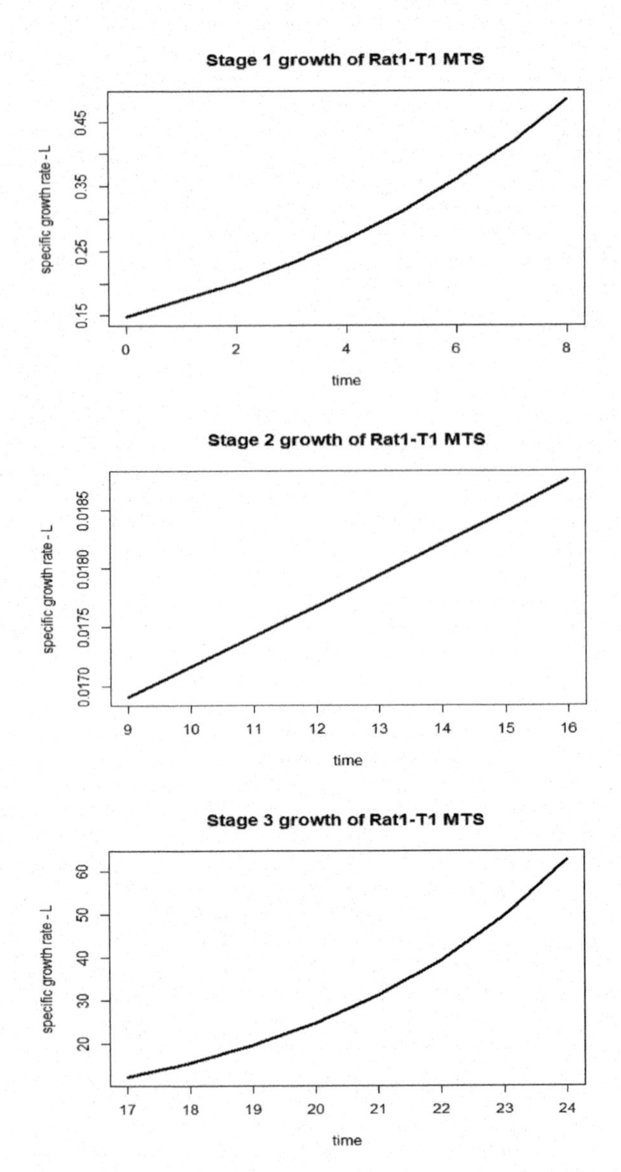

Fig. 12.11: Stages of Rat1-T1 MTS data.

In Figure 12.11,the Rat1-T1 MTS shows smooth exponential increase in the specific growth rate during stage 1 and stage 3, yet a linear growth in stage 2. With the highest growth rate around 24th days time. The perturbation of the curve could be due to various internal factors which is yet to be researched. 9L MTS growth rate in Figure 12.13 is exponential in all the three stages. With the highest growth rate peak around 75–80 days time. Even though exponential growth is seen in the specific growth rate of the data, Gompertz function has shown almost 99% goodness of fit with RMSE ranging from 8.2–9.9 for each MTS dataset. Even though the best fitting of the Gompertz equation is on Rat1-T1 with R squared value about 0.9975,

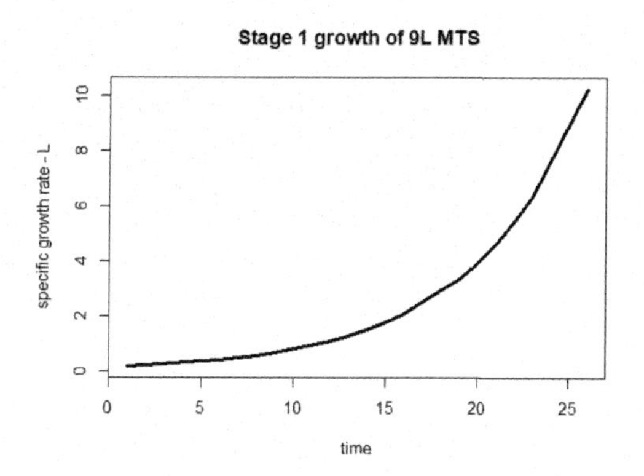

Fig. 12.12: stages of 9L MTS data.

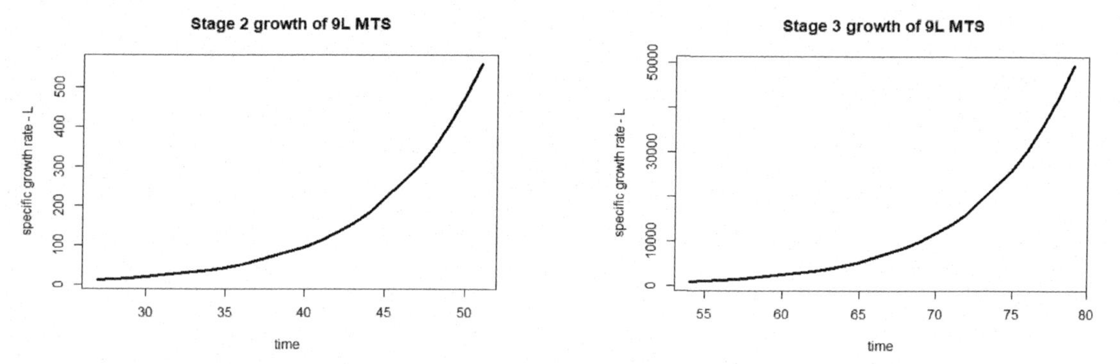

Fig. 12.13: Stages of 9L MTS data.

Table 12.4: Model fitting evaluation.

Dataset	RMSE	R	R squared
9L	9.968	0.9129	0.9173
U87	9.886	0.9901	0.9921
Rat1-T1	8.294	0.9978	0.9975

the study of residual is needed to be sure about the results. The RMSE tells us the standard deviation of the residuals. As Rat1-T1 has lowest RMSE value, the data points must be not that far from the regression line compared to 9L and U87 data set in Table 12.4.

12.5 Conclusion

In this work, we deduce that multicellular tumor spheroid (MTS) datasets follows the Gompertz function's properties. That is, assuming the host survives beyond the days specified in the data, the growth will approach a saturation point after which no more development will be possible. We magnified the tumor growth rate at three stages which gave better clarity in the understanding of growth pattern and variations for specific type of tumor. Also with the help of Lambert W function, approximating the growth rate and coefficient of growth rate measures found is useful for drug screening and doctors. As the growth rate is a crucial piece of information for the doctors to predict as well as choose the best course of treatment. Our future research will be focused on developing a strategy for predicting the pace of growth of any type of tumor.

References

[1] Laird, A.K. 1964. Dynamics of Tumor growth. British Journal of Cancer, 13(3): 490–502.

[2] Ruiz-Arrebola, S., D. Guirado, M. Villalobos, M. Lallena and M. Antonio. 2021. Evaluation of classical mathematical models of Tumor growth using an on-lattice agent-based Monte Carlo model. Applied Sciences, 11(11): 5241.

[3] Valluri, S.R., R.M. Corless and D.J. Jeffrey. 2020. Some applications of the Lambert W function to physics. Canadian Journal of Physics, 78(9), 823–831, 2020.

[4] Goličnik, M. 2012. On the Lambert W function and its utility in biochemical kinetics. Biochemical Engineering Journal, 63: 116–123.

[5] Anisha Radhakrishnan and M. Divya. 2015. Survey of data fusion and tumor segmentation techniques using brain images. International Journal of Applied Engineering Research, 10: 20559–20570.

[6] Anjana, J., V.K. Rajan, R. Biswas and R. Jayakumar. 2017. Controlled delivery of bioactive molecules for the treatment of chronic wounds. Curr. Pharm. Des., 23(24): 3529–3537.

[7] Puvaneswari, P. and K. Shailendhra. 2020. Viscoelastic dream pipe with triangular pressure gradient wave form for substantial enhancement of heat transfer. Journal of Non-Newtonian Fluid Mechanics, 278: 104247.

[8] Mao, J.J., G.G. Pillai, C.J. Andrade, J.A. Ligibel, P. Basu, L. Cohen, I.A. Khan and L.A. Salicrup. 2022. Integrative oncology: Addressing the global challenges of cancer prevention and treatment. CA Cancer Journal for Clinicians, 72(2): 144–164.

[9] Vadivelu, R.K., H. Kamble, M.J.A. Shiddiky and N.T. Nguyen. 2017. Microfluidic technology for the generation of cell spheroids and their applications. Micromachines, 8(4): 94.

[10] Brady, R. and H. Enderling. 2019. Mathematical models of cancer: When to predict novel therapies, and When Not to. Bull. Math. Biol., 81: 3722–3731.

[11] Przemyslaw Waliszewski and Jerzy Konarski. 2003. The Gompertzian curve reveals fractal properties of Tumor growth. Chaos, Solitons and Fractals, 16(5): 665–674.

[12] Wallace, D.I. and X. Guo. 2013. Properties of tumor spheroid growth exhibited by simple mathematical models. Front. Oncol., 3: 51.

[13] Aggrey, S.E. 2002. Comparison of three nonlinear and spline regression models for describing chicken growth curves. Poult. Sci., 81(12): 1782–1788.

[14] Edmondson, R., J.J. Broglie, A.F. Adcock and L. Yang. 2014. Three-dimensional cell culture systems and their applications in drug discovery and cell-based biosensors. Assay Drug Dev. Technol., 12(4): 207–218.

[15] Chignola, R., A. Schenetti, E. Chiesa, R. Foroni, S. Sartoris, A. Brendolan, G. Tridente, G. Andrighetto and D. Liberati. 1999. Oscillating growth patterns of multicellular tumour spheroids. Cell Prolif., 32(1): 39–48.

[16] Tjørve, K.M.C. and E. Tjørve. 2017. The use of Gompertz models in growth analyses, and new Gompertz-model approach: An addition to the Unified-Richards family. PLOS ONE, 12(6): e0178691.

[17] Lee, K.H. and T.H. Kim. 2021. Recent advances in multicellular Tumor spheroid generation for drug screening. Biosensors, 11(11): 445.

[18] Kunz-Schughart, L.A., M. Kreutz and R. Knuechel. 1998. Multicellular spheroids: A three-dimensional in vitro culture system to study tumour biology. Int. J. Exp. Pathol., 79(1): 1–23.

[19] Mascheroni, P., C. Stigliano, M. Carfagna, D.P. Boso, L. Preziosi, P. Decuzzi and B.A. Schrefler. 2016. Predicting the growth of glioblastoma multiforme spheroids using a multiphase porous media model. Biomech. Model Mechanobiol., 15(5): 1215–1228.

[20] Kamatar, A., G. Gunay and H. Acar. 2020. Natural and synthetic biomaterials for engineering multicellular Tumor spheroids. Polymers, 12(11): 2506.

[21] Cooper, G.M. 2000. The Cell: A Molecular Approach, 2nd edition, Sunderland (MA): Sinauer Associates. The Development and Causes of Cancer.

[22] Dániel András Drexler, Johanna Sápi and Levente Kovács. 2017. Modeling of Tumor growth incorporating the effects of Necrosis and the effect of Bevacizumab. Complexity, 1–10.

[23] Brohem, C.A., L.B. Cardeal, M. Tiago, M.S. Soengas, S.B. Barros and S.S. Maria-Engler. 2011. Artificial skin in perspective: Concepts and applications. Pigment Cell Melanoma Res., 24(1): 35–50.

Index

G

H

I

J

L

M

N

O

P

R